Handbook of Renal and Pancreatic Transplantation

Companion website

This book is accompanied by a companion website:

www.wiley.com/go/macphee/transplantation

The website includes:

- 60 full-colour figures to accompany Chapters 7 and 10

- Video clips of live donor nephrectomy to accompany Chapter 7

Handbook of Renal and Pancreatic Transplantation

EDITORS

Iain A. M. MacPhee

Division of Clinical Sciences: Renal Medicine, St. George's, University of London;
Department of Renal Medicine and Transplantation, St. George's Hospital, Blackshaw
Road, London, UK

Jiří Froněk

Transplant Surgery Department, Institute for Clinical and Experimental Medicine,
Prague, Czech Republic;
2nd Medical Faculty, Charles University, Prague, Czech Republic

WILEY-BLACKWELL

A John Wiley & Sons, Ltd., Publication

Library of Congress Cataloging-in-Publication Data

Handbook of renal and pancreatic transplantation / editors, Iain A. M. MacPhee, Jiří Froněk.
    p. ; cm.
    Includes bibliographical references and index.
    ISBN 978-0-470-65491-0
    I. MacPhee, Iain A. M.   II. Froněk, Jiří, 1970–
    [DNLM: 1. Kidney Transplantation.   2. Pancreas Transplantation. WJ 368]
    617.4'610592–dc23
                                                            2011049799

A catalogue record for this book is available from the British Library.

Set in 9.25/11.5 pt Minion by Toppan Best-set Premedia Limited
Printed and bound in Malaysia by Vivar Printing Sdn Bhd

1   2012

For: Paula, Laura, Lucy, Madeleine, Eliška, Kristýna and Mája.

Contents

List of Contributors, ix
Preface, xiii
Abbreviations List, xv

1 History of transplantation, 1
Jiří Froněk and Iain MacPhee

2 Assessment of the potential renal transplant recipient, 9
Patrick B. Mark and Alan G. Jardine

**3 Pre-transplant assessment and medical evaluation
of potential live kidney donors**, 33
Jonas Wadström

4 Histocompatibility and immunogenetics, 55
Susan V. Fuggle and Craig J. Taylor

**5 Donor management: care of the heartbeating brain-dead
multi-organ donor**, 77
Paul G. Murphy

6 Deceased donor retrieval, 91
*Albert M. Wolthuis, Diethard Monbaliu, Willy Coosemans
and Jacques Pirenne*

7 Live donor nephrectomy, 109
Jiří Froněk and Nicos Kessaris

**8 Organisation of transplant services, organ sharing and organ
allocation: A perspective from the UK and Eurotransplant**, 141
James Neuberger and Axel Rahmel

9 Deceased donor kidney transplantation, 159
Luisa Berardinelli

10 Living donor kidney transplantation, 173
Jiří Froněk and Nicos Kessaris

11 Pancreas transplantation, 191
Guido Woeste and Wolf O. Bechstein

12 Pancreatic islet transplantation, 203
František Saudek

13 Anaesthesia for renal transplantation, 219
Nicoletta Fossati

14 Anaesthesia for pancreatic transplantation, 227
Kai Zacharowski and Hans-Joachim Wilke

15 Anaesthesia for live donor nephrectomy, 235
Rehana Iqbal and Karthik Somasundaram

16 Immunosuppression, 243
Iain A.M. MacPhee and Teun van Gelder

17 Antibody-incompatible kidney transplantation, 271
Nicos Kessaris and Nizam Mamode

18 Renal transplantation in children, 287
Luisa Berardinelli and Luciana Ghio

19 Post-transplant diagnostic imaging, 297
Lakshmi Ratnam and Uday Patel

20 Transplant histopathology, 317
Eva Honsová

21 Infection, 335
Rachel Hilton and Martin W. Drage

22 Management during the first three months after renal
transplantation, 381
Iain A.M. MacPhee, Joyce Popoola and Daniel Jones

23 Management of long-term complications, 403
Paul N. Harden, Richard Haynes, Iain A.M. MacPhee and Jiří Froněk

24 Living donor follow-up, 437
Robert Elias and Jiří Froněk

25 Ethics of transplantation, 447
Robert Elias and Rehana Iqbal

Index, 461

Companion website

This book is accompanied by a companion website:
www.wiley.com/go/macphee/transplantation

List of Contributors

Wolf O. Bechstein
Department of General and Visceral Surgery, Johan Wolfgang Goethe University Frankfurt, Germany.

Luisa Berardinelli
General Surgery and Kidney Transplantation Unit, Policlinico University Hospital IRCCS, Milan, Italy.

Willy Coosemans
Department of Thoracic Surgery, University Hospitals Leuven, Belgium.

Martin W. Drage
Renal, Urology and Transplantation Directorate, Guy's Hospital, London, UK.

Robert Elias
Renal Unit, King's College Hospital, NHS Foundation Trust, London, UK.

Nicoletta Fossati
Department of Anaesthesia, St. George's Healthcare NHS Trust, London, UK.

Jiří Froněk
Transplant Surgery Department, Institute for Clinical and Experimental Medicine, Prague, Czech Republic.
2nd Medical Faculty, Charles University, Prague, Czech Republic.

Susan V. Fuggle
Transplant Immunology and Immunogenetics, Oxford Transplant Centre, Churchill Hospital, Oxford, UK.

Luciana Ghio
Department of Pediatrics, Policlinico University Hospital IRCCS, Milan, Italy.

Teun van Gelder
Nephrology and Clinical Pharmacology, Erasmus Medical Centre, Rotterdam, Netherlands.

Paul N. Harden
Renal Medicine and Transplantation, St. George's Healthcare NHS Trust, London, UK.

Richard Haynes
Renal Medicine and Transplantation, St. George's Healthcare NHS Trust, London, UK.

Rachel Hilton
Renal, Urology and Transplantation Directorate, Guy's Hospital, London, UK.

Eva Honsová
Clinical and Transplant Pathology Department, Institute for Clinical and Experimental Medicine, Prague, Czech Republic.

Rehana Iqbal
Anaesthesia Department, St. George's Healthcare NHS Trust, London, UK.

Alan G. Jardine
BHF Glasgow Cardiovascular Research Centre, University of Glasgow, Glasgow, UK.

Daniel Jones
Renal Medicine and Transplantation, St. George's Healthcare NHS Trust, London, UK.

Nicos Kessaris
Department of Renal Medicine and Transplantation, St. George's Healthcare NHS Trust, Blackshaw Road, London, UK.

Iain A.M. MacPhee
Division of Clinical Sciences: Renal Medicine, St. George's Healthcare NHS Trust, University of London, London, UK.
Department of Renal Medicine and Transplantation, St. George's Healthcare NHS Trust, Blackshaw Road, London, UK.

Nizam Mamode
Renal, Urology and Transplantation Directorate, Guy's Hospital, London, UK.

Patrick B. Mark
BHF Glasgow Cardiovascular Research Centre, University of Glasgow, Glasgow, UK.

Diethard Monbaliu
Department of Abdominal Transplant Surgery, University Hospitals Leuven, Belgium.

Paul G. Murphy
National Clinical Lead for Organ Donation, NHS Blood and Transplant and Department of Neuroanaesthesia and Critical Care, Leeds Genereal Infirmary, Leeds, UK.

James Neuberger
Liver Department, University Hospitals Birmingham. NHS Foundation Trust, Birmingham, UK.

Uday Patel
Radiology Department, St. George's Healthcare NHS Trust, London, UK.

Jacques Pirenne
Department of Abdominal Transplant Surgery, University Hospitals Leuven, Belgium.

Joyce Popoola
Renal Medicine and Transplantation, St. George's Healthcare NHS Trust, London, UK.

Axel Rahmel
Eurotransplant International Foundation, Leiden, Netherlands.

Lakshmi Ratnam
Radiology, St. George's Healthcare NHS Trust, London, UK.

František Saudek
Diabetes Center, Institute for Clinical and Experimental Medicine, Prague, Czech Republic.

Karthik Somasundaram
Anaesthesia Department, St George's Healthcare NHS Trust London, UK.

Craig J. Taylor
Transplant Immunology and Immunogenetics, Oxford Transplant Centre, Churchill Hospital, Oxford, UK.

Jonas Wadström
Departments of Transplantation Surgery and Transfusion Medicine, Karolinska University Hospital, Huddinge, Stockholm; Department of Transplantation Surgery, Karolinska University Hospital, Sweden.

Hans-Joachim Wilke
Clinic of Anesthesiology, Intensive Care Medicine and Pain Therapy University Hospital Frankfurt am Main, Germany.

Guido Woeste
Department of General and Visceral Surgery, Johan Wolfgang Goethe University Frankfurt, Germany.

Albert M. Wolthuis
Department of Abdominal Surgery, University Hospitals Leuven, Belgium.

Kai Zacharowski
Clinic of Anesthesiology, Intensive Care Medicine and Pain Therapy University Hospital Frankfurt am Main, Germany.

Preface

When we set out on planning this book there was no contemporary handbook for the practice of renal and pancreatic transplantation that was focussed on a European rather than North American approach. There are significant differences in transplant practice internationally and there is a need for a practical guide to application of the current evidence base.

This book aims to cover all aspects of transplantation from organ donation through long-term follow-up. We have aimed to provide information useful to all members of the multidisciplinary transplant team. This is not intended as a comprehensive textbook and readers are referred to the number of excellent existing works that serve this role.

We are delighted with the panel of experts from across Europe who agreed to contribute chapters and are extremely grateful for the time that they have contributed in putting the book together. We have learned a lot about transplantation in the editing process and hope that the reader will find the information equally useful. The videos demonstrating surgical technique for laparoscopic donor nephrectomy were developed from a successful course based on live surgical demonstrations. The drug treatment regimens described represent the authors' assessment of the available evidence and actual use in practice rather than adhering strictly to licensed indications and doses.

We are deeply grateful for the support of our families in tolerating the time required to put the book together.

Iain MacPhee
Jiří Froněk
February 2012

Abbreviations List

ACE	angiotensin-converting enzyme
ACMR	acute cell-mediated rejection
ADPKD	autosomal dominant polycystic kidney disease
ALG	anti-lymphocyte globulin
AMR	antibody-mediated rejection
ANCA	antineutrophil cytoplasmic antibody
APC	activated protein C
APTT	activated partial thromboplastin time
ARB	angiotensin II receptor blocker
ATIII	antithrombin III
aTCMR	acute T-cell-mediated rejection
ATG	antithymocyte globulin
AVF	arteriovenous fistula
BMI	body mass index
BP	blood pressure
BSA	body surface area
CABG	coronary artery bypass graft
CAD	coronary artery disease
CCMR	chronic active cell-mediated rejection
CDC	complement-dependent cytotoxicity
CDC-XM	complement-dependent lymphocytotoxic crossmatch
CDU	colour Doppler ultrasound
CITR	Collaborative Islet Transplant Registry
CKD	chronic kidney disease
CMV	cytomegalovirus
CMVIg	cytomegalovirus hyperimmunoglobulin
CNI	calcineurin inhibitor
CREG	cross-reactive group
cRF	calculated reaction frequency
CSE	combined spinal–epidural anaesthesia
CT	computerised tomography
CVD	cardiovascular disease
CVP	central venous pressure
DBTL	double-balloon triple-lumen
DCD	donor after circulatory death
DD	deceased donor
DES	drug eluting stent
DFPE	double filtration plasma exchange

DSA	digital subtraction angiography; donor-specific antibody
DTT	dithiothreitol
EBV	Epstein–Barr virus
ECD	expanded criteria donor
ECG	electrocardiogram
ECMO	extracorporeal membrane oxygenation
ELISA	enzyme-linked immunosorbent assay
ESRD	end-stage renal disease
FBC	full blood count
FC-XM	flow cytometric crossmatch
FMD	fibromuscular dysplasia
FSGS	focal and segmental glomerulosclerosis
G6PD	glucose-6-phosphate dehydrogenase
GFR	glomerular filtration rate
HAART	highly active antiretroviral therapy
HACA	human anti-chimeric antibody
HBD	heartbeating donor
HBV	hepatitis B virus
HCV	hepatitis C virus
HDU	high-dependency unit
HHV-8	human herpesvirus 8
HIV	human immunodeficiency virus
HLA	human leucocyte antigen
HR	hyperacute rejection
HSV	herpes simplex virus
HTK	histidine-tryptophan-ketoglutarate
HTLV1	human T-lymphotropic virus
HUS	haemolytic uraemic syndrome
IA	immunoadsorption
IBMIR	instant blood-mediated inflammatory reaction
ICP	intracranial pressure
IDDM	insulin-dependent diabetes mellitus
IFG	impaired fasting glucose
IgAN	immunoglobulin A nephropathy
IGT	impaired glucose tolerance
IHD	ischaemic heart disease
IL-2	interleukin 2
INF-γ	interferon-γ
IVIg	intravenous immunoglobulin
IVU	intravenous urogram
KT	kidney transplantation
LDK	living donor kidney
LVH	left ventricular hypertrophy
LVSD	left ventricular systolic dysfunction
MCGN	mesangiocapillary glomerulonephritis
MCP	membrane co-factor protein
MFI	median fluorescence intensity
MN	membranous nephropathy

MPGN	mesangioproliferative glomerulonephritis
MR	magnetic resonance
mTOR	mammalian target of rapamycin
NHBD	non-heartbeating donor
NODAT	new-onset diabetes after transplantation
NS	normal saline
OGTT	oral glucose tolerance test
PAK	pancreas after kidney
PALK	pancreas after living donor kidney
PAT	pancreas alone transplantation
PCA	patient-controlled analgesia
PCI	percutaneous coronary intervention
PCR	polymerase chain reaction
PEEP	positve end-expiratory pressure
P-gp	P-glycoprotein
PJ	*Pneumocystis jiroveci*
PONV	post-operative nausea and vomiting
PP	plasmapheresis
PSV	peak systolic velocity
PT	prothrombin time
PTC	peritubular capillaries
PTH	parathyroid hormone
PTLD	post-transplant lymphoproliferative disorder
PVN	polyomavirus nephropathy
RAS	renal artery stenosis
RRT	renal replacement therapy
RSI	rapid sequence intubation
RTR	renal transplant recipient
SAB	single antigen bead
SCD	sudden cardiac death
SPK	simultaneous pancreas kidney
TEA	thoracic epidural analgesia
TEE	transoesphageal echocardiography probe
TMA	thrombotic microangiopathy
TNF	tumour necrosis factor
TPMT	thiopurine-S-methyltransferase
TTP	thrombotic thrombocytopaenic purpura
UTI	urinary tract infection
VZV	varicella zoster virus

1 History of transplantation

Jiří Froněk and Iain MacPhee

In setting the scene for this handbook, we would like to acknowledge the contribution of the masters on whose backs we all climb. This book is written as a practical guide to the contemporary practice of transplantation. This is a brief account of how we got to where we are now. Early (but unsuccessful) attempts at transplantation have been documented for centuries. Advances in basic science allowed transplantation to become reality within the 20th century. Nowadays organ transplantation is accepted as a standard treatment for end-stage failure of a number of organs. The pioneers of transplantation medicine in the 20th century had to overcome substantial obstacles, including developing new surgical techniques, understanding transplant immunology and defining areas in which transplantation is of benefit. Nor was this era easy for public understanding of the fundamental issues involved. It was not simple to explain and achieve widespread acceptance of the concept of 'brainstem death' as distinct from 'cardiovascular death'. Transplantation has raised a vast number of ethical, philosophical and legal issues. Achievement of societal 'buy in' to difficult issues such as removal of organs after one's death or donation of an organ by a living donor were essential barriers to be overcome. Transplantation development is a result of the effort of many people from all over the world, who worked together and cooperated with the same aim and who participated in generating and applying new knowledge. Here we summarise the key events that led to the widespread adoption of kidney and other organ transplantation in the form we know it today.

1901 – Karl Landsteiner described the existence of **blood groups**. In 1930 he became a Nobel Prize Laureate.

1902 – Alexis Carrel published an end-to-end **vascular anastomosis** technique, which became a fundamental technique for vascular surgery and at the same time enabled the development of organ transplantation. Carrel received the Nobel Prize in Physiology or Medicine in 1912.

1902 – Emerich Ullmann carried out the **first experimental kidney transplantation**. He sewed the kidney onto a dog's neck. The kidney functioned for 5 days.

Handbook of Renal and Pancreatic Transplantation, First Edition. Edited by Iain A. M. MacPhee and Jiří Froněk.
© 2012 John Wiley & Sons, Ltd. Published 2012 by John Wiley & Sons, Ltd.

1906 – Mathieu Jaboulay made a **first xenotransplantation attempt in human medicine**. Pig or goat kidneys grafted onto the forearm of patients worked for around 1 hour.

1908 – Alexis Carrel and Charles Claude Guthrie pointed out the possibility of **use of organ hypothermia** for its long-term storage.

1912 – Görge Schöne was the first to state the suspicion that **graft rejection** has an immunological basis.

1913 – Abel, Rowntree and Turner created the **first 'artificial kidney'** and became the fathers of dialysis. Their machine was never used in human medicine.

1923 – The **first human peritoneal dialysis**.

1933 – Ukrainian surgeon Yu Yu Voronoy carried out the **first human cadaveric kidney transplant** on 3 April 1933. The donor was an elderly man, who died after a head injury, and the recipient was a 26-year-old woman with quicksilver poisoning. He carried out the operation under local anaesthesia and sutured the kidney onto the thigh blood vessels of the recipient, leading the ureter out through the skin. The kidney graft did not produce urine and the patient died 2 days after the operation.

1943 – Willem Kolff created the **first functioning dialysis machine**, thanks to the discovery that heparin is able to prevent blood coagulation.

1943 – Thomas Gibbon and Peter Medawar published their **first experience with skin allografts**, used in the treatment of burned World War II pilots. Peter Medawar was awarded the Nobel Prize in 1960.

1948 – Gorer, Lyman and Snell described a **dominant histocompatible locus** on a mouse. In 1980 Snell, together with Dausset and Benacerraf, became Nobel Prize Laureates.

1951 – René Küss described a kidney transplantation technique that is still used today.

1952 – Michon and Hamburger were the first to use a **kidney from a living related donor** in Paris. The kidney, transplanted from mother to son, functioned for 22 days.

1954 – On 23rd December, Joseph Murray, John Merrill and Hartwell Harrison carried out the first successful kidney transplantation between identical twins in Boston. The recipient, Richard Herrick, lived with a functioning kidney from his brother for 8 years, he died of a heart attack in 1962 with recurrence of his original illness (chronic glomerulonephritis) in the graft. Joseph Murray became a Nobel Prize Laureate in Medicine in 1990.

1955 – First heart valve transplants: Gordon Murray of Toronto, Ontario, used the main aortic valve of a male automobile accident victim to perform the world's first heart valve transplant on a patient with a severely leaking aortic valve. The transplanted valve functioned well for over 8 years.

1958 – Jean Dausset described the first **HLA antigen**.

1959 – Murray and Merrill carried out the **first kidney transplantation between non-identical twins**.

1962 – The **first dialysis centre** was established in Seattle.

1963 – First liver transplant: Thomas E. Starzl of the University of Colorado in Denver attempted the first liver transplant, but the patient died within a few days.

1963 – First lung transplant: James D. Hardy of the University of Mississippi in Jackson performed the first single human lung transplant, but the patient died within days.

1964 – Starzl described **ABO-incompatible kidney hyperacute rejection** caused by antibodies against the graft.

1965 – Paul Terasaki, T. L. Marchioro and Thomas Starzl described a **hyperacute kidney rejection**.

1966 – Paul Terasaki and Thomas Starzl reported the results of **prospective donor selection according to HLA standardisation level.**

1966 – First pancreas transplant: Richard C. Lillehei and William D. Kelly of the University of Minnesota, Minneapolis, transplanted a pancreas into a 28-year-old woman; the graft did work, but she died 3 months later from pulmonary embolism.

1967 – First successful liver transplant: Thomas E. Starzl of the University of Colorado in Denver performed the first successful liver transplant. The liver functioned for 13 months.

1967 – First successful heart transplant: Christiaan Barnard, at Groote Schur Hospital in Cape Town. The recipient died 18 days later of pneumonia.

1967 – Starzl and Iwasaki published Immunosuppression induction of **antilymphocyte globulin** and subsequently azathioprine and prednisone as maintenance treatment.

1969 – Discovery of mould *Beauveria nivea* (Tolypocladium infantum Gams), which produces **ciclosporin**.

1972 – Stähelin and Borel described **immunosuppressive qualities of ciclosporin.**

1974 – **First islet cell transplant:** David Sutherland of the University of Minnesota in Minneapolis performed the world's first islet cell transplant. The procedure worked for only a short time.

1978 – Roy Calne was the first to use **ciclosporin in human medicine**.

1979 – David Sutherland of the University of Minnesota in Minneapolis performed the **first living-related pancreas transplant**.

1981 – Benedict Cosimi described for the first time the **use of monoclonal antibody** in human medicine.

1983 – **First successful single lung transplant:** Joel Cooper of the Toronto Lung Transplant Group, Toronto General Hospital (now part of the University Health Network), performed a single lung transplant. Patient lived for more than 6 years before dying of kidney failure.

1983 – **First multi-visceral transplant:** The first multi-visceral transplant was performed at the University of Pittsburgh Medical Center in Pennsylvania.

1984 – **First heart–liver transplant:** The first heart–liver transplant was performed at the University of Pittsburgh Medical Center in Pennsylvania.

1986 – **First successful double lung transplant:** Joel Cooper of the Toronto Lung Transplant Group, Toronto General Hospital performed a double lung transplant, patient lived until 2001, died of a brain aneurysm.

1988 – **First successful liver–bowel transplant:** David Grant of the University Hospital of London Health Sciences Centre in London, Ontario, transplanted a liver and small bowel into 41-year-old recipient, who had been unable to eat or drink after having her small bowel removed in 1987.

1988 – **First two-in-one liver transplant:** Two patients at Paul Brousse Hospital in Villejuif, France, received a liver transplant, when one donated organ was cut in half.

1989 – First successful living-related liver transplant: Christopher Broelsch of the University of Chicago Medical Center transplanted a portion of a mother's liver into her 21-month-old daughter. Both mother and daughter are still healthy today.

1989 – First combination heart, liver, and kidney transplant: Surgeons at Presbyterian Hospital in Pittsburgh, Pennsylvania, transplanted a heart, liver and kidney into a 26-year-old woman. She survived for 4 months.

1990 – First successful living-related lung transplant: Vaughn A. Starnes, at Stanford University Medical Center in Palo Alto, California, transplanted the lobe of one lung into a 12-year-old girl (the lobe was donated by her mother).

1992 – Thomas Starzl described chimerism by transplanted patients, a possible manifestation of allograft tolerance.

1995 – First **laparoscopic live donor nephrectomy:** In 1995 Lloyd Ratner and Louis Kavoussi descried the laparoscopic live donor nephrectomy technique, first performed at Johns Hopkins.

1998 – Hand-assisted laparoscopic live donor nephrectomy technique described by Wolf *et al.*

1998 – First combined liver and bone marrow transplant: Surgeons at King's College Hospital in London, performed the first combined liver and bone marrow transplant procedure on 18-year-old recipient, suffering from CD40-ligand deficiency.

2000 – Edmonton protocol: The technique of islet isolation from a deceased donor pancreas followed by portal vein administration was first adopted in 1999 and published on 2000 by Shapiro. Islet transplantation can be used as alternative technique to pancreas transplantaion.

2002 – Hand-assisted retroperitoneoscopic live donor nephrectomy technique described by Wadström and Lindström.

2005 – First living donor islet transplant: On 19 January, a team of surgeons at the Kyoto University Hospital in Japan, under the supervision of Dr James Shapiro, took islet cells from the pancreas of a 56-year-old woman and transplanted them into the liver of her 27-year-old diabetic daughter.

At the beginning of 20th century, the modern transplantation era started with an experiment on an animal model. Despite failures and pessimism in experimental transplantation, some surgeons persisted in trying to transplant kidneys into patients. Although these procedures were unsuccessful, owing to absence of immunosuppression, development of the surgical techniques, including heterotopic transplantation, was a key step on the pathway. Dialysis allowed transplantation to become an elective rather than emergency life-saving procedure. Advances in graft conservation, immunology, immunosuppression and the field of extracorporeal perfusion methods led to a rapid development of deceased donor transplantation programmes. The development of living donor transplantation was a little overshadowed by other exciting new developments until 1990s, when we saw an international revival of interest in living donation owing to the inadequate supply of deceased donors to meet the demand for transplantation and also better long-term results with transplants from live donors.

In spite of medical advances that have reduced the incidence of end-stage organ failure for some diseases, the demand for deceased donor organs continues to out-strip supply. Some organs, or their function, can be temporarily replaced by artificial ones, for example left ventricular assist devices, but this replacement is generally only temporary, providing a bridge to transplantation. The use of organs of other animal species (xenotransplantation) is a matter for the distant future – if at all – owing to a number of immunological, physiological and infectious barriers. Maximising the supply of organs for transplantation is now a key priority for development. One possibility is better organisation of deceased donor programmes, including legislative modifications. There has been renewed enthusiasm for the retrieval of organs from individuals who have died suddenly and unexpectedly [donors after circulatory death (DCDs), previously known as non-heartbeating donors (NHBDs)]. The boundaries of living donation are also being probed, including extending criteria for suitability to donate a kidney and extension of living donation to other organs, including lung segment, liver, pancreas or intestinal transplantation.

Advances in transplantation medicine have improved and lengthened the lives of many people. The number of deceased donors per year remains in many countries more or less stable, despite attempts to increase this number. By contrast, the number of patients on the waiting list is growing. The need for development of transplantation is no less now than it was several decades ago. This time we have to make sure that the public is presented with a realistic view of organ transplantation in support of appropriate policy decisions. Motivating society to support organ donation, altruism and understanding of the key challenges facing transplantation remain key activities for those of us involved in the field.

Key references

1. Calne RY. (1998) *The Ultimate Gift: The story of Britain's Premier Transplant Surgeon*. Headline Book Publishing, London.
2. Guttmann RD, Hayry P, Rapaport F. (1998) A half-century retrospective of transplantation as viewed by the protagonists. *Transplant Proc* **31**, 7–49.
3. Hakim NS, Danovich GM. (2001) *Transplantation Surgery*. Springer, London.

4. Laca L, Grandtnerova B. (2003) *Transplantacie obliciek od zijucich darcov.* Enterprise spol. s.r.o., Slovak Republic.
5. Starzl TE. (1992) *Puzzle People: Memoirs of a Transplant Surgeon.* University of Pittsburgh Press, Pittsburgh.
6. http://www.medhunters.com/Article/transplantTimelineHeartLung
7. http://www.medhunters.com/Article/transplantTimelineLiverPancreas
8. http://www.medhunters.com/Article/transplantTimelineOtherUnusual
9. Shapiro AMJ, Lakey JRT, Ryan EA, *et al.* (2000) Islet transplantation in seven patients with type 1 diabetes mellitus using a glucocorticoid-free immunosuppressive regimen. *N Engl J Med* **343**, 230–238.
10. Ratner LE, Ciseck LJ, Moore RG, *et al.* (1995) Laparoscopic live donor nephrectomy. *Transplantation* **60**: 1047.
11. Wolf JS Jr, Tchetgen MB, Merion RM. (1998) Hand-assisted laparoscopic live donor nephrectomy. *Urology* **52**: 885.
12. Wadstrom J, Lindstrom P. (2002) Hand-assisted retroperitoneoscopic living donor nephrectomy: initial 10 cases. *Transplantation* **73**, 1839.

2 Assessment of the potential renal transplant recipient

Patrick B. Mark and Alan G. Jardine

Background

For many patients with end-stage renal disease (ESRD), renal transplantation provides benefits in both survival and quality of life compared with maintenance dialysis therapy and is generally accepted to be the optimum treatment for ESRD. However, in assessing which patients are likely to benefit from renal transplantation, a number of issues arise.

First, it is imperative that the potential renal transplant recipient (RTR) does not exhibit such a burden of co-morbid disease (most often cardiovascular disease) that the transplant operation cannot be justified owing to risk of peri-operative mortality. Peri-operative mortality in most transplant centres is low, with 1-year patient survival following renal transplantation of the order of 97% in the UK. Therefore, in reality peri-operative mortality is a less common problem for the majority of patients where transplantation has been considered a viable option. Screening should aim to identify remediable disease before transplant listing. As in most countries, only a third of patients with ESRD in the UK are listed for renal transplantation; screening should improve outcomes for patients whether or not they go on to receive a transplant. The transplant operation itself should be technically feasible from a surgical point of view, without anatomical or vascular pathologies that make implanting the transplant impossible. The surgical aspects of renal transplantation are dealt with elsewhere. More detailed consideration will be given to the management of cardiovascular disease in potential RTRs as part of the assessment process as well as other specific conditions likely to be associated with increased peri-operative risk.

Second, following the transplant operation, both patient and graft survival should be such that the quality and/or duration of life should represent a significant improvement compared with that provided by dialysis therapy. Early graft loss where the graft fails because of predictable causes (e.g. some recurrent renal diseases or non-compliance with immunosuppressive therapy) is a potential waste of a resource in

Handbook of Renal and Pancreatic Transplantation, First Edition. Edited by Iain A. M. MacPhee and Jiří Froněk.
© 2012 John Wiley & Sons, Ltd. Published 2012 by John Wiley & Sons, Ltd.

short supply, which in the case of deceased donor kidneys may have been better allocated to another potential RTR. Issues that might lead to early graft loss should be identified during the assessment process. Given the shortage of deceased donor kidneys, available kidneys should be considered a resource to maximise the benefits of transplantation to the wider community of patients with ESRD.

Finally, renal transplantation commits the RTR to lifelong immunosuppression, with inherent risks of infection and malignancy, as well as an increased risk of cardiovascular disease related to both pre-existing disease and that associated with hypertension, new onset diabetes after transplantation (NODAT), hyperlipidaemia and renal impairment. During the assessment of the RTR, attention should be paid to potential risks of committing the patient to long-term immunosuppression. Specific diseases, such as previous cancer, will be examined later in the chapter.

Many excellent guidelines examining optimal assessment of potential RTRs have been published, either under the auspices of national societies of transplantation or as review articles examining specific co-morbidities that impact on the transplant process [1,2]. In all cases, guidelines – including this chapter – can only serve to indicate possible strategies that might be beneficial for managing RTRs. By their nature, guidelines cannot be exhaustive and deal with every eventuality. Each potential RTR will present unique challenges. With that in mind, this chapter will examine conditions likely to present concerns during the process of renal transplantation, grouped by disease and organ system.

Preparation of the potential transplant recipient

Timing of assessment

Ideally, before a patient with progressive renal disease requires renal replacement therapy (RRT), it should be established whether the patient would be a suitable candidate for renal transplantation. Most centres would consider it appropriate to list the suitable candidate for a deceased donor kidney transplant when they are within approximately 6 months of requiring dialysis. Pre-emptive transplantation (whether with a deceased donor or live donor kidney), where the patient receives a transplant before initiation of dialysis, has been associated with better patient and graft survival. Similarly, increasing time on dialysis has been shown to have a detrimental effect on both these outcomes [3]. Thus, early assessment for transplantation should be part of standard preparation for RRT. Early assessment allows both optimisation of the potential RTR's health in preparation for transplantation, as well as facilitating identification and work-up of live donors. In many cases where the patient attends a renal clinic, this timing should be fairly predictable, based on the trend of decline in glomerular filtration rate, combined with knowledge of the rate of progression of the specific renal disease. Unfortunately, early referral for transplant listing may not be possible in the patient who presents with advanced chronic kidney disease ('crash landers'). These patients may require a period of stabilisation before assessment for transplantation.

Contraindications to renal transplantation

Some pre-existing conditions mean that renal transplantation will never be feasible. Others may either require treatment before transplant listing or that multiorgan transplantation be pursued. Examples of these may include liver–kidney transplantation in cirrhosis or combined heart–kidney transplantation for end-stage heart failure when intrinsic renal disease is also present. Any severe irreversible extra-renal condition (e.g. progressive neurological disease, severe respiratory disease) is likely to be an absolute barrier to renal transplantation. Recurrent or metastatic malignancy should be considered a contraindication to transplantation. Severe intractable psychiatric disease likely to impair consent or compliance is often a contraindication to transplantation. Patients who continue to abuse illicit drugs should be abstinent prior to transplant listing, and similarly those with refractory treatment non-adherence should not be listed until this issue can be resolved.

Assessment of the potential renal transplant recipient

General history and examination

Patients should undergo standard clinical history and examination before consideration of more detailed screening as part of work-up for renal transplant listing. Specific points in the history should include the cause of the underlying renal disease. This may include reviewing whether a native renal biopsy has been performed or whether the diagnosis is presumptive. A detailed family history should be taken. These factors combined may consolidate knowledge of the cause of renal failure, along with assessing whether any relatives may be suitable live donors. The current urine output is useful to document and will give some guide as to relative output of the native and transplanted kidneys postoperatively. The history should include a detailed assessment of cardiovascular health, including previous cardiac events and any cardiac interventions. Risk factors for cardiovascular disease such as family history, diabetes and cigarette smoking should be identified. Exercise tolerance should be discussed. Detailed focus should also be on any history of, and treatment for, previous malignancy. Similarly, any previous infections likely to impact on transplantation should be discussed. This should include any previous exposure to, or treatment for, tuberculosis or any period of residence in endemic areas.

Physical examination should identify the presence of congestive cardiac failure, bruits suggestive of underlying carotid arterial disease and murmurs to suggest valvular heart disease. Examination of the femoral pulses and peripheral vasculature will often demonstrate to the surgeon that the iliac vessels will be satisfactory for the transplant anastomosis. Reduced femoral pulses or signs of peripheral vascular disease suggest the need to carry out additional imaging. Abdominal examination will guide whether there is space to place the transplant kidney in patients with polycystic kidney disease or previous transplants.

Laboratory studies

Patients with advanced renal disease or ESRD routinely undergo blood sampling for assessment of kidney function or adequacy of dialysis, bone biochemistry, full blood count and parathyroid hormone. Blood sampling performed specifically as part of the transplantation process (many units will perform these as part of routine care), include coagulation screen, hepatitis B and C, HIV, Epstein–Barr virus (EBV), varicella zoster virus (VZV) and cytomegalovirus (CMV) screening. Vaccination should be offered to hepatitis B- and VZV-antibody-negative patients unless already vaccinated. Blood should be taken for blood grouping, tissue typing and HLA antibody testing.

Cardiovascular assessment

Cardiovascular disease (CVD) is the leading cause of death following renal transplantation, with death with a functioning graft the leading cause of graft loss. Moreover, nearly half the deaths with a functioning graft in the first month after transplantation are due to ischaemic heart disease [4]. Therefore, screening for underlying CVD is logical, with the intention that critical coronary artery lesions may be treated and optimal medical therapy employed prior to listing for renal transplantation [5]. However, controversy remains as to which patients should be screened; the optimal methods for carrying out screening and which patients are likely to benefit from medical therapy and/or coronary artery revascularisation with either percutaneous coronary intervention (PCI) and stenting or coronary artery bypass grafting (CABG). Furthermore – unlike the general population – in ESRD, CVD and coronary artery disease are not synonymous, with the majority of premature cardiovascular deaths occurring owing to sudden cardiac death rather than myocardial infarction. The current evidence base is limited and no trials have tested whether either cardiovascular screening itself, or specific cardiac interventions, benefit patients being assessed for transplantation. A suggested algorithm for screening based on currently available evidence is provided in Fig. 2.1.

Factors that predict post-transplant cardiovascular mortality are similar to those that predict death on the transplant list: age, diabetes mellitus, pre-existing coronary artery disease or vascular disease in other territories. An abnormal electrocardiogram, specifically ST changes representing left ventricular hypertrophy (LVH) with 'strain' have also

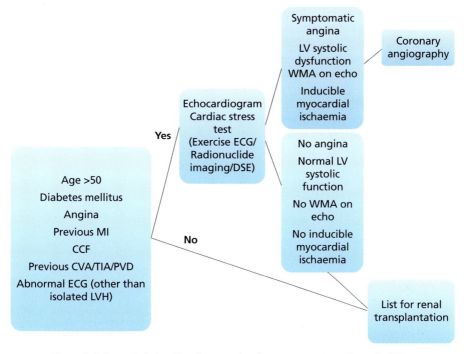

Figure 2.1 Suggested algorithm for screening for coronary artery disease in RTRs. CCF, congestive cardiac failure; CVA, cerebrovascular accident; DSE, dobutamine stress echocardiography; LVH, left ventricular hypertrophy; PVD, peripheral vascular disease; TIA, transient ischaemic attack; MI, myocardial infarction; WMA, wall motion abnormality.

been shown to be independent predictors of post-transplant cardiac death [6]. Therefore, more detailed cardiac assessment should be performed in patients who are 50 years or older, diabetics, patients with pre-existing ischaemic heart disease, an abnormal ECG (other than LVH without strain), congestive cardiac failure, and peripheral or cerebrovascular disease.

These patients should undergo echocardiography primarily to assess left ventricular function, document the presence of LVH and assess for the presence of valvular heart disease. Some form of non-invasive cardiac stress testing should be carried out, although local expertise and availability will dictate the exact modality used. Most centres will favour stress radionuclide myocardial perfusion imaging (thallium/sestamibi or similar) or dobutamine stress echocardiography. Exercise ECG testing has some limitations because of reduced exercise capacity in patients with ESRD. Nonetheless, it has the advantage as an objective validated method for documenting functional capacity in potential RTRs, and although many patients struggle to reach the maximum predicted heart rate, the ability to perform greater than 6 minutes of a Bruce protocol has been shown to be predictive of lower mortality [7].

All cardiac stress testing in potential RTRs is limited by the high prevalence of left ventricular abnormalities in this population. Approximately 70% of these patients will have LVH at echocardiography, with up 20% having left ventricular systolic dysfunction (LVSD). LVSD at echocardiography correlates with significant coronary artery disease and should prompt consideration of coronary angiography. Mild to moderate LVSD has been reported to improve following transplantation, presumably related to improvements in fluid status, and therefore should not be considered an absolute contraindication to transplantation [8]. Patients with severe LVSD are at considerably higher intraoperative, as well as long-term risk and careful consideration of the risk–benefit ratio of transplantation is required. In all patients with LVSD, treatment with angiotensin-converting inhibitors or angiotensin-receptor antagonists combined with beta blockade should be considered, although the evidence for the use of these agents in ESRD with heart failure is less well established than in the general population.

False positive stress tests with radionuclide imaging, exercise ECG and stress echocardiography may represent underlying structural heart disease but not necessarily critical coronary artery stenosis. In all cases a negative test is reassuring and has a high negative predictive value for cardiac events while the patient awaits transplantation. Similarly, a high-risk stress test, suggestive of critical coronary stenosis (left main stem disease, triple vessel coronary artery disease or a large area of vulnerable ischaemic myocardium), implies that the patient should undergo coronary angiography, to identify and potentially revascularise the at-risk myocardial territory prior to transplantation. The presence of a non-diagnostic or intermediate risk stress test (e.g. due to inability to reach maximal heart rate or underlying structural heart disease) in otherwise asymptomatic patients (free of angina, congestive cardiac failure or diabetes), should lead to consideration as to whether coronary angiography is likely to lead to revascularisation. If revascularisation is unlikely to result from angiography, it is usually reasonable to list the patient for renal transplantation without angiography, considering the overall risk–benefit ratio for that individual.

In our experience, in keeping with other large transplant centres in South America and the United States, even an aggressive policy of screening for cardiovascular disease has a low rate of actual coronary intervention, with as few as 6% of patients who undergo cardiovascular screening for renal transplantation undergoing coronary revascularisation with either PCI or with CABG [7,9,10]. Similarly, non-ESRD population studies have not shown benefits of PCI in patients with stable angina, nor are there benefits in prophylactic coronary revascularisation prior to vascular surgery [11]. Therefore, although it is logical to attempt to identify and treat patients with unstable symptoms and/or critical coronary lesions, who are at high risk of early post-transplant death, undue delay to listing for transplantation should not occur in those with low- to medium-risk stress tests. These guidelines are broadly in keeping with the American Heart Association guidelines for management of

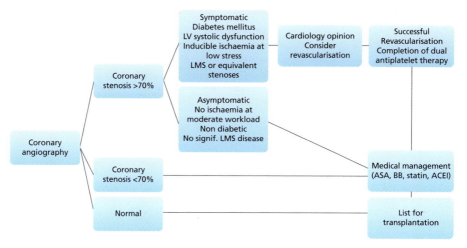

Figure 2.2 Suggested approach to managing the RTR with coronary artery disease. ACEi, angiotensin-converting enzyme inhibitor; ASA, aspirin; BB, beta-blocker; LMS, left main stem.

cardiovascular disease prior to non-cardiac surgery [12]. A suggested algorithm for further action after coronary angiography is shown in Fig. 2.2.

In all patients, consideration should be given to medical therapy to further reduce cardiac risk. Although no prospective trials have been performed in the ESRD population, most meta-analyses suggest that beta-blocker therapy used pre-operatively is likely to reduce the rate of peri-operative cardiac events in patients at high cardiovascular risk. In lower-risk patients, however, the converse is true and beta-blockers are unlikely to be protective. It is therefore unclear whether patients should be started on beta-blockers as prophylaxis while on the transplant list. If used, beta-blocker therapy should be commenced at least 1 month prior to transplantation to avoid hypotension and bradycardia. Similarly, in patients who are taking beta-blockers for hypertension, rather than ischaemic heart disease, beta-blocker therapy should be continued peri-operatively to avoid rebound tachycardia on withdrawal [12].

Patients who have undergone successful revascularisation with CABG or PCI should continue on long-term antiplatelet therapy. As the main effect of aspirin is by inhibiting platelet aggregation via thromboxane A2 but not thrombin, it is unlikely to aggravate peri-operative bleeding and may help reduce transplant renal vein thrombosis [13]. Many patients who have undergone PCI will be treated with drug eluting stents (DESs) coated with sirolimus, everolimus or paclitaxel. Treatment with clopidogrel is required for at least 3 months, or longer, depending on the clinical scenario, to allow endothelialisation and prevent in-stent thrombosis. Thereafter, all patients require long-term aspirin. Clopidogrel has been associated with increased bleeding following surgery and therefore should be discontinued 5 days prior to elective surgery. This is not possible while awaiting a deceased donor kidney, and it may be prudent to suspend the patient for 3 months post-drug-eluting stent insertion while clopidogrel therapy is required.

In addition to ischaemic heart disease, valvular heart disease is more common in ESRD compared with the general population, mainly because of valvular calcification, present in up to 40% of patients. Valvular calcification is associated with similar risk factors to ischaemic heart disease, such as advancing age and higher serum calcium. Although valvular heart disease is likely to progress more slowly following transplantation compared with dialysis, care should be given to valvular lesions of haemodynamic significance. In appropriate patients, successful repair of valvular heart disease should not be a bar to transplantation, although consideration will be required to any anticoagulation strategy in patients with prosthetic valves on anticoagulant therapy. The same is true in patients with chronic atrial fibrillation, which is a risk factor for stroke. The benefits of long-term warfarin therapy in ESRD are probably less marked than in the general population, owing to increased risks of both bleeding and calciphylaxis. Atrial fibrillation *per se* should not be a contraindication to transplantation. Anti-arrhythmic and or rate-controlling drugs should be continued peri-operatively to minimise any impact of tachyarrhythmia on the haemodynamic stresses of the transplant operation. The effect of rate-limiting calcium-channel-blocking drugs (verapamil and diltiazem) on metabolism of calcineurin inhibitors may entail dose adjustment.

Post-transplant cerebrovascular disease shares the same common risk factors as those for ischaemic heart disease – advancing age, atrial fibrillation, cigarette smoking, diabetes, hyperlipidaemia and hypertension. Overall, the risk of post-transplant cerebrovascular disease is relatively low (3.9% of a population of 1617 patients over a 4-year period) [14]. Patients with multiple risk factors, in particular those with previous stroke or transient ischaemic attack, should have targeted risk factor intervention and treatment with antiplatelet therapy or anticoagulation, used along similar lines as in the general population. It has been suggested that symptomatic patients from the general population with moderate to severe carotid stenosis may benefit from carotid endarterectomy or stenting. However, there is no evidence that screening potential RTRs with carotid ultrasound is likely to be beneficial.

Patients with peripheral vascular disease present specific challenges. Conventional risk factors for vascular disease are associated with peripheral vascular disease (increasing age, male gender, lipid abnormalities, smoking, vascular disease elsewhere, diabetes, lipid abnormalities). Diabetic patients and those with claudication or a history of ischaemic ulceration or amputation are at the highest risk. These patients may have underlying aorto-iliac disease, and symptomatic patients should have appropriate imaging to assess the technical feasibility of transplantation. The imaging will depend on local expertise and surgical preference, but usually aorto-femoral Doppler ultrasound may be used as a screening test with computed tomographic angiography and invasive angiography reserved for patients with abnormal Doppler studies or patients at highest risk. Extensive aorto-iliac disease may make renal transplant surgery technically impossible. Patients with lower limb amputations for peripheral vascular disease have been shown to have significantly poorer survival, and careful consideration should be given in individual cases prior to transplant listing.

Psychological aspects of ESRD and transplantation

ESRD is a chronic condition with associated psychological distress. Many patients with ESRD have underlying depression or anxiety either related to, or independent of, their renal disease. Although renal transplantation is a potentially exciting event, there is a degree of uncertainty at this period regarding the likely success of the graft, and additional stressors present such as delayed graft function, rejection, pain, loss of autonomy, high-dose steroid therapy and treatment in an unfamiliar centre. Psychological defence mechanisms such as humour are useful for dispelling anxiety, although maladaptive defence mechanisms may be problematic if they interfere with compliance. As compliance with immunosuppression is vital for successful long-term graft survival, all patients should have psychological assessment to assess for cognitive impairment, mental illness, likelihood of adherence to therapy and any ongoing issues with drug and alcohol misuse. The detail of assessment will be dependent on the individual patient.

Cognitive impairment is not necessarily an absolute bar to transplantation. However, care must be taken to ensure that informed consent is obtained and that a strategy to ensure compliance is in place. If the patient lacks capacity to make decisions regarding their health, a legally acceptable decision-maker should be identified to discuss potential benefits and risks associated with transplantation. Transplantation has been successfully performed in patients with major psychiatric illness, including psychosis, bipolar disorder and depression. These should be stable prior to transplantation. Patients and carers should be aware that perioperative events might act as stressors for mental illness, as well as the potentially hazardous impact of high-dose corticosteroid therapy on mental state. Patients on nephrotoxic psychiatric medication such as lithium should ideally be converted to an alternative agent prior to transplantation. In patients who have displayed non-adherent behaviour in the past, some transplant societies recommend that transplantation should be deferred until a 6-month period of acceptable compliance is complete. Similarly, kidney transplantation should be delayed until a 6-month period of abstinence can be displayed in patients with a history of substance abuse [15].

Transplantation in the elderly

The elderly patient with ESRD represents a unique challenge in assessment for transplantation. There is no formal age at which transplantation is absolutely contraindicated. Biological age is more important than chronological age, and there are some sprightly individuals with isolated renal disease in their early seventies who make better transplant candidates than patients with multiple co-morbidities in their fifties. Although overall life expectancy is likely to be reduced in elderly patients, patients greater than 60 years old who receive a transplant are likely to have better survival than matched controls. This trend is also true for patients greater than 70 years old, although data are conflicting. Data from the UK suggest a 66% 5-year patient survival in patients over 65 receiving a transplant [16]. Infections and malignancy tend to be more common, with fewer episodes of acute rejection, presumably related to the ageing immune system.

In appropriately selected elderly recipients, transplantation may offer lifetime dialysis-free survival, although the increased peri-operative hospital stay may be considered a higher price in those with a shorter life expectancy. With rising prevalence of malignancy and cardiovascular disease with age, screening should be rigorously applied. Both the patient and any live donor should have a realistic expectation that transplantation may reverse uraemia and hence need for dialysis but will not undo the effect of age on other systems, such as osteoarthritis and declining cognitive function.

Lifestyle in potential renal transplant recipients

With increased risks of both CVD and cancer, RTRs should be encouraged to pursue a healthy lifestyle with similar advice to that given to the general population. Suggestions should include avoidance of cigarette smoking, maintaining a normal body weight, appropriate dietary intake of fruit and vegetables and avoidance of physical inactivity. The demands of ESRD make these goals difficult to achieve owing to fluid and dietary restrictions as well as renal bone disease limiting physical activity. The transplant assessment period offers a chance to impress on the potential recipient the importance of these measures. Obesity and cigarette smoking are addressed directly.

Obesity

Obesity presents unique problems in the ESRD population. Malnutrition in patients with ESRD is strongly associated with premature mortality. Although body mass index (BMI) has some limitations as a marker for obesity, it is the most widely used measure. Obesity as defined as BMI>30 has been associated with poorer long-term graft survival following transplantation. Using UNOS data, BMI >35 have been associated with greater risks of delayed graft function, wound complications, acute rejection and prolonged hospital stay [17]. It appears that as BMI exceeds 40 any survival benefit provided by transplantation is likely to be lost. Some centres suggest that BMI greater than 35 may be considered a contraindication for these reasons, although it should be explained to patients that obesity *per se* should not be considered an obstacle to transplantation but more a potentially modifiable risk factor for increased complications. In patients, where obesity contraindicates transplantation, a strategy for planned weight loss should be instigated with a plan to review transplant listing when target BMI has been achieved. This advice, including the desired BMI (or weight-loss pattern), should be tailored to the individual. There is only very limited data on bariatric surgery pre-transplantation, but USRDS data suggest that median excess body weight loss of 31–61% has been achieved in a small cohort of patients [18].

Cigarette smoking

Cardiovascular disease and cancer represent the two leading causes of death in transplant recipients. Cigarette smoking is a major risk factor for cancer and CVD in the general population, and therefore it is imperative that patients are strongly encouraged to discontinue smoking prior to transplantation. In the few studies assessing the influence between smoking and outcome, cigarette smoking has been shown to be associated with poorer patient and graft survival, independently of other factors. The excess graft loss is generally due to death with a functioning graft, with excesses in both cardiovascular events and malignancy in smokers [19]. The existing evidence is less clear regarding whether smoking cessation during the pre-transplant assessment period is associated with a reduction in risk. Nonetheless, it would be inappropriate to advocate anything other than encouragement to help patients to stop smoking as part of transplant assessment.

Respiratory disease

The major concern with severe respiratory disease, which contraindicates renal transplantation, is increased peri-operative risk, including pulmonary oedema, infection and difficulty in weaning from ventilation. Specific aspects of provision of safe anaesthesia for renal transplantation are provided elsewhere in this book. Patients with severe pulmonary disease requiring oxygen therapy are unlikely to be renal transplant candidates owing to poor rehabilitation potential and probable reduced survival due to non-renal disease.

Gastrointestinal disease

Before widespread use of histamine antagonists and proton pump inhibitors, peptic ulceration was a common post-transplant complication. There is no indication for screening for peptic ulcer disease in asymptomatic transplant recipients, nor for routine screening for *Helicobacter pylori*. Symptomatic patients with dyspeptic symptoms should be managed as per usual local practice, considering that high-dose corticosteroids will be required in the post-transplant period. Although diverticulitis is the commonest cause of colonic perforation in transplant recipients, there is no evidence that screening for this alters outcome. Gallbladder stones are fairly common post-renal transplantation, occurring in 28% of patients in one series, but there is no evidence to support screening for cholelithiasis in renal transplant candidates.

Viral hepatitis and transplantation

In hepatitis B surface-antigen-positive patients, specific assessment by a hepatologist is suggested. Liver biopsy may be considered. Active viral replication, chronic active hepatitis or cirrhosis has a poor prognosis if untreated prior to transplantation. Lamivudine is well tolerated and appears to have good virological efficacy both in renal transplant recipients and patients on dialysis, although resistance has been reported. Fewer data are available on the use of adefovior or entecavir in renal transplantation. Patients with chronic hepatitis C infection benefit from renal transplantation compared with dialysis. Hepatology advice should be considered as part of transplant listing. Patients with mild to moderate chronic hepatitis on liver biopsy can proceed to renal transplantation, whereas those with cirrhosis may be considered for combined liver-kidney transplantation rather than isolated kidney transplantation. In cirrhotic patients, with maintained hepatic synthetic function, the risk of combined liver–kidney transplantation should be balanced with that of remaining on dialysis. Treatment of hepatitis C virus (HCV) infection with ribavarin and interferon has been used in dialysis patients, although it is poorly tolerated because of haemolysis. Post-transplant treatment with interferon is not possible owing to the risk of graft loss associated with the immunomodulatory actions of these agents. HCV infection is a risk factor for new onset diabetes after transplantation, and long-term graft survival is poorer in HCV-positive patients.

Recurrent renal disease

The cause of the original renal disease has a significant outcome on long-term transplant survival. Certain renal diseases require specific treatment strategies either prior to, or immediately post, transplantation. Others influence the potential choice of either deceased or living donor or related compared with unrelated donors. Furthermore, in certain diseases renal transplantation alone is inappropriate and combined liver–kidney or bone marrow–kidney transplantation may be considered.

Glomerulonephritis represents the underlying cause of ESRD in approximately 30–50% of RTRs. Recurrence of glomerulonephritis in the transplanted kidney occurs in approximately 10–20% of patients with glomerulonephritis as their cause of ESRD. Of these, 50–70% will lose their graft during long-term follow-up [20,21]. Difficulty exists in ascertaining the impact of recurrent glomerulonephritis on long-term graft survival for a number of reasons. First, a significant proportion of patients with glomerulonephritis have not undergone native renal biopsy to confirm the cause of ESRD. Therefore, when glomerulonephritis is identified on a post-transplant biopsy it may be recurrent disease or a distinct *de novo* glomerulonephritis, but without an original native biopsy this distinction cannot be made. The native biopsy is also less likely to be diagnostic in patients who present late with advanced chronic kidney disease. Variations in post-transplant practice (protocol vs. indication transplant biopsies) may lead to over-representation of histological recurrence of glomerulonephritis, which may not be clinically significant for some time. Many immunosuppressant drugs can cause haemolytic uraemic syndrome/thrombotic thrombocytopaenic purpura (TTP), which can be histologically indistinguishable from that caused by recurrent HUS/TTP or by humoral allograft rejection. Similarly, the differences between transplant glomerulopathy and recurrent membranoproliferative glomerulonephritis can be impossible to decipher, particularly without biopsy samples being processed for immunofluoresence and electron microscopy, which are not necessarily routinely performed on all transplant biopsies. Finally, immunoglobulin A (IgA) can be found deposited in some donor kidneys prior to transplantation, making true recurrent IgA nephropathy difficult to diagnose. Nonetheless, despite all these caveats, recurrent renal disease, in particular glomerulonephritis, is a not uncommon finding and is a significant cause of graft loss. Some effort can be made pre-transplant to both quantify this risk and in specific cases pre-emptively provide strategies to reduce early graft loss. A summary of data on recurrence of renal disease post transplantation is shown in Table 2.1.

Immunoglobulin A nephropathy

Immunoglobulin A nephropathy (IgAN) is the commonest glomerulonephritis worldwide and is the cause of ESRD in approximately 20% of transplant recipients. The pathogenesis is incompletely understood, and IgAN clinically manifests as hypertension, proteinuria with microscopic haematuria and progressive renal dysfunction. Macroscopic haematuria occasionally occurs. Men are affected more frequently than women. Recurrent IgAN is common after transplantation, recurring in between 15 and 50% of patients biopsied for clinical rather than protocol indications. The clinical manifestations of IgAN in transplants are similar to those in native kidneys. The 10-year incidence of graft loss due to recurrent IgAN has been suggested to be 9.7% from the largest registry report of IgAN cases [21]. During the first 5 years post transplant there appears to be no renal allograft survival disadvantage in IgAN compared with other causes of renal failure, and there may be some protective effect, perhaps due to alloreactive IgA anti-HLA antibodies that may abrogate the effect of IgG and IgM antibodies on the transplant. Long-term graft survival at 10 years is comparable to or possibly slightly worse than other renal diseases. Multiple reports have

Table 2.1 Recurrence rate of primary renal disease following renal transplantation graft. Data mainly generated from references [20,21].

Renal disease	Recurrence rate after transplantation (%)	Risk of graft failure at 5–10 years post transplant (%)	Factors associated with increased risk of recurrence	Strategies to avoid/treat recurrence
IgAN	20–50	Approx. 10	Previous graft loss due to IgAN	ACEi/ARB for hypertension± proteinuria
FSGS	20–50	13–20	Previous graft loss due to early recurrence	Plasmapheresis (PP) for recurrent disease Peri-operative (PP) for high risk of recurrence Maintain CNI-based immunosuppression?
MPGN				
Type I	20–50	Approx.15	Possibly HLA-B8DR3 and live donor	No effective treatment; exclude secondary causes
Type II	80–100	15–30		No effective treatment; exclude secondary causes
Membranous	10–30	10–15		Defer transplant until disease clinically inactive
Lupus nephritis	3–10	<5		Defer transplant until disease clinically inactive; treatment with PP, corticosteroids and cyclophosphamide in recurrent disease
ANCA-associated GN	<20	6–8		Defer transplant until disease clinically inactive; treatment with PP, corticosteroids and cyclophosphamide in recurrent disease
AGBM disease	<1 if AGBM negative; 50 if AGBM detectable			Careful genotyping in live donation; combined liver-kidney transplant in CFI/CFH mutation?
aHUS		80 at 2 years if CFH/CFI mutation		Combined liver–kidney transplantation
1° oxalosis	80–100			

questioned whether there is an interaction between related live donors and the recurrence of IgAN in the recipient. Overall, it appears that although there may be an increased risk of histological recurrence, this has not translated to an apparent risk of long-term graft loss. However, it is clear that IgAN should be excluded in potential live donors prior to transplantation, as familial forms of IgA have been described. Henoch-Schönlein purpura is the systemic variant of IgAN. Its behaviour with respect to transplantation appears to be similar to that of IgAN. In patients who have lost their first graft to IgAN, the rate of recurrence is much higher. A graft loss of 60% with a follow-up duration of 21–51 months has been reported [22], although other case series report good graft function at over 7 years follow-up despite biopsy-proven recurrent IgAN.

There is no effective treatment for preventing recurrent IgAN, and management of recurrences should be similar to that in primary IgAN as a native renal disease. Focus should be on treatment of hypertension, using where possible inhibition of the renin angiotensin system to reduce proteinuria. Therefore, patients with IgAN should be counselled as to the risk of histological recurrence on renal transplant biopsy. They should be aware that this may be a potential cause of graft failure, but in the majority of cases the long-term graft outcomes for patients with IgAN as the cause of ESRD are good. Live related donation should be avoided in the rare cases of familial IgAN and in cases where the first graft has been lost early owing to recurrent IgAN.

Focal and segmental glomerulosclerosis

Although focal and segmental glomerulosclerosis (FSGS) represents the histological lesion that is present in both primary FSGS as well as in a variety of secondary causes, including any cause of glomerular hyperfiltration, viral infections and other toxic insults leading to sclerosis of the glomerulus. Recurrence of the secondary lesion depends on the presence or treatment of the underlying disorder. Recurrent primary FSGS occurs in approximately 20–50% of transplants, leading to graft failure in 13–20% of patients at 10 years post transplant [21]. Difficulty exists in distinguishing histological features of early recurrent FSGS, which can be subtle and prone to sampling bias. Recurrence of FSGS is heralded by early-onset massive proteinuria usually in the first year post transplant. The pathogenesis is unclear but is thought to relate to a circulating factor, which increases glomerular permeability to albumin. Conflicting reports suggest that it is unclear if this is a permissive factor for glomerular permeability or the loss of an inhibitory regulator. In 10–15% of cases of primary FSGS, there is an additional genetic component, with mutations of genes encoding for nephrin, podocin, α-actinin 4 and CD2AP. Essentially, the likelihood of recurrence in the transplant is influenced by the aggressiveness of the original renal disease, with patients who progressed quickly to ESRD at greatest risk of recurrent disease. Patients who have lost previous grafts due to recurrent FSGS are at greater risk of recurrent disease. Patients who lost their first graft due to recurrent FSGS during the first year post transplant are at extremely high (>80%) risk of recurrence in subsequent transplants. Although the reports on risk in live versus deceased donor transplants do not clearly point to a specific risk with related donors, it would seem prudent to avoid living donor transplantation in patients with early graft loss due to recurrent FSGS.

Treatment is aimed at either removing the circulating factor, or replacing the inhibitory factor regulating glomerular permeability, by plasmapheresis. This should be instigated early once recurrent disease has been identified as the chance of success diminishes as the number of sclerosed glomeruli increases with progression of disease. Although pre-emptive plasmapheresis has been advocated for children and high-risk recipients, this has not been tested in a clinical trial. The approach for lower-risk individuals is less clear. There is some suggestion that ciclosporin may be beneficial in treating recurrent FSGS, compared with newer immunosuppressants such as sirolimus. Patients with primary FSGS should be counselled regarding the risk of post-transplant recurrence of FSGS, including the need for intense treatment regimens during the post-transplant period.

Membranoproliferative (mesangiocapillary) glomerulonephritis

Membranoproliferative glomerulonephritis (MPGN) has a high rate of recurrence in renal transplants. Type 1 MPGN (with mesangial and subepithelial deposits) recurs in 20–50% of allografts and presents as proteinuria and declining graft function. The overall rate of graft loss at 10 years due to recurrent type 1 MPGN is approximately 15%, with a much higher rate (80%) of graft loss due to recurrence in the second transplant, in patients who lost their first renal transplant owing to recurrent disease [21]. Additionally, receiving a live related kidney and HLA-B8DR3 are also risk factors for recurrence. In type 2 MPGN (dense deposit disease), recurrence is even more common, affecting 80–100% of patients. Recurrent disease manifests as non-nephrotic range proteinuria and declining graft function. Graft loss occurs in 15–30% of patients at 5 years. There is no effective therapy for either prevention or treating recurrent MPGN, and although a significant proportion of patients with MPGN will have perfectly acceptable outcomes following transplantation, potential recurrence should be highlighted as part of preparation for transplantation. Secondary causes of MPGN, including hepatitis B and C and other systemic diseases, should be managed by directing treatment at the underlying cause to reduce risk of recurrent disease.

Membranous nephropathy

Recurrent idiopathic membranous nephropathy (MN) occurs in 10–30% of patients and presents as proteinuria, often towards the end of the first year post transplantation. Secondary causes of MN should be excluded, and as MN is the commonest *de novo* glomerulopathy in renal transplants, recurrent disease should therefore be differentiated from *de novo* lesions. Graft failure from recurrent MN occurs in approximately 10–15% of cases at 10 years. No specific risk factors or treatment strategies have been defined, and it seems reasonable to list patients with idiopathic MN as cause of ESRD for transplantation without excessive caution.

Systemic lupus erythematosus

As patients with active lupus nephritis tend to be systemically unwell, transplantation should usually be deferred until there has been a period of disease inactivity for approximately 6 to 9 months. Although histological recurrence has been described in up to 30% of grafts, graft loss due to recurrent lupus nephritis is rare. Serological markers of disease activity do not appear to be particularly helpful at predicting recurrence. Patients with systemic lupus erythematosus should be checked for the presence of antiphospholipid antibodies to assess thrombotic risk. Overall, as graft survival is similar for patients with lupus nephritis as cause of ESRD compared with matched controls, these patients can be listed for transplantation when the systemic disorder appears relatively quiescent.

Antineutrophil cytoplasmic antibody-associated glomerulonephritis (pauci-immune glomerulonephritis)

Recurrent glomerulonephritis in renal transplants has been described in all the antineutrophil cytoplasmic antibody (ANCA)-associated glomerulonephritides (Wegner's granulomatosis, microscopic polyangiitis and idiopathic necrotising crescentic glomerulonephritis). Transplantation should be deferred until disease is clinically inactive. There is no evidence that ANCA titre at time of transplantation predicts likelihood of relapse. Recurrent systemic vasculitis may occur, as well as renal vasculitis in the transplant. The largest registry of recurrent glomerulonephritis in transplants suggests 10-year incidence of graft loss of 7.7% in ANCA-associated glomerulonephritides [21].

Anti-glomerular basement membrane disease

Current practice dictates that transplantation should be postponed in patients with antiglomerular basement membrane disease until circulating antiglomerular basement membrane antibodies are undetectable for at least 12 months. Thereafter, disease recurrence is rare. Recurrence has been reported in up to 50% of patients transplanted when antiglomerular basement membrane antibodies are present.

Atypical haemolytic uraemic syndrome

Haemolytic uraemic syndrome (HUS) is characterised by renal failure, thrombocytopaenia and microangiopathic haemolytic anaemia. HUS is commonly associated with a diarrhoeal illness, often shiga and shiga-like toxin producing *Escherichia coli* and *Streptococcus pneumoniae*. Typically, diarrhoea-associated (D+) HUS is a self-limiting disease (albeit with significant morbidity and mortality) with recovery of renal function in >90% of cases. In non diarrhoeal (D–) HUS, or atypical HUS, it is now recognised that a number of genetic mutations may be present affecting either factor H (CFH), membrane co-factor protein (MCP) or factor I (CFI) as well as factor B and C3 mutations. Although rare (incidence ~2 per million population per year), atypical HUS recurs rapidly after renal transplantation in 50% of patients. In patients with a CFH or CFI mutation, renal transplantation has a poor outcome, with graft loss due to recurrent disease in 80% of cases at 2 years. By contrast, patients with an isolated MCP mutation do relatively well post transplant, as the graft replaces the defective protein. Live related transplantation carries similar risks of recurrence for these groups, respectively, and additionally risks atypical HUS to the donor if they carry the same mutation. In general, live related transplantation should be avoided in atypical HUS. In patients with CFH or CFI mutations, combined liver–kidney transplantation may be considered in a centre with appropriate expertise [23].

Primary oxalosis and oxaluria

Primary oxalosis, a rare autosomal recessive cause of ESRD, leads to recurrent oxalate deposition in the graft post-renal-transplantation, leading to such swift graft loss that conventional renal transplantation is usually inappropriate. The disorder is due to a deficiency in hepatic alanine glyoxylate aminotransferase, which leads to increased urinary calcium oxalate excretion and nephrocalcinosis. Medical management with oral phosphate therapy to minimise oxalate deposition combined with pyridoxine therapy to act as a coenzyme in converting glyoxylate to lysine can be tried but is rarely effective, whereas combined liver–kidney transplantation is curative, as the transplanted liver replaces the absent enzyme.

Secondary oxaluria is usually due to intestinal resections, e.g. Crohn's disease or intestinal bypass for obesity, and leads to recurrent oxalate stones in the transplanted kidney. Although urinary oxalate excretion prior to transplantation guides the risk of recurrent disease, this may not be possible in the anuric ESRD patient. Where feasible, surgical correction should be considered to prevent recurrent oxaluria.

Adult polycystic kidney disease

Patients with massive polycystic kidneys occasionally require nephrectomy pre-transplantation to allow room for the transplanted kidney. Nephrectomy may additionally be required for bleeding, infection or discomfort. There is no evidence for routine screening of patients with polycystic kidney disease for cerebral aneurysms, although this should be performed in patients with previous intracerebral aneurysm rupture or with a strong family history of intracranial aneurysm rupture.

Alport syndrome

Alport syndrome is a genetic abnormality of type 4 collagen leading to nephritis and ESRD, usually associated with deafness. It is X-linked recessive in 80% of cases, with the remainder autosomal recessive (15%) or autosomal dominant (5%). As an inherited kidney disease, careful screening is required to avoid transplanting a potentially affected sibling as a live donor. Theoretically, following successful transplantation, antiglomerular basement antibodies may form in response to the donor kidney collagen. Clinically significant *de novo* anti-glomerular basement membrane disease is, however, rare. Overall outcomes of transplantation in Alport syndrome are good.

Amyloidosis

Patients with systemic primary amyloidosis are at increased risk for renal transplantation, usually owing to cardiac disease. Mortality in renal transplantation has been reported to be as high as 50% at 1 year, and careful consideration should be given prior to transplant listing with primary amyloidosis unless the presence of extra-renal disease is minimal. Bone marrow biopsy prior to renal transplantation may be considered. In rare hereditary systemic amyloidosis, combined liver–kidney transplantation has been reported to be curative. Secondary amyloidosis may recur in the graft, but patients with secondary amyloidosis may be good transplant candidates if the primary condition is well controlled. Colchicine is required in amyloidosis due to familial Mediterranean fever to prevent amyloid deposition in the graft.

Multiple myeloma

Traditionally myeloma has been considered a contraindication to renal transplantation, as patients with ESRD due to myeloma tend to have poor survival on dialysis, usually owing to infection. Advances in chemotherapy have improved this somewhat, but generally speaking patients with multiple myeloma are not transplant candidates. However, there are recent reports of exceptional results in highly selected individuals treated with bone marrow and renal transplantation from HLA-identical siblings [24]. Patients who have had successful bone marrow transplantation for myeloma could therefore be considered transplant candidates.

Patients with previous malignancy

Patients with ESRD have increased risk of cancer compared with the general population. Immunosuppressive therapy for renal transplantation subsequently dramatically raises this risk further. The overall risk is higher in younger patients and diminishes with age. Renal and bladder tumours are particularly increased. Risk factors for developing malignancy in ESRD patients include prior immunosuppressive therapy (either for previous transplantation or as treatment for glomerulonephritis), previous failed transplantation, transplantation of another non-renal organ and exposure to oncogenic viruses (EBV, HBV, HCV). All patients who receive a renal transplant should be counselled of the increased risk of malignancy following renal transplantation.

Patients who have had successful treatment for a previous malignancy may be suitable candidates for a renal transplant. It is usually appropriate to have a disease-free waiting period to ensure no emergence of occult metastatic disease. This is often a minimum period of 2 years, although it is highly dependent on the nature, grade, staging and treatment of the previous tumour. Overall, in patients transplanted following treatment of cancer, 53% of recurrences have been demonstrated if the interval between treatment was less than 2 years, 34% of recurrences in patients 2–5 years after treatment falling to 13% in patients who have waited over 5 years [1]. Close collaboration with the patient's oncologist should be encouraged when listing a patient with treated malignancy for renal transplantation. The Israel Penn International Tumour Transplant Registry (http://www.ipittr.org) is an invaluable source of information on malignancies in solid organ transplant recipients. However, as with all registries, reported data are likely to underestimate cases of post-transplantation malignancies owing to non-reporting of cases from some centres [25]. Suggested guidelines for minimum recurrence-free waiting times following treatment for malignancies are suggested in Table 2.2.

Table 2.2 Suggested waiting time for transplantation following successful treatment of cancer. Tumour, grade, staging, treatments and time post completion of therapy will need to be taken into account in individual cases. Data are mainly generated from references [1,2,25].

Tumour type	Suggested minimal wait time	Additional factors to consider before transplantation
Breast cancer		
In situ	2 years	Recurrence stage I and II
Invasive	5 years	disease in 5-8% recurrence post tx. Stage III disease recurrence 64%. Limited data on recurrence on in situ lesions or invasive lesions transplanted at 2-5 years
Colorectal		
Dukes A or B1	At least 2 years	Recurrence rate over all
>Duke's B2	5 years	12-21%. Recurrence rate from Duke's A or B1 is 14-20% and 42% in more advance disease. Most recurrences occur at 2-5years post tx.
Lung	At least 2 years	Limited data available. Histology, grade and stage of tumour likely to be important
Urogenital		
Renal		
Incidental	None	Recurrence <1% in incidental
<5 cm	2-5 years	tumours. Overall recurrence
>5 cm	5 years	30%. Evidence less clear for smaller tumours. Recurrence 61% before 2 years, 33% at 2-5 years and 6% at >5years post tx

Table 2.2 *Continued*

Tumour type	Suggested minimal wait time	Additional factors to consider before transplantation
Wilm's tumour	2 years	Should be a least 1year post completion of chemotherapy
Bladder		
Superficial lesions	None	High-risk local recurrence but low risk of invasive disease. Carcinoma in situ more aggressive. Recurrence rate 18-26% overall
Invasive	2 years	
Prostate	2 years	Localised disease (T1-2) recurrence rate 14-16%. Patients with disease outside prostate capsule should not be transplanted
Testicular	2 years	Recurrence rate 3-12% post transplant. Little data on 2-5 year wait.
Cervix		
In situ	None	In situ lesions will require ongoing gynaecological screening/treatment. Limited data to support management in invasive lesions
Localised cervical invasive	At least 2 years	
Skin		
Melanoma	5 years	83% recurrence reported if tx <5 years post treatment
Squamous cell carcinoma	No specific guidelines	Local recurrence 48-62%. Longer wait decreases recurrence (61% recurrence <2 years post tx, 35% at 2-5 years, 4% at >5years)
Basal cell carcinoma	None	
Haematological		
Leukaemia/ lymphoma (Hodgkin/NHL)	2 years	Most data on patients waiting >5 years. Recurrence rate 11% following transplant
PTLD	2 years	Overall recurrence rate 3%.
Thyroid	2 years	7–8% rate of recurrence post tx. Low grade incidental tumours favourable

Tx, transplant/transplantation.

Management of the potential transplant recipient on the waiting list

The wait for a deceased donor kidney is uncertain, with a median wait in the UK of 3 years. Some factors that influence patient and graft survival following successful transplantation are fixed, such as the underlying renal disease or HLA-tissue type. However both the cardiomyopathy and arteriopathy associated with ESRD progress with increasing time since the initial transplant assessment. These factors may increase in severity to the point that the transplant operation is riskier in the case of cardiac disease, or surgically more challenging with increasing arterial calcification. All dialysis patients irrespective of their transplant status should receive appropriate care to optimise their cardiovascular health, and this is equally true of those on the transplant list, irrespective of the expected waiting time for a kidney. There is a case for repeating cardiovascular assessment in patients on the transplant list. There is no evidence to guide how often, and which investigations should be repeated in otherwise asymptomatic patients, an exercise that could become both expensive and unwieldy for all the patients in any given centre. Nonetheless, it seems reasonable to re-evaluate the need for repeating investigations on an annual basis, with the strategy in an individual patient guided by the results of the initial screening investigations.

Key references

1. Kasiske BL, Cangro CB, Hariharan S, *et al.* (2001) The evaluation of renal transplantation candidates: clinical practice guidelines. *Am J Transplant* **1** (Suppl 2), 3–95.
2. Knoll G, Cockfield S, Blydt-Hansen T, *et al.* (2005) Canadian Society of Transplantation consensus guidelines on eligibility for kidney transplantation. *CMAJ* **173**, 1181–1184.
3. Meier-Kriesche HU, Kaplan B. (2002) Waiting time on dialysis as the strongest modifiable risk factor for renal transplant outcomes: a paired donor kidney analysis. *Transplantation* **74**, 1377–1381.
4. Ojo AO, Hanson JA, Wolfe RA, *et al.* (2000) Long-term survival in renal transplant recipients with graft function. *Kidney Int* **57**, 307–313.
5. Pilmore H. (2006) Cardiac assessment for renal transplantation. *Am J Transplant* **6**, 659–665.
6. Woo YM, McLean D, Kavanagh D, *et al.* (2002) The influence of pre-operative electrocardiographic abnormalities and cardiovascular risk factors on patient and graft survival following renal transplantation. *J Nephrol* **15**, 380–386.
7. Patel RK, Mark PB, Johnston N, *et al.* (2008) Prognostic value of cardiovascular screening in potential renal transplant recipients: a single-center prospective observational study. *Am J Transplant* **8**, 1673–1683.
8. Wali RK, Wang GS, Gottlieb SS, *et al.* (2005) Effect of kidney transplantation on left ventricular systolic dysfunction and congestive heart failure in patients with end-stage renal disease. *J Am Coll Cardiol* **45**, 1051–1060.

9. De Lima JJ, Gowdak LH, de Paula FJ, *et al.* (2010) Treatment of coronary artery disease in hemodialysis patients evaluated for transplant-a registry study. *Transplantation* **89**, 845–850.

10. Kasiske BL, Malik MA, Herzog CA. (2005) Risk-stratified screening for ischemic heart disease in kidney transplant candidates. *Transplantation* **80**, 815–820.

11. McFalls EO, Ward HB, Moritz TE, *et al.* (2004) Coronary-artery revascularization before elective major vascular surgery. *N Engl J Med* **351**, 2795–2804.

12. Fleischmann KE, Beckman JA, Buller CE, *et al.* (2009) ACCF/AHA focused update on perioperative beta blockade: a report of the American college of cardiology foundation/American heart association task force on practice guidelines. *Circulation* **120**, 2123–2151.

13. Robertson AJ, Nargund V, Gray DW, *et al.* (2000) Low dose aspirin as prophylaxis against renal-vein thrombosis in renal-transplant recipients. *Nephrol Dial Transplant* **15**, 1865–1868.

14. Aull-Watschinger S, Konstantin H, Demetriou D, *et al.* (2008) Pre-transplant predictors of cerebrovascular events after kidney transplantation. *Nephrol Dial Transplant* **23**, 1429–1435.

15. Prendergast MB, Gaston RS. (2010) Optimizing medication adherence: An ongoing opportunity to improve outcomes after kidney transplantation. *Clin J Am Soc Nephrol* **5**, 1305–1311.

16. Oniscu GC, Brown H, Forsythe JL. (2004) How great is the survival advantage of transplantation over dialysis in elderly patients? *Nephrol Dial Transplant* **19**, 945–951.

17. Gore JL, Pham PT, Danovitch GM, *et al.* (2006) Obesity and outcome following renal transplantation. *Am J Transplant* **6**, 357–363.

18. Modanlou KA, Muthyala U, Xiao H, *et al.* (2009) Bariatric surgery among kidney transplant candidates and recipients: Analysis of the United States renal data system and literature review. *Transplantation* **87**, 1167–1173.

19. Kasiske BL, Klinger D. (2000) Cigarette smoking in renal transplant recipients. *J Am Soc Nephrol* **11**, 753–759.

20. Choy BY, Chan TM, Lai KN. (2006) Recurrent glomerulonephritis after kidney transplantation. *Am J Transplant* **6**, 2535–2542.

21. Briganti EM, Russ GR, McNeil JJ, *et al.* (2002) Risk of renal allograft loss from recurrent glomerulonephritis. *N Engl J Med* **347**, 103–109.

22. Ohmacht C, Kliem V, Burg M, *et al.* (1997) Recurrent immunoglobulin A nephropathy after renal transplantation: A significant contributor to graft loss. *Transplantation* **64**, 1493–1496.

23. Taylor CM, Machin S, Wigmore SJ, *et al.* (2010) Clinical practice guidelines for the management of atypical haemolytic uraemic syndrome in the United Kingdom. *Br J Haematol* **148**, 37–47.

24. Fudaba Y, Spitzer TR, Shaffer J, *et al.* (2006) Myeloma responses and tolerance following combined kidney and nonmyeloablative marrow transplantation: In vivo and in vitro analyses. *Am J Transplant* **6**, 2121–2133.

25. Penn I. (2000) Cancers in renal transplant recipients. *Adv Ren Replace Ther* **7**, 147–156.

3 Pre-transplant assessment and medical evaluation of potential live kidney donors

Jonas Wadström

Introduction

Kidney transplantation is the best treatment for patients with end-stage renal disease (ESRD), and a kidney from a living donor, transplanted pre-emptively, gives the best outcome in terms of patient and graft survival [1,2]. Society and the medical community thus have to rely on the willingness of healthy individuals to donate kidneys in order to offer patients with ESRD the optimal treatment.

This chapter deals with the assessment of potential kidney donors. The main focus and objective of such assessment is to ensure that donor risks are minimised, both short term in the peri-operative period and long term living with one kidney. The assessment should also ensure that as little harm as possible is caused from a psychosocial and socioeconomic perspective. Finally, the assessment should also ensure that the recipient is not subjected to unreasonable risks and that the transplantation is likely to be as successful as possible.

The assessment is rigorous and extensive, which makes it costly and takes many more resources than is normally justified in a normal health-care setting. However, donors are not patients. They are healthy volunteers who help patients in need – and thereby help society to provide optimal and a cost-effective care for patients with ESRD. We should therefore always act as donor advocates and perform an optimal assessment without setting any priority on cost savings.

Particular aspects of live donor kidney transplantation

Donor nephrectomy is a major surgical procedure that is carried out on a healthy person, who receives no direct therapeutic benefit. The benefit accrues to the recipient and not the donor. The principle of *Primum non nocere* is challenged, so this requires particular considerations in terms of safety and informed consent. The particular safety aspects have been

Handbook of Renal and Pancreatic Transplantation, First Edition. Edited by Iain A. M. MacPhee and Jiří Froněk.
© 2012 John Wiley & Sons, Ltd. Published 2012 by John Wiley & Sons, Ltd.

mentioned above and will be discussed in more detail later on in this chapter. Informed consent can be seen as adhering to the principle of autonomy, respecting the wish to donate a kidney, which balances and justifies the violation of the *Primum non nocere* principle. The information a potential donor should receive before consenting needs to be more extensive and more far-reaching than the level of information that is normal for a surgical procedure. It should include the spectrum and frequency of peri-operative morbidity and the risk of mortality, which has remained constant over time and is about 0.03% [3,4]. It should also include the fact that on the one hand the assessment may reveal previously undiagnosed diseases that might influence future possibilities of obtaining health and life insurance, but on the other hand might have the advantage of early detection and treatment. There should also be information about potential negative psychosocial and socioeconomic consequences, as well as the expected outcome in terms of recipient survival and graft function. It is important to provide specific information if there are any increased risks to either donor or recipient. The information should be given both verbally and in writing, and in cases where you suspect that there are language difficulties, it is important that an independent translator is used from the very first encounter. Many donors appreciate the opportunity to meet someone who has donated, and it is desirable that the transplant team can provide such an opportunity. After a potential donor has been given all the relevant information it is important that adequate time is given to reflect on the decision to donate.

Informed consent does to some extent come into conflict with confidentiality. In order to give information about risks and expected outcome, some information must be shared between the recipient and donor. This information is often in the best interest of both parties. To avoid any misunderstandings and conflicts, it is advisable to have a discussion about confidentiality at an early stage. Another particular aspect related to the two people involved in one procedure is that the health-care professionals taking care of the donor should be separate from those taking care of the recipient, in order to ensure that the assessment and treatment is unbiased and in the best interest of the respective party.

If the donor is found to be unsuitable for medical reasons or withdraws, the transplant team should offer the donor adequate medical and/or psychological assistance.

Approaching and informing potential donors

A large majority of potential donors take the initial step and volunteer to become a donor. Not infrequently, however, donors are approached by the recipient or members of the recipient's family. A third alternative is that potential donors are approached by a member of the transplant team or the person is involved in the care of the recipient. This approach has several advantages, as it allows the donor to be approached by a third party who is a professional and who from the very beginning can give correct information about options for the recipient, steps of the evaluation process and risks associated with donor nephrectomy (from a medical, psychosocial and economic standpoint). The third-party approach also relieves pressure on the recipient to ask, and on the donor to say no if he or she is unable or unwilling to donate. If more than one potential donor has come forward and is suitable, the transplant team can assist in the decision process and guide the most suitable donor from a medical point of view, for example in case of HLA-identical siblings. Finally, there are situations in which the recipient is reluctant to accept an offer from a potential donor. Early contact with health-care professionals and the transplant team is then of great value in sorting out possible misunderstandings and avoiding future conflicts between the potential donor and recipient.

Who can be a donor?

Historically donors were blood-group-compatible members of the immediate family of the patient with ESRD. Now, with modern immunosuppressants and protocols for desensitisation, almost any competent person can be a donor. Although this is a very positive development, it also makes it difficult for a potential donor or the transplant team to give a medical excuse when a potential donor is unwilling to donate. The expansion of the donor pool also increases the workload of the transplant team, especially potential non-directed donors who often in the end are found unfit or decide not to donate. Finally, since practically any healthy individual can be a donor, at times it can be difficult to rule out paid donors. Paid donation is illegal in most countries.

Donor evaluation

The purpose and overall goal of the donor medical evaluation is to ensure that the donor is suitable and that the nephrectomy can be carried out with little risk. This involves the identification of contraindications and unreasonable medical risks. The main medical risks to be assessed and evaluated are twofold: risks related to surgery and the peri-operative period, and those related to the long-term consequences of donating a kidney. To a certain extent these risks overlap. If a risk is identified it has to be put into context and discussed with the donor to ascertain whether it is an acceptable risk and whether it can be reduced by taking appropriate prophylactic or therapeutic measures. Examples of such risks are borderline hypertension and impaired glucose tolerance associated with a body mass index (BMI) over 30. By losing weight it is likely that the potential donor will normalise their blood pressure and impaired glucose tolerance. This will lower both the short- and long-term risks of donation, provided the donor does not regain weight after the donation.

The donor evaluation also serves to identify and minimise risks for the recipient, such as transmittable infections and malignancies, as well as to ensure that the donated kidney has adequate function and can be transplanted without technical difficulties that might unreasonably compromise the success of the transplantation.

It is recommended that the evaluation is carried out according to a standardised protocol. That way the investigations can be made in a logical sequence without risk of omission, and unnecessary investigations can be avoided should a contraindication be revealed at some time point during the evaluation process. There should not be too many steps, however. It is reasonable that after initial contact and screening the evaluation be carried out in two to three steps. The most common donor complaint regarding the evaluation period is that it takes too long and involves too many hospital visits that interfere with work and social life. It can also lead to a prolonged period of worry and uncertainty about the outcome of the evaluation and the timing of the transplant.

There is a fairly good agreement between different national and international recommendations regarding the routine screening tests that should be carried out in the evaluation [5–7].

Initial steps

The aim of the initial assessment is to identify any obvious medical or psychosocial contraindications to donation, avoiding further unnecessary investigations. In this regard the medical history is important. The UK guidelines list a large number of issues that are of particular interest in the medical history (see Box 3.1). The initial clinical examination should be thorough and include BMI and blood pressure. The preliminary laboratory evaluation may vary from centre to centre and depends on findings in the patient and family history as well as in the clinical examination but should as a minimum include serum creatinine, urea, blood glucose, urine dipstick, ABO typing and HLA typing as well as a blood sample for crossmatching. A complete screening as recommended by UK guidelines is given in Box 3.2 and a more extensive thrombophilia screening according to Swedish guidelines is given in Box 3.3.

It is important that donors get realistic and correct information about the time necessary for the different investigations in the evaluation process and for surgery. They should be given the opportunity to plan work and social activities, and appointments for investigations should be offered accordingly.

Complete medical evaluation

If the initial medical and psychosocial evaluation reveals no contraindications to donation, the next step is to perform a complete medical evaluation. Some of the medical examinations carried out to

> **Box 3.1 Issues of particular interest in the medical history.**
> - Haematuria
> - Oedema
> - Urinary tract infection
> - Nephrolithiasis
> - Ischaemic heart disease
> - Cardiovascular risk factors
> - Hypertension
> - Diabetes mellitus, including family history
> - Previous jaundice
> - Thromboembolic disease
> - Previous malignancy
> - Chronic infections such as tuberculosis
> - Systemic disease that may involve the kidney
> - Family history of a renal condition that may affect the donor
> - Smoking
> - Problems with alcohol or drug dependence
> - Psychiatric history
> - Obstetric history
> - Residence abroad
> - Specific geographical risk factors
> - History with respect to transmissible infections
> - Belonging to high-risk groups of hepatitis B and C, HIV, HTLV1 and HTLV2 infection
> - Previous medical assessments for life insurance

evaluate the suitability of a potential donor have been mentioned above in the section 'Initial steps'. In the following, some examinations and conditions of special relevance for the specific risks of kidney donation will be discussed in more detail. As already mentioned, there are three main types of risk that the complete medical evaluation serves to assess: 1) peri-operative risks, 2) long-term risks of unilateral nephrectomy and 3) risks that the recipient might be subjected to. Many of these risks overlap. I make no pretention that the issues brought forward in this section are complete, and recommendations on what examinations should be carried out differ somewhat from centre to centre and between countries, depending on local conditions. Examples of different recommendations and guidelines are given in the references [5–8].

Assessment of renal function and anatomy

Renal function
A thorough assessment of kidney function and anatomy is essential to guarantee long-term adequate renal function in the donor and optimal outcome in the recipient. Immediately after nephrectomy kidney function is reduced by 50%, but there is a rapid functional adaptation with

Box 3.2 Routine screening investigations for the potential donor.

Urinalysis
- Dipstick for protein, blood and glucose
- Microscopy, culture and sensitivity
- Measurement of protein excretion rate

Blood tests
- Haemoglobin and full blood count
- Coagulation screen (prothrombin time (PT) and activated partial thromboplastin time (APTT))
- Glucose-6-phosphate dehydrogenase (G6PD) deficiency (where indicated)
- Sickle cell trait (where indicated)
- Haemoglobinopathy (where indicated)
- Thrombophilia screen (where indicated, according to Swedish guidelines – see Box 3.3)
- Serum creatinine, urea and electrolytes
- Liver function tests
- Bone profile (calcium, phosphate, albumin and alkaline phosphatase)
- Fasting plasma glucose
- Glucose tolerance test (if fasting plasma glucose 6–7 mmol/L)
- Fasting lipid screen (if indicated)
- Urate
- Thyroid function tests (if strong family history)
- Pregnancy test (if indicated)
- Men >60 years prostate-specific antigen (PSA)
- Virology and infection screen (see Box 3.5)

Cardiorespiratory system
- Chest X-ray
- Electrocardiogram
- Cardiovascular stress test (as routine or where indicated)
- Echocardiogram (where indicated)

Box 3.3 Detailed thrombophilia screening according to Swedish guidelines.
- Prothrombin time (PT), activated partial thromboplastin time (APTT)
- Antithrombin III (ATIII)
- Protein C
- Protein S
- Activated protein C (APC) resistance (screens for abnormalities including factor V Leiden)
- PT mutation
- Lupus anticoagulant
- Anti-phospholipid antibodies

hyperfiltration in the remaining kidney. Several studies have had surprisingly similar results and have demonstrated that kidney function returns to about 72% and stays so over time compared with age-matched controls [9–12]. Some more recent studies indicate that renal function might even improve over the first couple of years after donation.

It is also important for the recipient that the transplanted kidney has a sufficient functional capacity, as immunosuppressants and other drugs commonly used after transplantation are nephrotoxic.

Kidney function is usually defined as glomerular filtration rate (GFR). One would expect that in the 21st century measuring GFR and deciding on acceptable values for an individual donor would be an easy task. On the contrary, they are associated with a number of pitfalls, and accepting or rejecting a donor based on the result from a kidney function test requires well-considered decisions. It is important that health-care professionals involved in the evaluation of donors are aware of the difficulties and the pitfalls. Some of these are associated with the different methodologies for measuring GFR, units used to express it, differences in kidney function depending on age and size of donor and sometimes the matching between donor and recipient, depending on the estimated function of the kidney to be donated.

A broad spectrum of methods can be used to estimate GFR. The gold standard is inulin clearance. This method requires continuous intravenous infusion and measurements of inulin, which makes the method expensive and impractical in most clinical settings. All other methods used to estimate GFR, such as measurement of serum creatinine, creatinine clearance, formula equations, excretion of a bolus injected marker and a more recent marker – measurement of serum cystatin C – have their specific limitations and inaccuracy. Many of these methods show fairly good overall correlation. However, when compared to each other for a single individual measurement, the correlation can be very poor, and the estimated GFR might differ by up to 100% or even more in repeated measurements using the same method [13]. It is therefore recommended that GFR be estimated using several different methods, and at least one should be based on bolus injection of an excreting marker such as Cr EDTA, DTPA or Iohexol, which seem to the most accurate methods.

The units used to quantify GFR are either the absolute value expressed in mL/min or a corrected (relative) unit expressed in $mL/min/1.73\,m^2$. The latter is relative to the calculated body surface area (BSA). The relative value is the most commonly applied of the two and has the advantage that it makes it easier to assess kidney function independently from age, height and weight. The absolute values (mL/min) are predominantly used for dosing of medicines and for evaluation of an individual's total filtration capacity. Examples of GFR estimation methods that use different units are the Cockcroft-Gault formula and the MDRD Study formula, which express the estimated GFR in mL/min and $mL/min/1.73\,m^2$, respectively. The values can diverge significantly depending on the weight and height of the person being measured. For example, for two individuals with the same relative GFR of 40 the person

who is 140 cm tall and weighs 40 kg will have an estimated absolute GFR
of 29 whereas the other person, who is 200 cm tall and weighs 100 kg, will
have an estimated absolute GFR of 55. In extreme situations the
estimated absolute GFR may thus differ more than 100% despite a
similar estimated relative GFR. Almost universally, in all living donor
guidelines and recommendations the relative GFR is used to define
kidney function. The absolute values can, however, give valuable
information when there is a large size discrepancy between donor and
recipient and if there is a significant difference in the split function
between the kidneys. It is thus very important that health-care personnel
involved in the evaluation of potential kidney donors understand the
difference between absolute and relative estimated GFR and that the
values can differ substantially.

Deciding on an acceptable cut-off limit in kidney function for
accepting a donor can also be a difficult task. One complicating factor is
that kidney function declines with age and that an older person does not
require the same function as a young person. The decline in function
generally starts at the age of 40, and the decline rate is approximately 1
mL/min/1.73 m^2 per year [14]. The cut-off limits for acceptance thus
need to be individualised. The consensus guidelines from the Amsterdam
forum state that 'a GFR ≤80 mL/minute or 2 standard deviations below
normal (based on age, gender, and BSA corrected to 1.73/m^2) generally
precludes donation' [6]. Another way of defining the limit of acceptable
estimated GFR on an individual basis is to set a sufficient level of kidney
function before donation to have an effective GFR at the age of 80 years
and then to count backwards to set the limit for the acceptable estimated
GFR at the age of donation. Examples of such calculations are given in
the *UK Guidelines for Living Donor Kidney Transplantation* [5] and in the
textbook *Living Donor Kidney Transplantation: Current practices, emerging
trends and evolving challenges* [15].

Deciding if kidney function is acceptable can also be complicated if the
kidneys have different function. For most of the time this correlates with
the size of the kidneys. Split function can be measured by radioisotope
scan of the kidneys or by CT angiography [16,17].

When there is a significant difference in function between the two
kidneys, the kidney with lower function should be used for
transplantation. There is no general agreement on what is the lowest
acceptable GFR for a kidney to be transplanted. This has to be decided
upon on an individual basis and take into account the age of the
recipient, likelihood of rejection, alternative sources of donors, urgency
of the transplantation, etc.

Renal anatomy

The goal of assessment of the renal anatomy is twofold. One is to ensure
that the kidney to be donated is technically suitable for transplantation.
The other goal is to ensure that neither the donated kidney nor the
remaining kidney shows any pathology in the parenchyma, vessels or
collecting systems. To decide if a kidney is technically suitable for

transplantation, it is important to have detailed knowledge of the number, location and length of the renal arteries and veins as well as any abnormalities in the collecting system. If there are any relevant differences between the kidneys it is generally accepted that the best kidney should stay with the donor. When all factors, including function and quality, are equivalent, the kidney with the lowest risk for surgical complications in the recipient is selected – it is then generally preferable to remove the left kidney, as it has a longer renal vein, which makes the recipient operation easier. This is especially important for laparoscopic nephrectomy, in which the instruments used will 'consume' some of the vessel length. There also seems to be a lower risk for venous thrombosis when transplanting the left kidney, both from deceased and live donors [18]. If one or both kidneys have more than one artery the one with the least number of arteries is normally chosen. If there are single arteries but an early bifurcation this will de facto result in two or more arteries and should therefore be considered as two arteries. The number of veins rarely influences the choice of kidney since extra veins usually can be discarded and ligated.

Imaging techniques

As already discussed, it is very important to have detailed knowledge about both kidneys in order to accept a donor and to decide which kidney to remove. Traditionally this information has been collected by means of several different methods, such as intra-arterial angiography, either conventional or with digital subtraction angiography (DSA) for assessment of the renal vasculature. In addition, an intravenous urogram (IVU) has been used to assess the collecting systems and for the detection of urinary calculi. Finally, an ultrasound is used for assessment of the parenchyma and especially for diagnosis of cysts.

Today the preferred imaging technique is predominantly computerised tomography (CT) angiography (Fig. 3.1). The advantage of CT angiography is that in contrast to intra-arterial angiography, it is not invasive and obviates transfemoral catheterisation, with or without selective catheterisation of the renal artery(ies), which has associated complications such as bleeding, formation of aneurysms, dissection of the vessel intima and ultimately thrombosis.

Other advantages of CT are that it is rapid and relatively inexpensive when compared with other imaging modalities and involves significantly lower radiation exposure than conventional angiography. Provided that the scan is made with thin slices, the accuracy of vessel anatomy is excellent, and the possibility of making 3D reconstructions is very helpful when planning the surgery. The method allows proper evaluation of renal arteries and veins, renal parenchyma and also the urinary tract (late phase) during a single session. As already mentioned, the technique can also be used for measuring split function of the kidneys. On the negative side, the use of nephrotoxic contrast medium is still required.

An alternative method is magnetic resonance (MR) angiography. The advantage of MR angiography is the avoidance of exposure to ionising

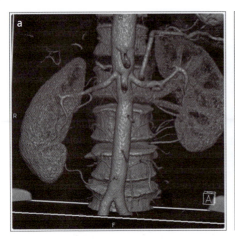 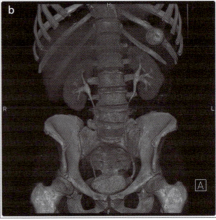

Figure 3.1 CT angiography reconstruction, showing (a) the vascular anatomy and (b) the collective system.

radiation and the use of non-nephrotoxic contrast medium. A disadvantage is that it is less accurate in detecting small arteries and stenoses and/or fibromuscular dysplasia (FMD) of the renal artery. In addition, it does not perform well for diagnosis of calculi in the renal tract and requires a donor who can hold their breath for significant period of time and is not claustrophobic.

Renal abnormalities

It is not uncommon for the imaging procedure to reveal anatomical variations, benign lesions, pathological lesions and even malignancies. Multiple arteries or complex venous anatomy is, as such, not associated with any morbidity and does not therefore constitute any risk for the donor. For the recipient, however, it is more risky to receive a kidney with several arteries and/or veins. While some studies have not demonstrated any difference in graft survival between kidneys with single vessels and kidneys with multiple vessels, it is not uncommon for a smaller artery to thrombose and as a consequence part of kidney function to be lost. It is therefore generally accepted that one should use the kidney with the least number of arteries if everything else is equal and that for all other types of abnormality the best kidney should stay with the donor. For certain abnormalities/pathological findings, such as atherosclerotic reno-vascular disease, there is a significant risk that the donor will develop hypertension, renal failure and cardiovascular disease in the future. This is a contraindication for donation. There are also a large number of abnormalities/pathological findings for which there is some risk in not removing the kidney from the donor but some risk for the recipient. Examples of such conditions are FMD, angiomyolipoma, renal artery aneurysms, renal calculi, etc. Finally, the evaluation can reveal a small incidental renal tumour that will require surgery for the donor. These kidneys can be used for transplantation provided that the tumour can be excised with a tumour-free margin. How to proceed in cases with abnormalities/pathological findings must be decided case by case, and both donor and recipient must be fully informed about the risks associated with the different possible solutions.

Assessment of renal risk factors

The evaluation of the renal status of a potential donor it is not limited to function and anatomy but also includes the assessment of any underlying renal disease or conditions that will put either the donor and/or the recipient at risk.

Proteinuria

Presence of abnormal urinary protein excretion is a marker for renal disease and is associated with cardiovascular disease. Measurement of urinary protein excretion is thus an important examination in the assessment of renal risk factors. The upper limit of protein excretion is <150 mg/day and albumin excretion <30 mg/day (microalbuminuria). A potential donor with diagnosed proteinuria is generally precluded from donation. Rare exceptions might be orthostatic and transient tubular proteinuria. To verify the underlying cause of proteinuria, a biopsy is often necessary.

There are several methods that can be used to test and quantify proteinuria.

- *Dipstick testing* is a semi-quantitative screening test. The stick generally detects albumin only. Microalbuminuria is a marker for glomerular damage. A weak positive result is usually indicative of microalbuminuria and a negative result tends to rule it out. The sensitivity, however, is not sufficient for the evaluation of potential kidney donors.
- *24-hour urine collection* is a much more accurate method for assessment of protein quantity. The urine electrophoresis gives a qualitative and quantitative assessment and can thus also detect extra renal conditions that preclude donation, such as myeloma, light chain disease and the fraction alpha 1-microglobulin (protein HC) as a marker for tubular damage. The Swedish guidelines require a serum and urine electrophoresis. A caveat is that incomplete 24-hour urine collections underestimate any protein leak.
- *Spot analysis of the albumin* is an alternative that removes the difficulties with 24-hour urine collection. The albumin/creatinine ratio on a first voided morning midstream urine specimen gives an accurate quantitative measurement. The definition of microalbuminuria in a spot analysis is a ratio of between 30 and 300 µg/mg (3 and 30 mg/ mmol).

Pyuria and bacteriuria

Significant pyuria is indicative of underlying renal disease or bacteriuria/urinary tract infections (UTIs). Asymptomatic bacteriuria is common in women. The cause of pyuria needs to be investigated. Sporadic uncomplicated UTIs, especially in women, need no further investigation, but recurrent or ascending UTIs require further examination with cystocopy and CT urography.

The diagnosis of pyuria and bacteriuria is made with:
- dipstick testing
- urinary microscopy
- urine culture.

Haematuria

Benign and transient haematuria has an incidence of approximately 5–10% and is more common in women. Persistent verified haematuria must, however, be investigated in order to rule out a malignancy, renal parenchymal diseases or nephrolithiasis. These conditions generally preclude donation.

Persistent haematuria is investigated with urinary microscopy/cytology, cystoscopy and CT urography. If these investigations are normal, it is recommended that a renal biopsy be done. However, the diagnostic value of a biopsy in such situations is fairly low, and there are risks associated with this invasive procedure that must be discussed with the potential donor. If a biopsy is carried out, it should be done on the kidney that is likely to be transplanted. A caveat is that if biopsy on that side would be technically difficult, it may be safer for the potential donor to biopsy the contralateral kidney. If all of the tests have been negative, it is regarded safe to go ahead with the donation.

The diagnosis of haematuria is made with the following.
- *Dipstick test*. The advantage of the dipstick test for haematuria is that it is simple with a very low false negative rate. False positives are not infrequent, however. In addition, benign transient haematuria is fairly common and repeated positive tests are needed to verify true haematuria, which needs further investigation.
- *Urinary microscopy*. This should be carried out on freshly voided urine with phase-contrast microscopy in order to be of diagnostic value.

Nephrolithiasis

Kidney stones are generally regarded as a contraindication for donation, as the recurrence rate is fairly high (30–50%) with future risk of infections, obstructions and related therapeutic procedures. In addition, there is also a risk to the recipient. A potential donor that has recently passed one or more stones or has developed stones due to metabolic risk factors, anatomical abnormalities or infections should be disqualified from being a donor. However, if the history of passing a stone is old, the stone is an asymptomatic incidental finding or if underlying metabolic, anatomic and infectious conditions have been ruled out, there is only a relative contraindication and there are no clear-cut recommendations. The situation then needs to be discussed with the donor and the recipient, and a donation should only be realised if both parties consent and are fully aware of the risks. They should be informed about measures that they should take to reduce the likelihood of recurrent stone formation (increase fluid intake to 3 L/day and decrease intake of animal protein, salt and oxalate).

There are several investigations for assessment of renal stone disease.
* *Spiral CT scan* is the method of choice. The initial unenhanced series of the CT angiography is a sensitive method of stone detection.
* *Plain X-ray* is the old gold standard and should be used if MR angiography is used, as MR is not sensitive for stone detection.
* *Metabolic risk assessments* should be carried out in potential donors with a history of stone formation or stones diagnosed on the radiologic examinations. The assessments should include investigation of serum calcium, parathyroid hormone (PTH), uric acid and 24-hour urine collection with examination of calcium, oxalate, uric acid, citrate and cystine.

Inherited kidney disease

There are a large number and variety of inherited kidney diseases, some of which may lead to kidney failure. If a potential donor is genetically related to the recipient with an inherited kidney disease or there is a family history, donor evaluation must include screening for the disease. The pattern of inheritance, age of onset and different patterns of clinical manifestations vary substantially depending on the type of disease. An exhaustive discussion of specific diseases is beyond the scope of this chapter, and members of a transplant team cannot be expected to possess an updated proficiency in this rapidly evolving field of clinical genetics. Therefore, each case has to go through a thorough examination, often involving other family members. In most cases an inherited kidney disease precludes donation.

The diagnostic tools for inherited kidney disease depend on the specific disease:
* detailed family history
* disease-specific investigations, such as ultrasound in case of autosomal dominant adult polycystic kidney disease (ADPKD)
* genetic testing, as recommended by the clinical genetics department.

Extra-renal factors and co-morbidity

Age

Minors (<18 years) are not allowed to donate, except in very special situations and in most countries only after a court decision. Most centres are also reluctant to use donors between 18 and 25 years of age, as they are often still very dependent on their families and it can be difficult for them to give autonomous consent. At the other end of the spectrum, there are no recommendations on an upper age limit for donation. Kidneys from older living donors are generally transplanted to older recipients and tend to be as successful as kidneys from younger donors provided renal function is good [19]. Old age, however, puts a focus on a very thorough assessment of cardiovascular and peri-operative risks as well as screening for malignancy.

Obesity

Obesity is considered to be a relative contraindication for kidney donation. The reasons for this are manifold. In the short term obesity is associated with increased peri-operative complications – mainly bleeding and wound infections, but also more severe complications, such as pulmonary embolism and respiratory complications. Obesity is also an independent risk factor for diabetes mellitus, hypertension, proteinuria and respiratory and cardiovascular disease. These risk factors thus need to be addressed specifically during work-up of an obese donor. In addition there is also a legitimate concern that obesity will increase the risk of developing chronic kidney disease (CKD) after nephrectomy, as shown by Praga *et al.* [20]. Although this finding has not been replicated in a study on obese donors with short-term follow-up [21], other studies have demonstrated that obesity leads to more rapid progression of CKD, probably mediated through cardiovascular disease risk factors [21–23]. When counselling an obese potential donor, one needs also to consider that long-term follow-up studies of donors have shown that donors gain weight after donation and experience an increased frequency hypertension, diabetes mellitus and proteinuria, which are associated with risk of cardiovascular disease and CKD [15,24]. Lifestyle risks and the impact of cumulative cardiovascular risk factors should thus be discussed with the donor.

Smoking

Smoking is one of the important lifestyle issues that needs to be addressed, as it has an impact on both short- and long-term transplantation risks, and cessation reduces these risks. In the short term smoking increases the risk for peri-operative complications, mainly cardiovascular and respiratory. In the long term it is associated with an increased risk for cardiovascular disease, hypertension, proteinuria and renal impairment.

Hypertension

Hypertension is a major risk factor for cardiovascular disease and can also be the cause of kidney failure on the one hand. On the other hand, kidney failure may be the cause of hypertension. Hypertension and kidney failure are thus intimately related, and hypertension is generally regarded as a contraindication for donation. There is, however, little evidence that unilateral nephrectomy in an otherwise healthy individual will cause hypertension. On average, one can expect a slight increase of about 2–3 mmHg. For donors with borderline or treated hypertension there is, however, evidence that unilateral nephrectomy may accelerate the development of hypertension. Hypertensive donors will require more hypertensive medication, and proteinuria will be aggravated, necessitating treatment with angiotensin-converting enzyme (ACE) inhibitors [15]. It is also a disturbing fact that in the majority of donors who later developed ESRD, the cause of kidney failure was nephrosclerosis [25–27]. Hypertension is therefore generally regarded as a contraindication for donation, although some centres accept potential donors with well-controlled hypertension. If there is any evidence of end-organ damage (hypertensive retinopathy or abnormal electrocardiogram, echocardiogram or chest X-ray), kidney donation is definitely contraindicated.

If a potential donor with borderline hypertension or well-controlled hypertension is to be accepted for donation it is recommended that:

- blood pressure and effectiveness of treatment is assessed by 24-hour ambulatory blood-pressure monitoring
- measures are taken to assess and minimise/treat other cardiovascular risk factors such obesity, hyperlipidaemia, impaired glucose tolerance, smoking, etc.
- the potential donor has access to lifelong checkups and treatment for his/her hypertension with ACE inhibitors and other drugs if required
- the potential donor is fully informed about the risks and has received information about lifestyle issues that might have a positive effect to mitigate the risks.

Diabetes mellitus

Similarly to hypertension, there is no clear evidence that unilateral nephrectomy will aggravate the course of diabetes and lead to a more rapid progression of secondary complications, including nephropathy. Lack of evidence, however, is not the same as evidence of no difference, and as diabetes mellitus is a risk factor for peri-operative complications and the development of chronic kidney disease, diabetes is regarded as an absolute contraindication for kidney donation [5–7,28].

The World Health Organization (WHO) definitions of diabetes and impaired glucose tolerance are given in Table 3.1.

It should be noted that any tests for the diagnosis of diabetes, impaired glucose tolerance (IGT) and impaired fasting glucose (IFG) have poor reproducibility. Repeat measurements are therefore necessary. Many centres feel that it is sufficient just to test for fasting glucose and that it is unnecessary to perform an oral glucose tolerance test (OGTT). However, the WHO definition of diabetes, IGT and IFG is based on the OGTT. The reasons for this are given in Box 3.4. OGTT is required in the Swedish guidelines [7].

Individuals with IGT/IFG are likely to develop manifest diabetes. The risk of developing diabetes within 5 years ranges approximately between 30 and 50%, depending on a variety of factors such as family history, ethnic group, age, obesity, history of gestational diabetes, etc. IGT and IFG are also associated with a higher risk of developing cardiovascular complications, so potential donors with IGT or IFG are generally not accepted as donors. In older potential donors, the lifetime risk of developing overt diabetes and subsequently secondary complications is very low, and they might therefore be accepted as donors. Just as for

Table 3.1 Summary of the 2006 WHO recommendations for the diagnostic criteria for diabetes mellitus and intermediate hyperglycaemia (data available at reference [29]).

Diabetes	Fasting plasma glucose 2-hour plasma glucose*	≥7.0 mmol/L (126 mg/dL) or ≥11.1 mmol/L (200 mg/dL)
Impaired glucose tolerance (IGT)	Fasting plasma glucose 2-hour plasma glucose*	<7.0 mmol/L (126 mg/dL) and ≥7.8 and <11.1 mmol/L (140 mg/dL and 200 mg/dL)
Impaired fasting glucose (IFG)	Fasting plasma glucose 2-hour plasma glucose*	6.1 to 6.9 mmol/L (110 mg/dL to 125 mg/dL) and (if measured) <7.8 mmol/L (140 mg/dL)

Currently haemoglobin A1c is not considered a suitable diagnostic test for diabetes or intermediate hyperglycaemia.
*Venous plasma glucose 2 hours after ingestion of 75 g oral glucose load. If 2-hour plasma glucose is not measured, status is uncertain, as diabetes or IGT cannot be excluded.

Box 3.4 Oral glucose tolerance test.

The oral glucose tolerance test (OGTT) should be retained as a diagnostic test for the following reasons:

- fasting plasma glucose alone fails to diagnose approximately 30% of cases of previously undiagnosed diabetes
- OGTT is the only means of identifying people with impaired glucose tolerance (IGT)
- OGTT is frequently needed to confirm or exclude an abnormality of glucose tolerance in asymptomatic people
- an OGTT should be used in individuals with fasting plasma glucose 6.1–7.0 mmol/L.

---

potential donors with borderline or well-controlled hypertension, these potential donors need to be fully informed about the risks and have received information about lifestyle issues that might have a positive effect to mitigate the risks. Measures should also be taken to assess and minimise/treat other cardiovascular risk factors such obesity, hyperlipidaemia, smoking, etc.

Assessment of peri-operative risks

In surgery there is never a zero per cent risk. The focus of the assessment of peri-operative risk factors is to identify and evaluate them. Some risks may be unacceptably high, whereas others can be attenuated with prophylaxis or treatment before surgery. If risk factors have been identified, these, and any prophylactic measures, need to be discussed with the potential donor, who should also be involved in the final decision.

A personal and family history is important to reveal any risk factors. Specifically, adverse reactions in connection with previous surgery or dental treatment can give valuable information. These include difficulties during intubation, unexpected bleeding, thrombosis and allergic, hyperthermic or anaphylactic reactions.

Donors should generally be Class I according to the American Association of Anesthesiologists (ASA) physical status classification. In this group of patients, peri-operative complications are rare and there is only a very small chance of detecting any abnormality in the evaluation that signifies increased risk. However, donors are not patients, and given the special circumstances that surround live donor nephrectomy, most centres follow a meticulous pre-operative assessment as part of the donor evaluation. Some aspects will be discussed more in detail here.

Cardiovascular disease is intimately associated with renal disease, and this has been discussed already. Clearly, cardiovascular disease is also associated with increased peri-operative risks. Latent or clinically silent disease will not be revealed without screening tests, and these should be used on broad indications. For instance, the guidelines of Sweden and Norway require that exercise electrocardiography or stress scintigraphy – alternatively stress echocardiography – should be carried out in all potential donors above the age of 50 years, even if they are asymptomatic and without risk factors.

Pulmonary embolism is the single most common cause of peri-operative death in live donors. Risk factors for thromboembolic events must, therefore, be investigated thoroughly as part of the pre-operative assessment. Some risk factors are rare but important to check for because they are associated with a high risk of venous thromboembolism, whereas others are frequent but carry a lower risk. It should further be noted that the presence of two risk factors need not be just additive but can significantly increase the hazard of thromboembolic events. For instance, the combination of prothrombin gene mutation and oral contraceptives dramatically increases risk for cerebral venous thrombosis 149-fold even though the relative risk of each individual factor is much smaller. Thromboembolic risk factors that are screened for according to the Swedish guidelines are given in Box 3.3. How much the risk is increased in a specific case is difficult to establish, as it will also depend on age, BMI, type and length of surgery, etc. How much increased risk is acceptable will also have to be decided on an individual basis, depending on the type of prophylaxis given and for how long, etc. At the present author's institution, Uppsala University Hospital in Sweden, a marginally increased risk such as heterozygous carrier of activated protein C resistance is not regarded as a contraindication. The donor would receive a higher dose of low-molecular-weight heparin, and prophylaxis would be prolonged for 6 weeks after surgery in combination with compression stockings and an ultrasound of the leg before discharge in order to rule out any deep venous thrombosis of the leg [30].

Factors with risk of transmission form the donor

Donor malignancy

Malignancies of numerous types are known to have been transmitted in connection with transplantation and to develop manifest disease in the recipient. The frequency of transmission has historically been very low, but with the increasing use of marginal and older donors, this issue has become more relevant for the evaluation of potential donors. Tumour screening should be performed as recommended for the general population and on indication based on family history and other risk factors for malignancy. For deceased donors there are general recommendations that donors with a history of malignant disease should normally not be used. In a living donor situation, more time is available to assess the donor and screen for recurrence appropriately. Some tumours, such as melanoma, have a very high risk of recurrence and transmission whereas others, such as non-melanoma skin cancer and carcinoma in situ of the uterine cervix, do not. Although it is difficult to make a precise prediction of the risk of disease transmission, the risk/ benefit balance for the recipient must be quantified and discussed with the donor and the recipient.

Infections

It is in the best interest of both donor and recipient not to proceed with a donation if the donor has an active infection. For the donor there is an increased peri-operative risk for undergoing surgery with an active infection and for the recipient there is a risk of transmission. There are also a number of infections that might not be overt or known of by the donor and therefore need to be screened for. Screening of living donors should follow the same principles that apply to deceased donors and blood donors. A detailed clinical history is important and should include a psychosocial and sexual history as well as details of residence in geographical areas where there is a high prevalence of infections that are relevant in a transplant setting. Particular attention should also be paid to the possibility of past tuberculosis when examining the chest radiograph.

If a positive result is obtained for an infection that is transmitted sexually or by intravenous drug use, this might raise complex ethical problems. It is important that there is comprehensive and open discussion with the prospective donor before testing for viral infections, particularly for HIV, hepatitis C virus (HCV) and hepatitis B virus (HBV). A strategy for dealing with a positive result should be formulated before testing.

If transplantation is being considered from a donor with a history of HCV or HBV infection, the risks must be carefully explained to the donor and recipient. Advice from a virologist should be sought under these circumstances.

Serological testing for transmittable infectious deceases according to UK guidelines is given in Box 3.5.

> **Box 3.5 Donor and recipient screening.**
> * Human immunodeficiency virus (HIV) 1 and 2
> * Cytomegalovirus (CMV)
> * Varicella zoster virus (VZV)
> * Epstein–Barr virus (EBV)
> * Hepatitis C virus (HCV)
> * Hepatitis B virus (HBV)
> * Syphilis
> * Toxoplasmosis
> * *Human herpesvirus 8 (HHV-8)
> * *Human T-lymphotropic virus (HTLV1)
> * *Schistosomiasis
> * *Strongyloides stercoralis*
> * *Malaria (blood film)
> * *Trypanosoma cruzi*
> *Where clinically indicated, e.g. specific endemic (geographical) risks.

Key references

1. Wolfe RA, Ashby VB, Milford EL, *et al.* (1999) Comparison of mortality in all patients on dialysis, patients on dialysis awaiting transplantation, and recipients of a first cadaveric transplant. *N Engl J Med* **341**, 1725–1730.
2. Meier-Kriesche HU, Port FK, Ojo AO, *et al.* (2000) Effect of waiting time on renal transplant outcome. *Kidney Int* **58**, 1311–1317.
3. Najarian JS, Chavers BM, McHugh LE, *et al.* (1992) 20 years or more of follow-up living kidney donors. *Lancet* **340**, 807–810.
4. Matas AJ, Bartlett ST, Leichtman AB, *et al.* (2003) Morbidity and mortality after living donor kidney donation, 1999–2001: Survey of United States transplant centres. *Am J Transplantation* **3**, 830–834.
5. British Transplantation Society. (2011) *UK Guidelines for Living Donor kidney Transplantation.* Available online from: http://www.bts.org.uk/transplantation/standards-and-guidelines/.
6. Delmonico F; Council of the Transplantation Society. (2005) A report of the Amsterdam Forum on the care of the live kidney donor: Data and medical guidelines. *Transplantation* **79**, S53–S66.
7. Swedish Transplantation Society. (2007) *Evaluation Protocol for Living Kidney Donors.* Available online from: http://www3.svls.se/sektioner/tp/fnytt/Evaluation%20Dec2007.pdf.
8. Marson LP, Lumsdaine JA, Forsythe JLR, *et al.* (2005) Selection and evaluation of potential living kidney donors. In: Gaston RS and Wadström J (eds), *Living Donor Kidney Transplantation. Current practices, emerging trends and evolving challenges,* pp. 33–55. Taylor & Francis, London.
9. Fehrman-Ekholm I, Duner F, Brink B, *et al.* (2001) No evidence of accelerated loss of kidney function in living kidney donors: Results from a cross-sectional follow-up. *Transplantation* **72**, 444–449.
10. Fehrman-Ekholm I, Thiel GT. Long-term risks after living kidney donation. In: Gaston RS and Wadström J (eds). *Living Donor Kidney Transplantation. Current practices, emerging trends and evolving challenges,* pp. 99–113. Taylor & Francis, London.

11. Goldfarb DA, Matin SF, Braun WE, *et al.* (2001) Renal outcome 25 years after donor nephrectomy. *J Urol* **166**, 2043–2047.

12. Ramcharan T, Matas AJ. (2002) Long-term (20–37 years) follow-up of living kidney donors. *Am J Transplant* **2**, 959–964.

13. Biglarnia AR, Wadström J, Larsson A. (2007) Decentralized glomerular filtration rate (GFR) estimates in healthy kidney donors show poor correlation and demonstrate the need for improvement in quality and standardization of GFR measurements in Sweden. *Scand J Clin Lab Invest* **67**, 227–235.

14. Grewal GS, Blake GM. (2005) Reference data for 51Cr-EDTA measurements of GFR derived from live kidney donors. *Nucl Med Commun* **26**, 61–65.

15. Thiel GT, Nolte C, Tsinalis D. (2005) Living kidney donors with isolated medical abnormalities: the SOL-DHR experience. In: Gaston RS and Wadström J (eds). *Living Donor Kidney Transplantation: Current practices, emerging trends and evolving challenges*, pp. 55–75. Taylor & Francis, London.

16. Shokeir AA, Gad HM, el-Diasty T. (2003) Role of radioisotope renal scans in the choice of nephrectomy side in live kidney donors. *J Urol* **170**, 373–376.

17. Nilsson H, Wadstrom J, Andersson LG, *et al.* (2004) Measuring split renal function in renal donors: Can computed tomography replace renography? *Acta Radiol* **45**, 474–480.

18. Bakir N, Sluiter WJ, Ploeg RJ, *et al.* (1996) Primary renal graft thrombosis. *Nephrol Dial Transplant* **11**, 140–147.

19. Foss A, Heldal K, Scott H, *et al.* (2009) Kidneys from deceased donors more than 75 years perform acceptably after transplantation. *Transplantation* **87**, 1437–1441.

20. Praga M, Hernandez E, Herrero JC, *et al.* (2000) Influence of obesity on the appearance of proteinuria and renal insufficiency after unilateral nephrectomy. *Kidney Int* **58**, 2111–2118.

21. Reese PP, Feldman HI, Asch DA, *et al.* (2009) Short-term outcomes for obese live kidney donors and their recipients. *Transplantation* **88**, 662–671.

22. Othman M, Kawar B, El Nahas AM. (2009) Influence of obesity on progression of non-diabetic chronic kidney disease: a retrospective cohort study. *Nephron Clin Pract* **113**, 16–23.

23. Foster MC, Hwang SJ, Larson MG, *et al.* (2008) Overweight, obesity, and the development of stage 3 CKD: The Framingham Heart Study. *Am J Kidney Dis* **52**, 39–48.

24. Fehrman-Ekholm I, Elinder CG, Stenbeck M, *et al.* (1997) Kidney donors live longer. *Transplantation* **64**, 976–978.

25. Fehrman-Ekholm I, Nordén G, Lennerling A, *et al.* (2006) Incidence of end-stage renal disease among live kidney donors. *Transplantation* **82**, 1646–1648.

26. Kido R, Shibagaki Y, Iwadoh K, *et al.* (2009) How do living kidney donors develop end-stage renal disease? *Am J Transplant* **9**, 2514–2519.

27. Ellison MD, McBride MA, Taranto SE, *et al.* (2002) Living kidney donors in need of kidney transplants: a report from the organ procurement and transplantation network. *Transplantation* **74**, 1349–1351.

28. Kasiske BL, Ravenscraft M, Ramos EL, *et al.* (1996) The evaluation of living renal transplant donors: Clinical practice guidelines. *J Am Soc Nephrol* **7**, 2288–2313.

29. WHO. (2006) *Definition and Diagnosis of Diabetes Mellitus and Intermediate Hyperglycemia: Report of a WHO/IDF consultation.* Available online from: http://whqlibdoc.who.int/ publications/2006/9241594934_eng.pdf.

30. Biglarnia A, Bergqvist D, Johansson M, *et al.* (2008) Venous thromboembolism in live kidney donors–a prospective study. *Transplantation* **86**, 659–661.

4 Histocompatibility and immunogenetics

Susan V. Fuggle and Craig J. Taylor

Histocompatibility and immunogenetics

Transplants from genetically different donors are recognised as foreign by the recipient's immune system and are rejected unless the recipient receives immunosuppression. This immune response is largely attributable to recognition of mismatched donor Human Leukoycte Antigens (HLAs). The normal function of HLA, the major histocompatibility complex in humans, is in immune recognition and defence against foreign pathogens and neoplasia. HLA glycoproteins expressed on the cell surface act as self-recognition molecules by binding short fragments of self proteins (peptides) derived from within the cell (endogenous) and surrounding tissue (exogenous) that are presented to self-HLA-restricted T lymphocytes. In the case of infection or neoplasia, however, altered and foreign peptides bound to HLA are recognised as 'non-self' by host T lymphocytes and stimulate a powerful immune response. HLA class I and II genes are highly polymorphic, and as a consequence the HLA glycoprotein products are able to bind and present peptides derived from the diverse array of potential pathogens. In the context of transplantation, mismatched donor HLA (non-self) both stimulate a rejection response and are themselves targets of the alloimmune response [1].

The HLA system

The genes encoding HLA are located on the short arm of chromosome 6 in a region that spans 4 Mb and contains more than 250 expressed genes, around 28% of which have immune-related functions. The genes and their glycoprotein products can be divided according to their structure and function into two groups: HLA class I and HLA class II. A group of genes termed 'class III genes' are located between class I and II and encode a number of immune-related proteins, including tumour necrosis factor (TNF), complement factors C2, C4, C4B and properdin factor B, heat-shock proteins and the steroid 21-hydoxylase.

Handbook of Renal and Pancreatic Transplantation, First Edition. Edited by
Iain A. M. MacPhee and Jiří Froněk.
© 2012 John Wiley & Sons, Ltd. Published 2012 by John Wiley & Sons, Ltd.

HLA class I

The major HLA class I genes considered in kidney transplantation are *HLA-A, HLA-B* and *HLA-C*. These genes encode a 44 kD glycoprotein heavy chain consisting of three extracellular immunoglobulin-like domains (α1, α2, α3), a hydrophobic transmembrane region and a cytoplasmic tail. Most of the amino acid polymorphism of HLA class I resides within the α1 and α2 domains, which fold to form a peptide-binding cleft that accommodates a peptide of eight to ten amino acids in length, usually derived from endogenous cytoplasmic proteins. The amino acid polymorphism controls the sequences of peptides accommodated within the peptide binding cleft and therefore governs the peptide repertoire presented by class I proteins. By contrast, the α3 domain is highly conserved and is the ligand for CD8 on T lymphocytes. On the cell surface the class I heavy chain is stabilised by non-covalent association with β2 microglobulin, a 12 kD glycoprotein encoded on chromosome 15. The HLA class I proteins are expressed on virtually all nucleated cells.

HLA class II

The main HLA class II loci are *HLA-DR, HLA-DQ* and *HLA-DP*. The glycoprotein products are heterodimers of non-covalently associated α (33 kD) and β (28 kD) chains, both consisting of two extracellular immunoglobulin-like domains, a transmembrane region and a cytoplasmic tail. In the case of the class II molecules, the α1 and β1 membrane distal domains combine to form the peptide-binding cleft. The β chain is highly polymorphic, and this governs the repertoire of peptides bound, whereas the HLA-DR and HLA-DP α chains are relatively conserved. The bound peptides vary in length between 10 and 20 amino acids and are mostly derived from endocytosed or phagocytosed proteins. The β2 domain associates with CD4 on T lymphocytes, conferring class II restriction in antigen presentation.

HLA class II molecules are constitutively expressed on cells with immune function including B lymphocytes, macrophages and dendritic cells, but can be induced on T lymphocytes upon activation and on many other cells during an inflammatory response. In a transplanted kidney, HLA class II expression can be induced on vascular endothelium and renal tubules, potentially increasing the immunogenicity of the organ and acting as a target for allograft rejection.

HLA polymorphism and nomenclature

The first HLA specificity (MAC, now termed HLA-A2) was described by Jean Dausset in 1958, for which he was awarded the Nobel Prize in 1980 [2]. Investigations into HLA polymorphism were originally undertaken using serological techniques and the field advanced rapidly, and continues to advance, through collaborative International Histocompatibility Workshops involving exchange of reagents and central analysis of the results. The application of DNA technology to HLA typing has demonstrated a greater degree of polymorphism than was originally anticipated; for example, at the *HLA-A* locus 28 specificities have been defined at the serological level, whereas recent nomenclature reports identifies approximately 1500 DNA variants (alleles) [3,4]. The WHO Nomenclature Committee for 'Factors of the HLA System' meet to assign official nomenclature to newly identified specificities/alleles. Further information about HLA polymorphism can be found at http://hla.alleles.org.

There are significant differences in the frequency of particular HLA types within a population and between different ethnic groups. For example, within a pool of 10,000 UK deceased solid organ donors, HLA-A2 is very common and found in approximately 50% of donors, whereas HLA-A29 is found in 8% of donors (Table 4.1). When considering donors by ethnicity, frequencies of certain specificities vary significantly; for instance, HLA-A36 is found in 12% of Black donors and in <0.05% of White donors. This variation has implications for the selection of a suitable donor for a particular recipient and is discussed below in the section 'Application of HLA to kidney and pancreas transplantation'.

In serological assays HLA-specific antibodies (either alloantisera or monoclonal antibodies) bind to tertiary epitopes of the HLA specificities expressed on the cell surface of viable peripheral blood lymphocytes. Epitopes may either be unique for a particular antigen (termed 'private' determinants) or can be shared between structurally similar antigens (termed 'public' or 'supertypic' determinants). Many HLA specificities share epitopes that give rise to cross-reactive groups (CREGs) of antigens, and knowledge of these patterns of serological reactivity is important when selecting donors for potential transplant recipients.

Further complexity in terminology has been introduced because as the study of HLA polymorphism progressed, alloantisera were found that were able to discriminate two or more specificities within certain previously defined antigens. The originally defined antigen is termed a 'broad' specificity and the subdivisions are termed 'splits'. For example, the broad specificity HLA-A28 can be subdivided into HLA-A68 and HLA-A69, which are annotated with the broad antigen in parenthesis: HLA-A68(28) and HLA-A69(28). Essentially, antibodies identifying the broad specificity bind to a public epitope common to the group of antigens, and the antibodies identifying the 'splits' are specific for 'private' epitopes.

HLA typing is now most frequently performed by analysis at the DNA level and reported using WHO nomenclature. In 2010 the WHO Nomenclature Committee introduced a new nomenclature system to accommodate all the known alleles and to allow further alleles to be included as they are discovered [3]. Each allele is given a unique identifier composed of up to four sets of digits, each separated by colons (see Box 4.1). The digits that precede the first colon describe the HLA type that corresponds most closely to the serologically defined HLA type.

Table 4.1 HLA phenotype prevalence in the UK organ donor population. Based on 10,000 UK deceased solid organ donors.

HLA-A		HLA-B		HLA-DR		HLA-Cw		HLA-DQ	
Antigen	%	Antigen	%	Antigen	%	Antigen	%	Antigen	%
A1	34	B5	9	DR1	19	Cw1	7	DQ1	58
A2	50	B51	8	DR2	29	Cw2	7	DQ5	27
A203	0	B52	1	DR15	28	Cw3	23	DQ6	41
A210	0	B5102	0	DR16	2	Cw9	8	DQ2	44
A3	26	B5103	0	DR3	27	Cw10	12	DQ3	53
A9	17	B7	27	DR17	26	Cw4	17	DQ7	34
A23	3	B703	0	DR18	<1	Cw5	21	DQ8	18
A24	14	B8	25	DR4	35	Cw6	18	DQ9	9
A2403	<1	B12	33	DR5	16	Cw7	56	DQ4	4
A10	9	B44	32	DR11	13	Cw8	7		
A25	4	B45	2	DR12	3	Cw12	6		
A26	4	B13	4	DR6	23	Cw13	0		
A34	<1	B14	7	DR13	19	Cw14	2		
A66	<1	B64	2	DR14	5	Cw15	3		
A11	12	B65	4	DR1403	<1	Cw16	7		
A19	19	B15	13	DR1404	<1	Cw17	1		
A30	5	B62	12	DR7	26	Cw18	<1		
A31	6	B63	<1	DR8	4				
A32	7	B75	<1	DR9	2				
A33	2	B76	0	DR10	1				
A74	<1	B77	0	DR103	4				
A29	8	B16	5						
A28	7	B38	2	DR51	29				
A68	6	B39	3	DR52	58				
A69	<1	B3901	<1	DR53	57				
A36	<1	B3902	0						
A43	0	B17	9						
A80	<1	B57	8						
		B58	1						
		B18	8						
		B21	4						
		B49	3						
		B50	2						
		B4005	<1						
		B22	4						
		B54	<1						
		B55	4						
		B56	1						
		B27	9						
		B2708	<1						
		B35	13						
		B37	3						
		B40	13						
		B60	11						
		B61	2						
		B41	1						
		B42	<1						
		B46	<1						
		B47	1						

Table 4.1 *Continued*

HLA-A		HLA-B		HLA-DR		HLA-Cw		HLA-DQ	
Antigen	%	Antigen	%	Antigen	%	Antigen	%	Antigen	%
		B48	<1						
		B53	1						
		B59	0						
		B67	<1						
		B70	1						
		B71	<1						
		B72	<1						
		B73	<1						
		B78	<1						
		B81	<1						
		B82	<1						
		B83	0						

Bold, broad HLA specificities; non-bold, split HLA specificities and associated antigens.

Box 4.1 Example of HLA nomenclature used to identify serologically defined HLA specificities and their associated DNA-defined alleles.

HLA-B*44:02:01:02S:

HLA	The gene cluster.
HLA-B	The HLA locus.
HLA-B*	* denotes information at the DNA sequence level.
HLA-B*44:	First field: 44: the allele group that correlates most closely with the serological specificity, HLA-B44(12).
HLA-B*44:02	Second field: 02: the allele at amino acid sequence level that encodes the specific HLA polymorphism.
HLA-B*44:02:01	Third field: 01: synonymous substitution within the coding region that does not change the amino acid sequence of the expressed protein.
HLA-B*44:02:01:02	Fourth field: DNA sequence polymorphism in non-coding regions.
Additional suffixes:	
S	Protein found only in a secreted form
N	Null allele, gene not transcribed or translated and protein not expressed on cell surface
L	Allele encoding protein with low or significantly reduced cell surface expression
Q	'Questionable', an allele with a mutation previously shown to have a significant effect on expression, but where the level of expression has not been confirmed.

For example, the DNA sequence encoding the serologically defined HLA-A68(28) specificity is denoted 'HLA-A*68:01' and the serologically defined specificity HLA-69(28) is denoted 'HLA-A*69:01'.

Inheritance of HLA

HLA glycoprotein products are co-dominantly expressed and inherited according to Mendelian principles, and therefore individuals express two HLA specificities at each locus. The HLA class I and class II genes encoded by either the maternal or paternal chromosome are generally inherited together en bloc as one 'haplotype'. When considering living donor transplantation within a family, parents will be one haplotype matched with their children, and siblings will have a 50% chance of having a one haplotype match and a 25% chance of being HLA identical or completely mismatched. Genetic recombination does occur between *HLA-A*, *HLA-B* and *HLA-DR* loci but at a relatively low frequency.

HLA typing methodology

An HLA type can be performed either serologically or using DNA-based methods capable of different levels of resolution. The resolution needed will depend on the requirements of the particular clinical application.

Serological HLA typing
Serological HLA typing is performed using the complement-dependent cytotoxicity (CDC) assay, also known as lymphocytotoxicity, in which viable lymphocytes, usually isolated from peripheral blood, are incubated with a panel of selected HLA-specific alloantisera or monoclonal antibodies pre-aliquoted into a microtitre plate. Following addition of rabbit serum (used as an exogenous source of complement) and staining with vital dye the microtitre plates are examined microscopically for cell death. The serological HLA type can be deduced from the pattern of HLA-specific antibody reactivity.

DNA-based HLA typing
HLA typing using DNA methodology is more accurate than serological typing and additionally defines alleles that are not distinguished by serology. Three different methods are in routine use for HLA typing, and all are based on the polymerase chain reaction (PCR).

PCR-SSP typing
In PCR typing using sequence-specific primers (PCR-SSP), large panels of PCR oligonucleotide primers specific for particular HLA alleles or groups of alleles are used to amplify the target DNA sequence that is subsequently visualised by gel electrophoresis. The HLA type is derived from the pattern of amplified DNA bands of the correct molecular

weight. This method is robust, can be completed within 3.5 hours and is frequently used to HLA-type deceased organ donors.

PCR-SSOP

PCR typing using sequence-specific oligonucleotide probes (PCR-SSOP) involves a generic PCR amplification of a given HLA exon encoding the hypervariable region followed by hybridisation with sequence-specific oligonucleotide probes. In the current PCR-SSOP technology, the individual probes are each bound to a multiplex of 100 microspheres coloured with different ratios of two fluorescent dyes, designed such that each microsphere can be uniquely identified under laser excitation. Hybridised PCR products are detected through fluorescent tagging of biotin incorporated into the PCR product and the HLA type is derived from analysis of the positive microspheres. This methodology is best suited to high volume HLA typing, but may also be applied to HLA typing of deceased organ donors.

PCR-SBT

PCR with sequence-based typing (PCR-SBT) generates high-resolution HLA types by DNA sequencing of the polymorphic regions of the genes and is most often used for HLA typing donors and recipients for haematopoietic stem cell transplantation. For solid organ transplantation, however, HLA typing at the highest serological equivalent resolution appears to confer the maximum benefit, and therefore PCR-SBT is not routinely used.

HLA typing of solid organ transplant donors and recipients

Organ donors and their prospective recipients are routinely typed for HLA-A, HLA-B, HLA-C, HLA-DR and HLA-DQ using DNA-based methods. In some centres additional serological HLA typing may be performed, although DNA typing is necessary to achieve the required level of resolution for HLA matching and donor organ exchange. In many centres donors and recipients may also be typed for HLA-DP as antibodies to HLA-DP are frequently identified in sensitised patients awaiting kidney and pancreas transplantation.

Application of HLA typing to kidney and pancreas transplantation

The level of HLA matching between the donor and recipient is determined by comparing their respective HLA types and is usually expressed as a 'mismatch grade', to reflect the HLA incompatibilities capable of eliciting an alloimmune response. A transplant between a donor and recipient having no HLA-A, HLA-B and HLA-DR incompatibilities is reported as a '0.0.0' HLA-A,-B,-DR mismatch grade, and, for example, a single mismatch at both HLA-A and HLA-B and two mismatches at HLA-DR would be denoted as a '1.1.2' mismatch grade. If a donor is homozygous at HLA-A, HLA-B and HLA-DR, a transplant recipient may have a '1.1.1' mismatch grade, but not share any HLA specificities with the donor. In many centres the mismatch grade is one of the factors used to guide the immunosuppressive regimen for a transplant recipient, with more poorly matched transplants receiving more potent immunosuppression. The HLA mismatch grade is often incorporated into local and national kidney and pancreas organ allocation algorithms.

HLA matching can be reported at different levels of resolution depending on the requirements of the organ exchange programme or the transplant unit. In haematopoietic stem cell transplantation, HLA matching is performed at the four digit allele level at HLA-A, HLA-B, HLA-C, HLA-DR and HLA-DQ, whereas for solid organ transplantation the mismatch grade is based on low-resolution HLA typing, often equivalent to the serologically defined broad and/or split specificity level. Thus a donor and recipient could have a 0.0.0 mismatch grade at the serological broad level, but have one or more mismatches if 'splits' are taken into account.

HLA matching and kidney transplant outcome

HLA matching between donor and recipient was first shown to have a beneficial effect on renal transplant survival more than 30 years ago [5,6]. In the early reports HLA-A and HLA-B matching improved allograft survival, but matching for HLA-DR had a more powerful effect [5]. The significant developments in immunosuppressive agents and patient management have led to improvements in transplant survival and a decrease in the effect of HLA matching in terms of graft survival. Although a recent analysis of data from the United Network for Organ Sharing did not show a benefit of HLA matching [7], an analysis of data from the Collaborative Transplant Study (CTS) continues to show a strong and significant effect of HLA matching on outcome in transplants performed between 2000 and 2004 [8]. Recent analyses of kidney transplant outcome in the UK showed no effect of HLA-A mismatching, but a significant effect of two HLA-B mismatches and a stepwise effect of mismatching at HLA-DR [9]. In addition, even in successful kidney transplants functioning beyond 1 year, donor–recipient HLA-DR matching has been associated with a reduced incidence of acute rejection and a reduced requirement for immunosuppression [10]. Further analyses from the CTS have shown that increased immunosuppressive burden associated with increasing HLA-DR mismatching is associated with a higher incidence of non-Hodgkin lymphoma, osteoporosis and hip fracture, increased hospitalisation for infection within the first year of transplant and increased death rate within 3 years through infection

[11,12,13]. Most of this co-morbidity probably results from higher immunosuppression levels administered to combat graft rejection in poorly HLA-matched transplants.

Sensitisation to HLA alloantigens

Patients can develop alloantibodies to foreign HLA through exposure to alloantigens during pregnancy, transfusion of blood products and previous transplantation. Patients who have had previous transplants frequently develop HLA antibodies to the mismatched donor HLA. If the donor and recipient are very poorly matched and the transplant fails, the patient can develop a highly complex HLA-specific antibody profile that renders the recipient difficult to re-transplant. This is particularly important when considering transplantation for children and young adults, who may need a repeat transplant at some time in the future.

Detection of allosensitisation

In recent years there have been significant advances in the technology available for detection and characterisation of HLA-specific antibodies. The assay technology can be based on serological antibody detection using panels of HLA-typed lymphocytes and solid-phase assays using purified HLA bound to a synthetic surface, and was reviewed by Fuggle and Martin in 2008 [14].

Cell-based assays

Complement-dependent cytotoxicity

The CDC assay, in which patient sera are incubated with a panel of viable lymphocyte targets of known HLA type, was the first assay routinely used to detect and specify HLA antibodies. On addition of rabbit complement, bound antibody causes complement activation and cell death, which is detected by vital staining and visualisation using light microscopy. Lymphocyte panels used for antibody screening can either be 'random' or 'selected'; random panels are comprised of unselected volunteer blood donors bearing HLA types that are representative of the local population and therefore indicate the proportion of deceased donors with which the patient would have HLA-specific antibodies; in selected panels, the volunteer blood donors are chosen to include all common and rare HLA specificities, often where the HLA specificities are not in the usual linkage, so that antibody specificities can be defined more accurately. The results from CDC assays are frequently reported as '% panel reactive antibodies', or '%PRA', but this is a misleading term because of the variability in panel composition, dependant on whether the panel is random, selected or a combination of both. There are a number of disadvantages to the CDC assay, and two of the most important are that non-HLA-specific antibodies (often IgM autoreactive antibodies) are routinely detected and non-complement fixing antibodies are not detected.

Flow cytometry

Antibody screening can be performed by flow cytometry using lymphocyte targets, either assayed individually or as pooled cells obtained from multiple individuals. In this assay antibody bound to target lymphocytes are detected with a fluorescent conjugated anti-immunoglobulin (IgG) reagent followed by analysis in a flow cytometer. The technique is more sensitive than CDC and has the advantage that IgM autoreactive antibodies are not detected (although IgG autoreactive antibodies are detected), and that non-complement fixing IgG isotypes (IgG2 and IgG4) are detected. This assay, however, has now been superseded in routine antibody screening programmes by the solid-phase assays.

Solid-phase assays

The solid-phase assays represent a major advance in standardising HLA antibody detection and specification. Commercial products are available both to detect the presence of HLA class I- or class II-specific antibodies and to determine their specificity. Purified HLA are immobilised onto a solid matrix and bound antibody is detected using optical detection systems. The HLA glycoproteins can be purified from natural sources, such as platelets or lymphoblastoid cell lines, or produced as recombinant proteins. For the detection of antibody the solid matrix is coated with purified HLA obtained from a number of different donors, whereas for antibody specification the matrix is coated with class I or class II HLA obtained from an individual cell – or for specifying antibodies in patients with complex antibody profiles, recombinant protein of a single HLA specificity (known as 'single antigen beads', or SABs) is used.

Enzyme-linked immunosorbent assays

The first solid-phase assay used was the enzyme-linked immunosorbent assay (ELISA), in which purified HLA is used to coat the wells of the microtitre plate. Following incubation with a patient's serum, bound antibody is detected with an enzyme-conjugated secondary antibody that produces a colour change in an enzyme substrate, measured by optical density. The assay is semi-quantitative, more sensitive than CDC and can detect non-complement fixing antibodies.

Flow cytometry

In the flow cytometry assays the solid matrix are microparticles coated with purified HLA proteins and bound patient-HLA-specific antibody is detected using a secondary fluorescent conjugated anti-human immunoglobulin and analysed by flow cytometry. The assay has similar advantages to the ELISA assay, but in most laboratories has been superseded by Luminex technology.

X-map (Luminex)

Luminex technology is now widely used for antibody detection and specification, and because of its speed and specificity is particularly useful for post-transplant antibody monitoring as an aid to diagnosis of graft rejection, and monitoring antibody levels following antibody reduction therapy in antibody-incompatible transplant programmes. In the assay up to 100 bead populations, each uniquely identifiable by colouration with a combination of two dyes in different proportions, can be combined in a single test. Antibody bound to the microparticles is detected with a secondary antibody, an R-Phycoerythrin-conjugated anti-human immunoglobulin. The analysis is performed in a dedicated flow cytometer with lasers that excite both the internal dye and reporter on the secondary antibody. The results are reported as units of median fluorescence intensity (MFI) that can reflect the level of antibody to individual HLA specificities present in patient sera. However, there are a number of considerations when interpreting the results of Luminex assays: there is batch variation in the amount of antigen on the beads, beads often have both native and denatured antigen on the surface, IgM HLA antibodies in patient's serum may block binding of IgG antibodies leading to falsely low MFI values, and in patients with high levels of antibody the microspheres may be saturated and therefore the MFI may not reflect the true level of antibody [15]. Dilutions of serum may be required, particularly when the assay is used to assess patients for antibody incompatible transplants and when monitoring patients during antibody removal and following transplant.

Clinical application

Pre-transplant HLA-specific antibody screening

Kidney transplantation in recipients with pre-existing donor-HLA-specific antibodies confers an immunological risk that can range from a high risk of immediate hyperacute rejection (constituting a veto to transplantation); through intermediate risk of acute humoral and/or cellular rejection (requiring pre-emptive therapeutic intervention before or at the time of transplantation); to low risk requiring regular post-transplant antibody monitoring and therapeutic intervention as clinically indicated [15,16]. Knowledge of mismatched donor HLA specificities and the patient's pre-transplant allosensitisation status based on prior identification and specification of circulating HLA specific antibodies is essential to inform the decision to accept or decline a live or deceased donor kidney. High levels of IgG against specific HLA alleles, detected by complement-dependent lymphocytotoxicity and/or solid-phase single antigen binding assays (Luminex) are considered as a contraindication and recorded as an 'unacceptable' donor HLA mismatch (veto), whereas low levels or absence of antibody to a given HLA allele constitute an 'acceptable' donor HLA mismatch.

HLA-specific alloantibody levels and their alloantigen specificity may change over time, depending on the priming source (i.e. transfusion of blood products, pregnancy or previous allograft) and timing of alloantigen exposure (i.e. historic, periodic or continuous). In the case of patients requiring a repeat transplant, the antibody status may change markedly over a short time period, and this may be associated with immunosuppression withdrawal or ongoing acute and chronic rejection of in situ donor tissue. Furthermore, alloantibodies that have declined over time and are currently negative can spontaneously return following non-specific immune activation through recent infection. It is therefore essential to record the nature and timing of all potential alloantibody priming events and determine the recipient alloantibody status before registration of the patient on the transplant waiting list, and undertake regular antibody monitoring to ensure an up-to-date record of acceptable and unacceptable HLA mismatches. UK national guidelines recommend that routine antibody monitoring should be undertaken at least once every 3 months, and additionally between 2 and 4 weeks after transfusion of blood products. Recording of acceptable and unacceptable HLA mismatches to which a patient is sensitised serves to avoid inappropriate offers and subsequent shipping of deceased donor organs to the recipient transplant centre for patients with unacceptably high levels of donor-specific antibodies (DSA).

HLA polymorphism has evolved from common ancestral genes and has given rise to groups of HLA alleles that share antigenic protein epitopes that display a high degree of serological crossreactivity, whereby exposure to a single or limited repertoire of mismatched HLA alleles can result in broadly reactive HLA-specific antibodies to many different alleles. As a consequence, some sensitised patients awaiting kidney transplantation have high levels of antibody to a broad range of allogeneic HLA that constitute unacceptable mismatches to the majority of potential donor HLA types. Such patients are termed 'highly sensitised', and in the absence of prioritisation strategies, the likelihood of identifying a suitable HLA compatible donor is remote. The level of sensitisation and probability of an unrelated deceased donor kidney being compatible with HLA-specific antibody is determined by the percentage calculated reaction frequency (% cRF), which in the UK is defined as the proportion of 10,000 consecutive organ donors that carry one or more unacceptable HLA mismatches. Highly sensitised patients that have ≥85% cRF are expected to have HLA-specific antibodies against 85% or more of random deceased kidney donors and are therefore less likely to receive a transplant; such patients are therefore prioritised in local and national organ allocation policies for well-HLA-matched antibody-compatible donor kidneys [17].

Pre-transplant donor crossmatch
The purpose of the final pre-transplant donor crossmatch is to confirm the absence of donor-HLA-specific antibodies, or that DSA levels are

within an acceptable threshold that will not result in uncontrolled acute humoral rejection. The crossmatch results together with antibody screening data serve to inform an individual patient's immunological risk assessment and to guide appropriate pre-emptive therapeutic clinical strategies to treat and control graft rejection [15,16]. In the case of deceased donor kidney allocation, a short list of potential recipients is generated following exclusion of those with unacceptable donor HLA mismatches (vetoed based on the donor-recipient HLA type and pre-transplant antibody screening data) and ranked according to local or national organ allocation criteria (See Chapter 8). Recipient sera that are representative of the highest period of alloantibody sensitisation and the most recent sera (obtained within the last 3 months) are selected for crossmatching against donor lymphocytes. In addition, in cases of repeat transplantation and recent potential alloantibody priming events, inclusion of a current recipient serum obtained within 24 hours of the transplant operation is also recommended.

The crossmatch procedure is performed by incubating recipient serum with donor lymphocytes followed by the detection of antibody binding, and this can be achieved using the complement-dependent lymphocytotoxic crossmatch (CDC-XM) and/or flow cytometric crossmatch (FC-XM) assays. Pre-transplant crossmatch policies differ between transplant centres, depending on the pre-transplant antibody screening policy and the patient's sensitisation status. For non-sensitised patients receiving a first transplant, most centres would require a pre-transplant donor crossmatch to be undertaken using the CDC assay alone, whereas for sensitised patients and regrafts, many centres would also undertake a flow cytometric crossmatch. Moreover, for sensitised patients with HLA class I-specific antibodies a crossmatch may be performed against donor T lymphocytes or unseparated lymphocytes, whereas for patients with HLA class II-specific sensitisation additional crossmatching against isolated donor B lymphocytes may also be included.

Not all recipient antibodies that bind donor lymphocytes and give rise to a positive crossmatch are harmful to a transplanted kidney, and it is therefore important to differentiate between potentially damaging antibodies and non-damaging antibodies. It has long been recognised that most donor reactive IgM antibodies detected using the CDC assay are not HLA specific and give rise to a clinically irrelevant false positive crossmatch [18]. In addition, many centres also ignore IgM HLA-specific antibodies as there is little evidence of their pathogenic role in allograft rejection. IgM non-HLA-specific antibodies are characterised as having no discernable HLA specificity detected in panel screening, have low affinity binding and are often autoreactive, particularly against B lymphocytes [19]. There are several strategies applied to the CDC donor crossmatch test to differentiate between non-pathogenic IgM antibodies and clinically important IgG HLA-specific antibodies, and these include: 1) the 'Amos wash technique' in which donor lymphocytes are washed after incubation with recipient serum to remove antibodies with low binding affinity; 2) addition of a secondary anti-human globulin antibody after incubation of patient serum with donor cells in order to increase the sensitivity for IgG alloantibody binding; 3) pre-incubation of patient serum with dithiothreitol (DTT), a reducing agent that cleaves the sulph-hydral bonds that stabilise the pentameric structure of IgM antibodies, but leaves IgG relatively intact. A positive lymphocytotoxic crossmatch in the unmodified CDC assay that is negative following addition of DTT is indicative of IgM antibodies, whereas a positive crossmatch in both the absence and presence of DTT indicates IgG antibody binding. It should be noted, however, that cytotoxicity caused by weak IgG antibodies may be destroyed by addition of DTT, and it is therefore important to interpret such results in conjunction with antibody screening and flow cytometric crossmatch results.

Ensuring a negative donor–recipient pre-transplant crossmatch result using either CDC and/or flow cytometric techniques has virtually eradicated both hyperacute and acute humoral rejection, and undertaking a prospective pre-transplant crossmatch is considered mandatory. In the case of live donor kidney transplantation, the final pre-transplant crossmatch is usually scheduled within 14 days preceding the planned transplant operation date. For deceased donor kidney transplantation, however, the pre-transplant donor–recipient crossmatch must be performed using donor tissue obtained around the time of organ retrieval.

The logistics and technical aspects of undertaking the prospective pre-transplant donor crossmatch test take between 4 and 6 hours, and this process often delays the transplant operation, resulting in prolonged donor-organ cold-storage time and a concomitant increased incidence of delayed graft function. Until recently the most robust tissue required to obtain donor lymphocytes for crossmatching has been donor lymph node and spleen obtained at the time of organ retrieval. More recently, however, modern lymphocyte isolation techniques using immuno-magnetic beads and donor peripheral blood provide an alternative that enables conclusion of the recipient selection and crossmatch process before completion of the donor operation. Furthermore, some centres that employ comprehensive pre-transplant antibody screening regimens may choose to omit the prospective pre-transplant donor crossmatch test for selected non-sensitised recipients and for recipients with no unacceptable donor HLA mismatches. The policy of predicting a negative donor crossmatch and omitting the prospective pre-transplant donor crossmatch test (known as a 'virtual crossmatch') must, however, only be undertaken using stringent criteria where a negative donor–recipient crossmatch can be predicted with absolute confidence and there is direct clinical benefit to the patient through shortened organ cold ischaemia time [20].

Clinical application of donor crossmatch results and immunological risk assessment

In the past the pre-transplant donor crossmatch results have served to inform a binary decision to proceed or to veto kidney transplantation between a given donor and recipient pair. Based largely on historical evidence associating a positive donor lymphocytotoxic crossmatch with hyperacute (antibody-mediated) rejection [1], it became mandatory to ensure that only donor and recipient pairs with a negative pre-transplant donor lymphocyte crossmatch should proceed to transplantation. Where applied properly, this policy has virtually eliminated hyperacute rejection, and the majority of current clinicians will not encounter a genuine case throughout their career.

It is now clear, however, that not all positive donor lymphocyte crossmatches preclude successful transplantation; in addition, selective application of more sensitive antibody screening and crossmatch techniques to identify weaker donor HLA-specific antibodies may be of clinical benefit, particularly for sensitised patients and those awaiting repeat transplantation [21]. When relying solely on the donor CDC-XM result alone, it was noted that allosensitised recipients and those receiving a repeat transplant have a higher incidence of delayed graft function and reduced graft survival rates. The interpretation of the final pre-transplant donor crossmatch result does not stand alone and requires knowledge of potential allosensitisation priming events, historical and current antibody screening data, and the kidney donor and recipient HLA type to identify mismatched donor HLA specificities.

The clinical significance and concomitant immunological risk assessment of donor-HLA-specific antibodies and/or a positive donor lymphocyte crossmatch are dependent on interrelated factors, including:

- timing – historic (DSA detected in past sera)/current (DSA detected in recent sera)
- immunoglobulin class – IgM/IgG DSA
- antibody specificity
  HLA class I (HLA-A, -B, -C) DSA
  HLA class II (HLA-DR, -DQ, -DP) DSA
  non-HLA specific
- antibody level.

Timing
The presence of circulating donor-HLA-specific antibodies at the time of transplantation carries a risk of acute humoral and/or hyperacute rejection, whereas DSA present in the past (identified using historic sera), but not detectable on the day of transplant (known as 'peak positive – current negative') will not cause immediate antibody-mediated rejection, but may indicate an increased immunological risk of graft rejection.

Immunoglobulin class
The unmodified CDC-XM test detects both IgM- and complement-fixing IgG isotypes (IgG3 > 1 > 2 > 4), whereas the standard flow cytometric crossmatch assay (using anti-human IgG secondary antibody) will detect all human IgG isotypes. IgM and IgG DSA are indicative of a primary or secondary immune response, respectively, the latter acting as a marker for

T-cell help for B-cell immunoglobulin class switch and the probable presence of alloreactive memory T and/or B cells. In-vitro cell-culture studies have shown that alloreactive T-cell proliferation is readily controlled by calcineurin inhibitor (CNI) based immunosuppression for patients with primary IgM antibodies, but are refractory to suppression in sensitised and highly sensitised patients with IgG alloreactive antibodies [22,23]. Similar correlations have also been observed in clinical kidney transplantation where peak positive – current negative crossmatch grafts caused by IgG DSA are at increased risk of irreversible rejection that is refractory to CNI-based immunosuppression, whereas positive crossmatch transplants caused by IgM antibodies have good overall graft outcome [24].

Antibody specificity

A positive donor lymphocyte crossmatch can be caused by HLA class I (HLA-A, HLA-B, HLA-C) and/or HLA class II (HLA-DR, HLA-DQ, HLA-DP) -specific antibodies and non-HLA-specific antibodies. A positive donor T- and B-lymphocyte CDC crossmatch caused by IgM non-HLA-specific antibodies can be safely ignored. By contrast, a positive T- and B-lymphocyte crossmatch caused by IgG HLA class I DSA present in current sera carries a high risk of hyperacute rejection, whereas historical positive (current negative) IgG HLA class I DSA will not undergo hyperacute rejection but carries a high risk of an anamnestic (primed) cellular and/or humoral rejection response that is more likely to be refractory to conventional immunosuppressive regimens [24]. By contrast, a positive B-cell crossmatch caused by IgG HLA class II DSA is unlikely to cause hyperacute rejection, as this has only been reported in a small number of cases that had an exceptionally high antibody titre. Recent evidence suggests, however, that IgG HLA class II DSA are associated with longer-term graft attrition for which, at present, there is no proven therapeutic intervention to attenuate progressive and incipient graft damage [25].

Antibody levels

DSA levels can be broadly grouped as low, intermediate and high and are determined by testing patient sera at dilution or by comparing the results obtained using the donor CDC and FC crossmatch tests and solid-phase HLA-specific antibody-binding assays [15]. These methods used for antibody detection vary widely in terms of their sensitivity, with Luminex-based DSA detection being very sensitive (i.e. able to detect very low levels of antibody) compared with FC-XM (intermediate) and CDC-XM being least sensitive and therefore only detecting relatively high antibody levels. When information from these assays are applied together, DSA detected by Luminex SAB alone, or Luminex SAB and FC-XM (but CDC negative), or Luminex SAB, FC-XM and CDC-XM provide an approximation of low, intermediate and high antibody levels, respectively.

Towards individualised immunological risk assessment

The clinical usefulness of any laboratory test is determined by its sensitivity and specificity. The clinical value of antibody screening and donor lymphocyte crossmatch results are measured by their ability to accurately predict a particular clinical event (specificity) and the likelihood of a false positive and false negative prediction of that same event (sensitivity). In the context of renal transplantation, a positive pre-transplant donor CDC-XM due to IgG HLA class I-specific antibodies present in current serum has a high predictive value for hyperacute rejection, but a negative crossmatch fails to identify sensitised patients at increased risk of acute humoral rejection. Furthermore, a positive pre-transplant FC-XM (CDC-XM negative) is correlated with an increased incidence of humoral rejection, but may also be positive in patients that have an uneventful post-transplant clinical course [26]. By contrast, however, when FC-XM is selectively applied to allosensitised patients with known DSA only, both the test sensitivity and specificity for predicting humoral rejection is increased [27]. An additional emerging factor used to determine immunological risk is the level of DSA defined by the semi-quantitative MFI value obtained from Luminex-based single antigen bead assays [28]. It is not yet possible to provide precise 'cut-off' MFI values to predict humoral rejection and graft failure, nor is it possible to predict with a high degree of confidence the antibody level likely to give rise to a positive donor CDC-XM and/or FC-XM. However, as a general guide, many laboratories consider DSA MFI values of 1000–3000 to be low, 3000–6000 intermediate and >6000 high [29].

An illustrative guide to immunological risk assessment is shown in Table 4.2, and a more detailed version can be found in reference [16]. It should be noted that HLA-specific antibody-incompatible kidney transplantation in cases with intermediate and high immunological risk should be considered with caution and only undertaken in centres with clinical policies designed to prospectively identify and attenuate the risk, such as pre- and post-transplant antibody reduction therapy. Furthermore, other factors such as repeat donor HLA mismatches in DSA positive regrafts constitute an additional risk that may also influence the immunological risk stratification.

HLA-specific antibody monitoring after kidney transplantation

Recent evidence has highlighted a major pathophysiological role of HLA-specific antibodies after kidney transplantation and their association with graft loss. Graft biopsy pathology has highlighted tubulitis, transplant glomerulopathy and associated proteinuria in cases with post-transplant DSA, and this is correlated with incipient graft attrition [30]. Terasaki *et al.* reported graft attrition rates of 6.6% per annum in

Table 4.2 Immunological risk stratification according to antibody screening and donor crossmatch results.

DSA specificity	DTT-modified CDC-XM	FC-XM	DSA MFI	Timing	Immunological risk*
HLA-A,-B,-C	Positive	Positive	High	Current	High
HLA-A,-B,-C	Negative	Positive	Intermediate	Current	Intermediate
HLA-A,-B,-C	Negative	Negative	Low	Current	Low
HLA-A,-B,-C	Positive	Positive	High	Historical	High/Intermediate
HLA-A,-B,-C	Negative	Positive	Intermediate	Historical	Intermediate
HLA-A,-B,-C	Negative	Negative	Low	Historical	Low
HLA-A,-B,-C	Negative	Negative	Negative	H&C**	Standard
HLA-DR,-DQ,-DP	Positive	Positive	High	Current	High/Intermediate
HLA-DR,-DQ,-DP	Negative	Positive	Intermediate	Current	Intermediate
HLA-DR,-DQ,-DP	Negative	Negative	Low	Current	Low
HLA-DR,-DQ,-DP	Positive	Positive	High	Historical	High/Intermediate
HLA-DR,-DQ,-DP	Negative	Positive	Intermediate	Historical	Intermediate
HLA-DR,-DQ,-DP	Negative	Negative	Low	Historical	Low
HLA-DR,-DQ,-DP	Negative	Negative	Negative	H&C**	Standard

*High immunological risk – hyperacute rejection is likely and such transplants should only be undertaken after effective pre-emptive antibody reduction therapy; intermediate immunological risk – transplantation should be avoided if reasonably possible, but may be undertaken with appropriate clinical caution and/or pre-emptive antibody reduction therapy; low immunological risk – may be associated with an increased risk of acute rejection, but little or no overall influence of graft survival.
**H&C, historic and current.

cases with DSA compared with 3% when no DSA was present [25]. A direct cause and effect of DSA and resulting pathology has not been definitively proven, although Terasaki *et al.* reported that appearance of DSA precedes graft failure in around 80–90% of long-term survivors [25].

The presence of post-transplant antibodies may be caused by reactivation of previously undefined pre-transplant allosensitisation or reactivation of pre-existing low antibody levels. In addition, acute rejection may give rise to *de novo* appearance of DSA [31]. It is therefore recommended that post-transplant antibody monitoring should be undertaken for all patients with suspected acute rejection and also declining function with unknown cause. The response of recipient DSA levels to treatment (e.g. antibody reduction therapy) can be monitored using semi-quantitative Luminex-based SAB assays, and this correlates well with long-term outcome. Everly and colleagues have shown that for cases when DSA antibody levels are reduced to <50% of pre-treatment levels, outcome is good, but the prognosis is poor when DSA levels remain above 50% [32].

Summary

Although donor–recipient HLA matching may be beneficial in terms of reducing the incidence of rejection and improving graft outcome, the main role of histocompatibility testing is to identify and characterise allosensitisation through the identification of HLA-specific antibodies. Determination of donor specificity and antibody levels is used to assess the immunological risk of proceeding to transplant. Furthermore, monitoring donor-HLA-specific antibodies after transplant supports the diagnosis of humoral/cellular rejection and may guide clinical intervention strategies and indicate prognosis in the longer term.

Acknowledgements

Craig Taylor is supported by the National Institute for Health Research, Cambridge Biomedical Research Centre.

References
1. Kissmeyer-Nielsen F, Olsen S, Petersen VP, *et al.* (1966) Hyperacute rejection of kidney allografts, associated with pre-existing humoral antibodies against donor cells. *Lancet* **2**, 662–665.
2. Dausset J. (1958) Iso-leuko-antibodies. *Acta Haematol* **20**, 156–166.
3. Marsh SG, Albert ED, Bodmer WF, *et al.* (2010) Nomenclature for factors of the HLA system, 2010. *Tissue Antigens* **75**, 291–455.
4. Holdsworth R, Hurley CK, Marsh SG, *et al.* (2009) The HLA dictionary 2008: A summary of HLA-A, -B, -C, -DRB1/3/4/5, and -DQB1 alleles and their association with serologically defined HLA-A, -B, -C, -DR, and -DQ antigens. *Tissue Antigens* **73**, 95–170.
5. Ting A, Morris PJ. (1978) Matching for B-cell antigens of the HLA-DR series in cadaver renal transplantation. *Lancet* **1**, 575–577.
6. Persijn GG, Cohen B, Lansbergen Q, *et al.* (1982) Effect of HLA-A and HLA-B matching on survival of grafts and recipients after renal transplantation. *N Engl J Med* **307**, 905–908.
7. Su X, Zenios SA, Chakkera H, *et al.* (2004) Diminishing significance of HLA matching in kidney transplantation. *Am J Transplant* **4**, 1501–1508.
8. Opelz G, Döhler B. (2007) Effect of human leukocyte antigen compatibility on kidney graft survival: Comparative analysis of two decades. *Transplantation* **84**, 137–143.
9. Johnson RJ, Fuggle SV, O'Neill J, *et al.* (2010) Kidney Advisory Group of NHS Blood and Transplant. Factors influencing outcome after deceased heart beating donor kidney transplantation in the United Kingdom: An evidence base for a new national kidney allocation policy. *Transplantation* **89**, 379–386.
10. Taylor CJ, Welsh KI, Gray CM, *et al.* (1994) Clinical and socio-economic benefits of serological HLA-DR matching for renal transplantation over

three eras of immunosuppression regimens in a single unit. In: Terasaki PI, Cecka JM, (eds), *Clinical Transplants*, pp. 233–241. UCLA Tissue Typing Laboratory, Los Angeles, California.

11. Opelz G, Döhler B. (2010) Impact of HLA mismatching on incidence of post-transplant non-Hodgkin lymphoma after kidney transplantation. *Transplantation* **89**, 567–572.

12. Opelz G, Döhler B. (2010) Pediatric kidney transplantation: Analysis of donor age, HLA match and post-transplant non-Hodgkin lymphoma. *Transplantation* **90**, 292–297.

13. Opelz G, Döhler B. (2011) Association of mismatches for HLA-DR with incidence of post-transplant hip fracture in kidney transplant recipients. *Transplantation* **91**, 65–69.

14. Fuggle SV, Martin S. (2008) Tools for human leukocyte antigen antibody detection and their application to transplanting sensitized patients. *Transplantation* **86**, 384–390.

15. Taylor CJ, Kosmoliaptsis V, Summers DM, *et al.* (2009) Back to the future: Application of contemporary technology to long-standing questions about the clinical relevance of HLA-specific alloantibodies in renal transplantation. *Hum Immunol* **70**, 563–568.

16. British Society for Histocompatibility and Immunogenetics (BSHI) and British Transplantation Society (BTS). (2010) *Guidelines for the Detection and Characterisation of Clinically Relevant Antibodies in Allotransplantation.* Available online from: http://www.bshi.org.uk/pdf/BSHI_BTS_ guidelines_2010.pdf.

17. Johnson RJ, Fuggle SV, Mumford L, *et al.* (2010) Kidney Advisory Group of NHS Blood and Transplant. A New UK 2006 National Kidney Allocation Scheme for deceased heart-beating donor kidneys. *Transplantation* **89**, 387–394.

18. Ting A, Morris PJ. (1983) Successful transplantation with a positive T and B cell crossmatch due to autoreactive antibodies. *Tissue Antigens* **21**, 219–226.

19. Taylor CJ, Ting A, Morris PJ. (1991) Production and characterisation of human monoclonal lymphocytotoxic autoantibodies from a renal dialysis patient. *Tissue Antigens* **37**, 112–120.

20. Taylor CJ, Kosmoliaptsis, Sharples LD, *et al.* (2010) Ten year experience of selective omission of the pre-transplant crossmatch test in deceased donor kidney transplantation. *Transplantation* **89**, 185–193.

21. O'Rourke RW, Osorio RW, Freise CE, *et al.* (2000) Flow cytometry crossmatching as a predictor of acute rejection in sensitized recipients of cadaveric renal transplants. *Clin Transplant* **14**, 167–173.

22. van Kampen CA, Versteeg-van der Voort Maarschalk MF, Roelen DL, *et al.* (2002) Primed CTLs specific for HLA class I may still be present in sensitized patients when anti-HLA antibodies have disappeared: relevance for donor selection. *Transplantation* **73**, 1286–1290.

23. Oostingh GJ, Davies HFS, Bradley JA, *et al.* (2003) Comparison of allogeneic and xenogeneic in vitro T cell proliferative responses of sensitised patients awaiting kidney transplantation. *Xenotransplantation* **10**, 545–551.

24. Taylor CJ, Chapman JR, Ting A, *et al.* (1989) Characterisation of lymphocytotoxic antibodies causing a positive crossmatch in renal transplantation: Relationship to primary and regraft outcome. *Transplantation* **48**, 953–958.

25. Terasaki PI, Cai J. (2008) Human leukocyte antigen antibodies and chronic rejection: from association to causation. *Transplantation* **86**, 377–383.

26. Mahoney RJ, Norman DJ, Colombe BW, *et al.* (1996) Identification of high- and low-risk second kidney grafts. *Transplantation* **61**, 1349–1355.
27. Süsal C, Döhler B, Opelz G. (2009) Presensitized kidney graft recipients with HLA class I and II antibodies are at increased risk for graft failure: A Collaborative Transplant Study report. *Hum Immunol* **70**, 569–573.
28. Mizutani K, Terasaki P, Hamdani E, *et al.* (2007) The importance of anti-HLA-specific antibody strength in monitoring kidney transplant patients. *Am J Transplant* **7**, 1027–1031.
29. Lefaucheur C, Loupy A, Hill GS, *et al.* (2010) Preexisting donor-specific HLA antibodies predict outcome in kidney transplantation. *J Am Soc Nephrol* **21**, 1398–1406.
30. Loupy A, Suberbielle-Boissel C, Hill GS, *et al.* (2009) Outcome of subclinical antibody-mediated rejection in kidney transplant recipients with preformed donor-specific antibodies. *Am J Transplant* **9**, 2561–2570.
31. Li X, Ishida H, Yamaguchi Y, *et al.* (2008) Poor graft outcome in recipients with de novo donor-specific anti-HLA antibodies after living related kidney transplantation. *Transpl Int* **21**, 1145–1152.
32. Everly MJ, Everly JJ, Arend LJ, *et al.* (2009) Reducing de novo donor-specific antibody levels during acute rejection diminishes renal allograft loss. *Am J Transplant* **9**, 1063–1071.

5 Donor management: care of the heartbeating brain-dead multi-organ donor

Paul G. Murphy

Introduction

The ever-increasing demand for donor organs is a reflection of both the rising incidence of end-stage organ failure (related at least in part to the increasing prevalence of hypertension and diabetes mellitus) and the effectiveness of transplantation as the preferred and sometimes only treatment option for it. The principal restriction to transplantation in many countries, including the UK, is the availability of suitable donor organs, and although pragmatic and partial solutions to this lie in the continuing development and expansion of living donation programmes, organ transplantation in general continues to rely heavily on deceased donation. Furthermore, the availability of suitable deceased donor organs is declining, for various reasons:

- advances in the treatment of severe traumatic brain injury, ischaemic stroke and aneurysmal subarachnoid haemorrhage are resulting in a decline in the incidence of confirmed brain death
- the pool of potential heartbeating brain-dead donors is more elderly and has a raised incidence of medical co-morbidities that may represent a relevant contraindication to transplantation
- increasing emphasis on the limitation or withdrawal of treatments that appear to be of little or no overall benefit to patients with catastrophic brain injuries, thereby creating a cohort of patients who become suitable for Maastricht category III donation after circulatory death rather than potential heartbeating brainstem-dead donors.

Although efforts to increase the availability of donor organs have focused largely on increasing the number of organ donors (usually expressed for comparative purposes as the annual number per million of population), the primary objective is successful transplantation, not donation and retrieval. Furthermore, it can be argued that to allow uncorrected donor pathophysiology to unnecessarily restrict both the number and quality

Handbook of Renal and Pancreatic Transplantation, First Edition. Edited by Iain A. M. MacPhee and Jiří Froněk.
© 2012 John Wiley & Sons, Ltd. Published 2012 by John Wiley & Sons, Ltd.

(and therefore longevity) of organs that can be transplanted degrades the gift of donation and the trust that the donor and their family have placed in the donation process. It follows that, from the perspective of both the donor and the recipient, although donor numbers dominate the strategic attempts to increase transplantation rates, appropriate effort should also be directed towards maximising the number of organs retrieved from a heartbeating donor and providing those organs in the best possible condition. It similarly follows that the metrics used to track donation and transplantation should include not just donor numbers but also the number and type of organs per donor as well as population-adjusted rates of successful deceased donor organ transplantation. Data from NHS Blood and Transplant indicates that the average heartbeating brainstem dead donor in the UK donates an average of just under four organs, with the number of transplants performed and number of patients transplanted being somewhat fewer than this, compared with the theoretical maximum of eight (two kidneys, a liver, two lungs, a heart, a small bowel and a pancreas). Furthermore, the number of organ transplants per donor in the UK falls of sharply in donors over the age of 50 years. Overall, while most heartbeating brainstem-dead donors will donate liver and kidney, the proportion donating cardiothoracic organs is much smaller, and this has had a profound impact upon the number of heart and lung transplants being carried out in the UK currently. Although the solution to this lies in part in reviewing the criteria for donor selection as well as the development of *ex-vivo* organ perfusion systems that may allow the condition of an organ to be assessed and potentially improved before transplantation
(e.g. *ex-vivo* lung perfusion techniques), it is also the case that much can be done before organ retrieval to improve the likelihood of successful transplantation. Specifically, there is now considerable evidence that the application of standardised donor management protocols increases the number of retrieved organs, with a particular impact on retrieval of cardiothoracic organs. Conversely, persistence of physiological instability of the heartbeating brainstem-dead donor may establish within the donor organ(s) tissue injury that may subsequently degrade both the function and longevity of any subsequent graft, as shown semi-schematically in Fig. 5.1. Thus, the role played by intensivists in organ donation should not be limited to the identification and referral of potential donors; rather, it should also extend to maximising the number of organs offered for retrieval and to optimising their condition in order to give the best possible opportunity for a successful and long-lasting graft.

Donor management requires a proactive approach based upon a sound understanding of the physiological derangements exhibited by the heartbeating donor. Although some of these relate to the primary injury suffered by the patient or the generic complications of critical care, there are two other processes that are specific to the severely brain-injured patient: the adverse systemic effects of brain-directed critical care, and the pathophysiological consequences of brain death.

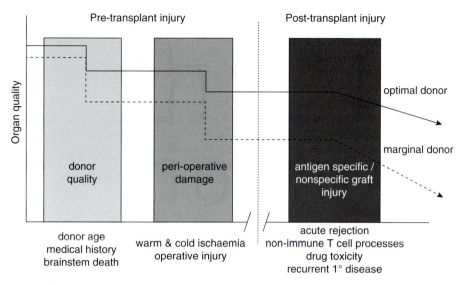

Figure 5.1 Schematic outline of timelines for tissue injury and graft loss following cadaveric organ transplantation.

The somatic complications of brain-directed therapies

Protocols for the management of severe brain injury frequently focus on maintenance of cerebral perfusion, often to the detriment of other organ function. For instance, respiratory failure is a common complication of neuro-critical care, and may result from the aspiration of gastric or orophayngeal contents at the time of the initial insult, or be (more frequently) a consequence of micro-aspiration, progressive sputum retention and dependent atelectasis in patients who are deeply sedated, pharmacologically paralysed and denied all but the most essential respiratory therapies and tracheal toilet during their critical care. Although cardiovascular impairment is perhaps less common, it can be equally catastrophic and has a multifactorial aetiology that derives from the aggressive approach to control of intracranial pressure (ICP) and the maintenance of cerebral perfusion (pressure). Thus, aggressive diuretic therapy using a combination of loop diuretics, mannitol and hypertonic saline solutions is a prominent feature of many treatment protocols, and may result in hypovolaemia, hypernatraemia and hypokalaemia. Vasopressor infusions are commonly used to support the circulation and maintain cerebral perfusion pressure in such circumstances, in part counteracting both the relative hypovolaemia that results from aggressive diuretic therapies as well as the hypotensive side effects of sedative agents employed to both facilitate controlled ventilation and manage intracranial hypertension. Anecdotally prolonged use of escalating doses of vasopressor drugs is associated with global subendocardial ischaemia of the myocardium, particularly when given in combination with the lipid-based sedative agent propofol, and any resulting organ ischaemia will be further exacerbated by uncorrected hypovolaemia.

More generally, the brainstem-dead donor is a critically ill patient who may have been cared for within an intensive-care unit environment for many days, and thereby may have been exposed to the generic iatrogenic complications of critical care, including hospital-acquired sepsis, the complications of invasive vascular access, endotracheal intubation and urinary catheterisation, poor nutrition and an increased risk of thromboembolic disorders. They may have suffered severe polytrauma and had a series of surgical interventions, and even in the absence of overt blood loss may have a mild anaemia associated with repeated blood sampling and critical illness.

Pathophysiology of brain death

General considerations

The pathophysiological features of brainstem death are specific, various and well described. Indeed, the systemic consequences of the condition that is now recognised as brainstem death were described in the first landmark description of the condition by Mollaret and Guillon in 1959. The severity of the various physiological derangements is proportional to the rate of rise in the ICP, and is typically worst therefore in children and young adults (who lack the additional compliance offered by the more atrophic brain), or in circumstances where the rise in ICP is very sudden (e.g. acute obstructive hydrocephalus). It should be emphasised that while these derangements are almost always correctable, untreated they may result in rapid deterioration and cardiac arrest. Correction of these physiological derangements can be time consuming and may require intensive interventions that may be viewed by some to be inappropriate given the nature of the primary pathology and the bleak prognosis for the patient. However, since it is frequently necessary to stabilise a patient's condition in order for a diagnosis of brainstem death to be properly made, subsequent donor optimisation is very often simply an extension of these strategies. Furthermore, there is no evidence that families of potential donors object to such interventions once permission for organ retrieval has been obtained; rather, they value the continued care and attention that their loved one is receiving and support the attempts to improve both the number and quality of organ transplants that might result.

Cardio-respiratory instability

Haemodynamic instability is a characteristic feature of brainstem death and occurs in the majority of donors, although it varies very considerably in its severity. Two phases of the haemodynamic response to brain death are recognised – an initial phase of hypertension and myocardial

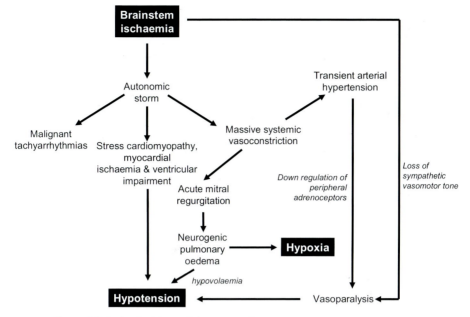

Figure 5.2 Pathophysiology of the autonomic storm.

irritability, often referred to as the autonomic storm, followed by a more prolonged phase of refractory vasodilatation ('vasoparalysis'), hypotension and organ hypoperfusion. When severe, it frequently coexists with an acute impairment of gas exchange that is the result of so-called 'neurogenic' pulmonary oedema.

The autonomic storm
Malignant rises in ICP result in progressive ischaemia of the brainstem, and lead to a period of systemic and pulmonary hypertension that is associated with myocardial irritability, arrhythmias and myocardial ischaemia (Fig. 5.2). Experimental models of brain death reveal that the autonomic storm is associated with high levels of circulating catecholamines and that it can be effectively obtunded by prior high spinal blockade. The autonomic storm associated with brainstem ischaemia is best considered to be an example of stress-induced cardiomyopathy (*takotsubo* cardiomyopathy), which although frequently catastrophic at presentation, is potentially fully recoverable with appropriate support. Electrocardiogram changes are common and are frequently accompanied by rises in cardiac troponins and echocardiographic evidence of regional or global myocardial impairment. Myocardial irritability may on occasion result in terminal tachyarrhythmias. Although this initial phase is usually temporary and self-limiting it can occasionally be profound and result in irreversible cardiovascular collapse.

Neurogenic pulmonary oedema

The filtration of fluid across a capillary barrier is determined by the hydrostatic and oncotic pressure gradients across the barrier, as well as the intrinsic permeability of the barrier. The catecholamine surge associated with the autonomic storm triggers a very sudden rise in left ventricular end diastolic and pulmonary capillary pressures, which in turn results in disruption of the integrity of alveolar-capillary barrier. Although pulmonary capillary pressures may subside as the left ventricle recovers, alveolar flooding persists while the passage of fluid into the lungs remains dependent upon the hydrostatic pressure gradient alone. Furthermore, the primary stress-related injury to the pulmonary microcirculation can establish an inflammatory process that may serve to both amplify and prolong this phase of 'high-permeability' pulmonary oedema. The loss of significant volumes of protein-rich fluid into the alveolar air spaces can cause both profound hypoxaemia and also hypovolaemic shock (the latter being accompanied by haemoconcentration and a relative polycythaemia).

Neurogenic hypotension

Death of the brainstem deprives the patient of all somatic sympathetic activity, the loss of which is revealed once the consequences of the autonomic storm have subsided. In addition, catecholamine receptors that have been exposed to supra-normal levels of endogenous agonists, subsequently demonstrate a lower responsiveness to any exogenous catecholamine. This loss of vasomotor tone and reactivity (so-called 'vaso-paralysis') results in profound hypotension that is often refractory to administered catecholamine-based vasoconstrictors such as norepinephrine (noradrenaline) and phenylephrine, but responsive to novel constrictors such as angiotensin and vasopressin. Clinically, it is important to recognise that hypotension and hypoperfusion in the brainstem-dead donor may be a complex consequence of a number of inter-related physiological derangements, including loss of vasomotor tone, myocardial impairment and hypovolaemia (Fig. 5.2), possibly compounded by electrolyte and acid–base disorders as well as hypothermia.

Hypothalamic failure

Brain (stem) death implies loss of hypothalamic function, and in practice, patients who are brainstem dead frequently exhibit one or both of the consequences of hypothalamic failure – hypothermia and failure of the neuroendocrine hypothalamo-pituitary axis.

Hypothermia

Hypothermia is almost invariable, and is primarily the result of vasodilatation and the consequent loss of heat to cooler surroundings, exacerbated by a reduction in metabolic rate and heat production due to loss of muscle tone. It is often overlooked during initial clinical assessment because the patient's peripheries feel warm (this being the primary cause of the hypothermia), and may take some hours to correct, particularly while the patient remains vasodilated. Hypothermia delays the diagnosis of brainstem death and may exacerbate haemodynamic and haemostatic instability.

Failure of the hypothalamo-pituitary axis

Failure of the hypothalamo-pituitary axis results most notably in diabetes insipidus through failure of the secretion of antidiuretic hormone (ADH, also known as vasopressin) from the neurohypophysis. Lack of ADH results in the excretion of large volumes of dilute urine, sometimes in excess of 1000 mL per hour, and if untreated leads to hypovolaemia, hypokalaemia and hypernatraemia, the latter being specifically associated with hepatic dysfunction and early graft failure. The diuresis is easily terminated with 1–2 mg of parenteral desmopressin, (1-desamino-8-D-arginine vasopressin), a synthetic analogue of ADH that has a longer half-life and which lacks the vasoconstricting properties of the endogenous hormone. It is equally important to correct the existing water deficit with rapid intravenous infusion of an equivalent volume of 5% dextrose.

Although hypothalamic failure also deprives the anterior lobe of the pituitary gland (adenohypophysis) of higher centre control, the clinical significance of this is unclear, particularly since the blood supply to the gland itself is largely extra-dural (implying that the intrinsic functions of the gland might be preserved in the brainstem-dead donor). There is a large and somewhat conflicting literature describing the significance or otherwise of any acute derangement in anterior lobe function in the brainstem-dead donor, particularly thyroid function, and although many donor management protocols include routine thyroid replacement therapy as a component of so-called triple hormone replacement therapy (i.e. in combination with vasopressin and methylprednisolone) for all potential donors, more recent studies suggest a lack of benefit from thyroid replacement when used as a routine.

Biochemical, haematological and metabolic disorders

Brainstem-dead donors frequently have profound and conflicting derangements of fluid and electrolyte balance that are the product of a variable combination of aggressive diuretic therapies, which may then be compounded by the onset of diabetes insipidus, the autonomic storm and the subsequent administration of both 5% dextrose and high-dose methylprednisolone. The brainstem-dead donor is usually hypovolaemic, with the common biochemical abnormalities being hypernatraemia, hyperglycaemia, hypokalaemia, hypomagnesaemia and hypophosphataemia.

As noted above, the brainstem-dead donor is commonly relatively anaemic (although this may be temporarily obscured by the haemoconcentration of neurogenic pulmonary oedema). In addition, the severely injured brain releases tissue thromboplastins that may provoke thrombolysis and a consumptive coagulopathy dissemination that may add to blood loss, whereas acidosis impairs coagulation and hypothermia and high levels of circulating catecholamines interfere with platelet function.

The combination of critical illness and the elements of the autonomic storm, particularly hypoperfusion and high circulating levels of catecholamines, have a profound effect on intermediate metabolism. Reduced myocardial energy stores contribute to myocardial impairment and are further worsened by exogenous catecholamine therapies, whereas progressive metabolic acidosis and rising blood lactate together with a reduced mixed venous oxygen saturation point to substantial anaerobic metabolism in the brainstem-dead donor.

Management of the multi-organ donor

Donor optimisation is the active correction of a specific constellation of physiological derangements associated with brainstem death, and requires the continuation and sometimes an escalation of critical care in the period between confirmation of death and organ retrieval. It carries the specific twin objectives of both increasing the number of organs that might be successfully retrieved (and transplanted) from a heartbeating brainstem-dead donor, and also improving the condition of those organs and therefore possibly their longevity. It in principle requires a switch in focus from therapies that are directed towards resuscitation of the injured brain (which is dead) to those that focus upon restoration of physiological and metabolic homeostasis of the transplantable somatic organs and tissues. Although the timely application of donor optimisation interventions should be seen as a standard of care that all potential donors should receive, it is of particular importance in circumstances where retrieval of the cardiothoracic organs is a possibility, and there is persuasive evidence that the number of retrieved hearts and lungs can be significantly increased by the early application of invasive haemodynamic monitoring and lung-protective ventilatory strategies.

Clinical staff will on occasion hesitate to follow donor optimisation protocols, particularly if they require the introduction of new invasive monitoring devices and deny a grieving family access to their loved one. It is vital that all staff are aware of the benefits of donor optimisation and that there are no ethical or legal obstacles to it, or to properly approved clinical trials that are directed towards improving donor management. The temptation to minimise further clinical interventions after the diagnosis of death should therefore be avoided, not least because this degrades the potential gift that a donor and his/her family may make. It is similarly important that the family of the potential donor understand the rationale for active donor management, the nature of the necessary interventions and their potential benefits, and its likely duration (particularly in circumstances where repeated assessments of, for instance, myocardial function may be required).

When planning donor management for an individual patient, it is useful to assess the potential for thoracic retrieval as early as possible, as

the organ-specific management protocols for the thoracic organs require a greater degree of intervention than those that guide splanchnic resuscitation. Schedules for the generic and system-specific elements of donor optimisation are given in Tables 5.1–5.4. Although the details are considerable, the fundamental principles of donor care are relatively few:
• Hypotension and hypovolaemia jeopardises the successful retrieval and transplantation of the liver, kidneys and other abdominal organs. Hypernatraemia is independently associated with hepatic dysfunction and graft loss.

Table 5.1 Donor management: general guidance and initial management.

Goals	Monitoring and investigations	Interventions
Continued support for donation from donor family	Clinical assessment Review of fluid balance charts	Offer full explanation of the rationale and nature of active donor management to the family of the potential donor.
Early recognition and correction of hypovolaemia	Urinary catheter Nasogastric tube Continuous ECG (3/5 lead) and pulse oximetry monitoring	Clinical and laboratory assessment of fluid status and early correction of hypovolaemia with 3–5 mL/kg boluses of crystalloid/colloid, repeated as indicated; note that
Early recognition and treatment of diabetes insipidus: urine output >4 mL/kg/h that is associated with a rising serum sodium (>145 mmol/L) or rising serum osmolality and falling urine osmolality (>300 and <200 mosM, respectively).	Invasive arterial and central venous pressure monitoring Core/peripheral temperature 12-lead ECG Chest X-ray Full blood count Clotting screen Blood urea and electrolytes Arterial blood gases Blood lactate and mixed venous oximetry	hydroxyethyl starch solutions have been associated with an increased incidence of delayed kidney graft function, and are best avoided if possible Correction of diabetes insipidus • Vasopressin 1–4 units/h and/or DDAVP, 1–4 µg IV, • Estimate and replace previous uncorrected diuresis in full with 5% dextrose until hypernatraemia is reversed Methylprednisolone, 15 mg/kg, given as soon as possible
Management of systemic inflammation Metabolic homeostasis Thromboprophylaxis Antimicrobial prevention and treatment		Initiate/continue enteral nutrition Continue parenteral nutrition Maintain tight glycaemic control (blood glucose 4–8 mmol/L) with intravenous insulin infusion as indicated Review medication chart; continue pharmacological thromboprophylaxis and antibiotics if indicated

Table 5.2 Donor management: haemodynamic optimisation.

Goals	Monitoring and investigations	Interventions
Improve organ perfusion • Correction of hypovolaemia • Restoration of vasomotor tone • Improvement of myocardial contractility General haemodynamic goals: • Heart rate 60–100 bpm • CVP <12 cmH_2O • Mean arterial pressure 70 mmHg • Systolic blood pressure >100 mmHg • Mixed venous saturation >60% Reduction of catecholamine infusion(s) Increase likelihood of heart retrieval and transplantation	12-lead ECG Chest X-ray Acid–base, blood lactate and mixed venous oximetry Serum electrolytes **Assessment of cardiac performance and injury:** Transthoracic echocardiogram Early cardiac output monitoring Cardiac troponin assay Coronary angiography (in selected cases/units)	**Initial therapy** a. early correction of hypovolaemia, diabetes insipidus and electrolyte and acid–base disturbances as directed above. b. vasopressin infusion, 1 unit followed by 1–4 units/h: • as initial therapy for fluid-unresponsive hypotension, or • to replace/reduce existing catecholamine infusions **Additional therapies in unresponsive cases** a. if the donor remains hypotensive or echocardiography indicates poor ventricular performance (ejection fraction <40%) initiate cardiac output monitoring, titrating fluid, vasoconstrictors or inotropic therapy to following end points: • cardiac index >2.4 L/min/m^2 • pulmonary artery occlusion pressure <12 cmH_2O • systemic vascular resistance 800–1200 dynes/s/cm^5 • left ventricular stroke work index >15 g/kg/min Use catecholamines as sparingly as possible, and consider dopamine or dobutamine before epinephrine, norepinephrine or phenylephrine. Low-dose dopamine (4 μg/kg/min) may reduce the incidence of delayed kidney graft function and the need for post-operative renal support. b. in refractory cases consider parenteral empirical thyroid replacement therapy • levothyroxine (tetra-iodothyronine, T_4), 20 μg IV bolus, followed by 10 μg/hour, or • liothyronine, (tri-iodothyronine, T_3), 4 μg IV bolus, followed by 3 μg/hour **Coronary angiography** May increase proportion of hearts retrieved from DBD donors. • To lower risk of contrast nephropathy, ensure normovolaemia and administer N-acetylcysteine 150 mg/kg IV in 150 mL normal saline over 30 minutes immediately prior to injection of contrast, followed by 50 mg/kg in 500 mL over following 4 hours).

Table 5.3 Donor management: respiratory optimisation.

Goals	Monitoring and investigations	Interventions
Correct the atelectasis that follows the apnoea tests Continue/reinstate the general respiratory care of the intubated and ventilated patient, and protect against risk of pulmonary microaspiration Identify and reverse specific pulmonary complications of critical care/brainstem death Introduce lung-protective ventilatory therapies (which have been shown to increase proportion of lung retrievals from heartbeating donors)	Chest X-ray Arterial blood gases Sputum Gram stain and culture Broncho-alveolar lavage	Give methylprednisolone, 15 mg/kg Reinstate routine chest physiotherapy, 2 hourly rotation to lateral position and regular endotracheal suction 30° head up tilt and firm inflation of endotracheal tube cuff to prevent microaspiration and bronchial soiling Intensive alveolar recruitment - e.g. periodic application of PEEP up to 15 cm H_2O, sustained inspiration to 30 cm H_2O for 30–60 seconds and diuresis where indicated. Ventilatory targets are as follows: • Tidal volume 6–8 mL/kg; PEEP 5–10 cm H_2O; PIP <30 cm H_2O • pH 7.35- 7.45, $PaCO_2$ 4.5–6 kPa, PaO_2 >11 kPa , SaO_2 >95% Initiate antibiotic therapy as directed by results of sputum/lavage microscopy and culture, avoiding nephrotoxic anti-microbials

• The ventricular impairment associated with stress-induced cardiomyopathy is usually reversible, although this may take 24 hours or more of intensive cardiovascular monitoring and support. Infusions of high doses of epinephrine and norepinephrine are often used in such circumstances and are associated with poor transplant outcomes. Cautious fluid resuscitation should be the initial approach to hypotension, whereas vasopressin should be the first-line vasoconstrictor.

• The extent of haemodynamic monitoring should parallel escalations of therapy. Although transthoracic 2D echocardiography may be of value in guiding therapy, assessment for transplantability may be better informed by measurements of flow that are independent of outflow resistance. The introduction of vasopressin as first-line vasoconstrictor frequently enables reduction or withdrawal of catecholamine infusions.

Table 5.4 Donor management: metabolic, biochemical and haematological optimization.

Goals	Monitoring and investigations	Interventions
Identify and correct the metabolic, biochemical and haematological derangements associated with the treatment of acute severe brain injury and brainstem death, particularly: • hypernatraemia • hypokalaemia • hyperglycaemia • anaemia • disseminated intravascular coagulation Markers of adequate perfusion include decreasing blood lactate, mixed venous saturation >60%, and urine output of 1–2 mL/kg/h (in absence of diabetes insipidus)	Full blood count Clotting screen and thromboelastography if available. Blood urea, creatinine and electrolytes Urine electrolytes and osmolality Liver function tests Repeated point of care measurements of blood glucose, arterial blood gases, serum lactate and mixed venous oximetry.	Correct diabetes insipidus and the associated hypernatraemia as indicated in Table 5.1. When low, administer parenteral electrolyte supplements to restore serum electrolyte concentrations to normal range. Continue/commence nutrition, and maintain blood glucose 4–8 mmol/L with intravenous insulin infusion Maintain haemoglobin at 9–10 g/dL. Treat derangements in coagulation with appropriate clotting factors and/or platelets if there is significant ongoing bleeding. Have clotting factors available for organ retrieval. If the potential donor is known to be CMV seronegative, only use screened blood products that are known to be CMV negative.

Invasive haemodynamic monitoring (e.g. pulmonary artery catheterisation) facilitates a more rational approach to the balancing of fluid, inotrope and vasopressor therapies, and improves the likelihood of successful heart and lung retrieval.

• Methylprednisolone and vasopressin are the cornerstones of hormonal resuscitation of the brainstem-dead donor. The former is targeted at the systemic inflammatory response associated with brainstem death, while the latter is a potent vasoconstrictor that also has useful antidiuretic actions. The role of thyroid hormone replacement is uncertain and should be reserved for refractory cases.

Conclusion

Donor optimisation is a labour-intensive task that is directed towards the reversal of a specific constellation of physiological derangements associated with brainstem death, and carries the clear objective to improve both the number and quality of organs that are made available for transplantation. Clinicians should be aware that the treatment period required to reverse organ dysfunction ranges from 12 to 24 hours, and that doing so more completely fulfils the wish of an individual to be an organ donor. Donor optimisation should therefore be seen as an integral component of the final acts of care for a deceased patient rather than an unwelcome intrusion on a family's grief. The outcome of donor optimisation interventions may be limited by a number of factors, including the nature of the condition leading to death, any complications of the treatments delivered during the patient's final illness and any pre-existing chronic co-morbidities that the patient may have had. Although retrieval teams should play no part in the diagnosis and confirmation of death, transplant coordinators have a crucial role to play in ensuring effective liaison between those caring for the potential donor in the intensive-care unit and those responsible for retrieval and transplantation.

Key references

1. Mollaret P, Goulon M. (1959) Le coma dépassé. *Revue Neurologique (Paris)* **101**, 3–15.
2. Akashi YJ, Nef HM, Mollmann, H, *et al.* (2010) Stress cardiomyopathy. *Ann Rev Med* **61**, 271–286.
3. NHS Blood and Transplant. (2011) *Annual UK Transplant Activity Report, 2009–2010*. Available online from: http://www.uktransplant.org.uk/ukt/ statistics/transplant_activity_report/transplant_activity_report.jsp.
4. Bederson J, Connolly EJ, Batjer H, *et al.* (2009) Guidelines for the management of aneurysmal subarachnoid hemorrhage: A statement for healthcare professionals from a special writing group of the Stroke Council, American Heart Association. *Stroke* **40**, 994–1025.
5. Cittanova, ML, Leblanc I, Legendre C, *et al.* (1996) Effect of hydroxyethyl starch in brain-dead kidney donors on renal function in kidney-transplant recipients. *Lancet* **348**, 1620–1622.
6. Dictus C, Vienenkoetter B, Esmaeilzadeh M, *et al.* (2009) Critical care management of potential organ donors: our current standard. *Clin Transplant* **23**, 2–9.
7. Kutsogiannis DJ, Pagliarello G, Doig C, *et al.* (2006) Medical management to optimize donor organ potential: review of the literature. *Can J Anaesth* **53**, 820–830.
8. NHS Institute for Innovation and Improvement. Map of Medicine clinical pathways: donor management. Available online from: http:// eng.mapofmedicine.com/evidence/map/index.html.
9. Mascia L, Pasero D, Slutsky AS, *et al.* (2010) Effect of a lung protective strategy for organ donors on eligibility and availability of lungs for transplantation: A randomized controlled trial. *J Am Med Assoc* **304**, 2620–2627.
10. McLean AD, Rosengard BR. (1999) Aggressive donor management. *Current Opin Organ Transplant* **4**, 130–136.
11. Novitsky D. (1997) Detrimental effects of brain death on the potential organ donor. *Transplant Proc* **29**, 3770–3772.
12. Novitzky D. (1998) Selection and management of cardiac allograft donors. *Current Opin Organ Transplant* **3**, 51–61.

13. Ramos HC, Lopez R. (2002) Critical care management of the brain-dead organ donor. *Current Opin Organ Transplant* **7**, 70–75.

14. Rosendale JD, Kaufmann HM, McBride MA, *et al.* (2003) Hormonal resuscitation yields more transplanted hearts with improved early function. *Transplantation* **75**, 1536–1541.

15. Salim A, Martin M, Brown C, *et al.* (2006) Complications of brain death: Frequency and impact on organ retrieval. *Am Surg* **72**, 377–381.

16. Schnuelle P, Gottmann U, Hoeger S, *et al.* (2009) Effects of donor pretreatment with dopamine on graft function after kidney transplantation. *J Am Med Assoc* **302**, 1067–1075.

17. Shemie SD, Ross H, Pagliarello J, *et al.* (2006) Organ donor management in Canada: Recommendations of the forum on Medical Management to Optimize Donor Organ Potential. *CMAJ* **174**, S13–S30.

18. Totsuka E, Dodson F, Urakami A, *et al.* (1999) Influence of high donor serum sodium levels on early postoperative graft function in human liver transplantation: Effect of correction of donor hyernatraemia. *Liver Transpl Surg* **5**, 421–428.

19. Venkateswaran RV, Patchell VB, Wilson IC, *et al.* (2008) Early donor management increases the retrieval rate of lungs for transplantation. *Ann Thorac Surg* **85**, 278–286.

20. Venkateswaran RV, Steeds RP, Quinn DW, *et al.* (2009) The haemodynamic effects of adjunctive hormone therapy in potential heart donors: A prospective randomized double-blind factorially designed controlled trial. *Eur Heart J* **30**, 1771–1780.

21. Venkateswaran RV, Townend JN, Wilson IC, *et al.* (2010) Echocardiography in the Potential Heart Donor. *Transplantation* **89**, 894–901.

22. Wheeldon DR, Potter CDO, Oduro A, *et al.* (1995) Transforming the "unacceptable" donor: Outcomes from the adoption of a standardized donor management technique. *J Heart Lung Transplant* **14**, 734–742.

6 Deceased donor retrieval

Albert M. Wolthuis, Diethard Monbaliu, Willy Coosemans and Jacques Pirenne

Organ retrieval

Although sometimes easily forgotten, every successful organ transplantation starts with the identification of a potential donor, followed by meticulous organ procurement. In the 1960s and 1970s, the first reports on kidney retrieval techniques were published [1–3]. A combination of abdominal and thoracic organ retrieval was first reported in the early 1980s [4,5]. A surgical technique for abdominal organ procurement (kidney, liver, pancreas and small bowel) was first described by Starzl and colleagues [6,7], and to date there is considerable variation in techniques [8–13].

The transplant coordinator plays a central role in the communication between the donor hospital and the organ procurement teams. Often, the multiorgan procurement – a logistically complex and demanding procedure – occurs in a non-academic hospital, which is infrequently involved in this process. Thorough guidance and explanation by both the transplant coordinator and the procurement surgeon(s) is of paramount importance to allow for a swift and uncomplicated procedure. If something unexpected happens, it is important that the teams adopt a courteous and considerate approach to maintain a professional demeanour. The procurement surgeon in charge is responsible for verification of the donor information (brain-death certification in case of heartbeating donor) and a rapid but thorough physical examination (abnormal bruises, melanoma, scars, etc). The donor is installed in supine position with the arms alongside the body and is shaved from chin to upper thigh. The skin is prepared from the neck to the suprapubic region with an antiseptic solution. Antibiotic prophylaxis is given, along with a neuromuscular blocking agent to prevent spinal reflexes.

Handbook of Renal and Pancreatic Transplantation, First Edition. Edited by Iain A. M. MacPhee and Jiří Froněk.
© 2012 John Wiley & Sons, Ltd. Published 2012 by John Wiley & Sons, Ltd.

Heartbeating donation

Multiorgan retrieval

A multiorgan procurement in a heartbeating donor can essentially be divided into four parts and should be done by an experienced procurement surgeon:

- preparing the donor organs for the cold flush by dissection and cannulation of the major thoracic and abdominal vessels
- *in situ* cold perfusion, which is the start of the cold ischaemia
- dissection and procurement of the organs according to urgency (heart, lungs, liver/pancreas and kidneys)
- preparing the organ for cold storage on the back-table.

Preparing the donor organs for the cold flush by dissection and cannulation of the major thoracic and abdominal vessels

Exposure through a standard sterno-laparotomy

A midline longitudinal incision is made from the suprasternal notch to the pubic symphysis. By this incision, exposure of all thoracic and abdominal organs together with optimal control of the great vessels can be achieved. A laparotomy is performed, and while protecting the liver with a large pack, the sternotomy can be done in the midline. A standard sternotomy is always recommended even in the case of procurement of abdominal organs only, for maximal exposure allowing a safe dissection of the upper abdomen, and to exclude any unknown thoracic malignancies. The pleurae are opened and both lungs are carefully inspected and palpated for emphysematous changes, infection, oedema and tumours.

Every procedure starts with the meticulous inspection of all thoracic and abdominal organs to identify anatomy (and anatomical variations) and to exclude any previously unknown concomitant pathology, such as neoplasm or infection. Unexpected lesions should be sent for immediate frozen section.

Preparations for *in situ* cooling

The essential preparations necessary for *in situ* cooling of the abdominal organs will be done first. The falciform ligament is divided. To facilitate access to the upper abdomen, the upper parts of the diaphragm are cut bilaterally. Care must be taken to keep both diaphragms as a barrier between abdomen and thorax to prevent overflowing of slushed ice saline and blood during the cooling process between the thorax and abdomen. Access to the distal aorta and inferior vena cava is then obtained by mobilising the caecum and the right colon upwards and medially. The retroperitoneum is incised at the base of the caecum and the right colon is released until the hepatic flexure, exposing the retroperitoneal structures, including aorta, vena cava, right ureter and kidney. This manoeuvre also includes the upright mobilisation of the distal part of the small bowel, followed and completed by an extended Kocher manoeuvre to free the duodenum and the head of the pancreas (Cattell Braasch manoeuvre). This mobilisation is stopped when the inferior vena cava is fully exposed just above the level of both renal veins and when the origin of the superior mesenteric artery is identified. At this point, the root of the superior mesenteric artery can be encircled with a vessel loop. This allows selective occlusion of this artery after 1 L of preservation fluid has been flushed to prevent overperfusion of the pancreas, and it may serve as a landmark for the dissection after the cold flush. The foramen of Winslow is easily accessible and the presence of an accessory right hepatic artery can be appreciated by palpation inferolateral to the common bile duct in the hepato-duodenal ligament.

Access to the infrarenal abdominal aorta and inferior vena cava

Further preparation for cannulation is subsequently achieved by preparing the distal abdominal aorta. First the inferior mesenteric artery is ligated and divided, followed by a dissection of the distal part of the aorta. Particular attention is given at this stage to identify any abnormal anatomy such as the presence of accessory infrarenal arteries arising from the aorta or the common iliac arteries, which should be identified and preserved accordingly. The distal part of the aorta is encircled just above the level of the iliac bifurcation and attention has to be paid during this manoeuvre to avoid accidental rupture of lumbar arteries. To prevent tearing off the lumbar arteries, they can be clipped and divided. At this time the abdominal aortic cannulation can be achieved safely. Cannulation in the aorta at this level should be avoided in case of abnormalities such as an aortic aneurysm, the possibility of an aortic tube graft or the presence of abnormal arterial anatomy, such as lower renal polar arteries, which originate from the iliac artery. In such cases, aortic cannulation can be replaced by iliac cannulation with ligation or clamping of the contralateral iliac artery. Also, the inferior vena cava is dissected free, isolated and encircled just above the level of both common iliac veins. In the case of retrieval of both thoracic and abdominal organs, venting of venous outflow via the inferior vena cava is preferred, but if only abdominal organs are to be retrieved, venous decompression can be obtained by incising the inferior vena cava in the pericardium at the beginning of the cold flush, thereby avoiding dissection and cannulation of the abdominal inferior vena cava. At this stage, the most important dissection in the lower abdomen is completed and the major vessels have been prepared for cannulation.

Access to the suprarenal abdominal aorta

Following the isolation of the distal aorta, proximal control of the aorta should be achieved, enabling a complete and closed perfusion circuit to cool and perfuse all abdominal organs. To reach the proximal aorta, the left triangular ligament of the liver is incised and the lesser omentum (omentum minus) is opened distal to the vagal branches of the liver. The upper part of the lesser omentum is palpated to detect the presence of an accessory left hepatic artery. The proximal abdominal aorta is reached through the muscular parts of the crura of the diaphragm and remains a challenging part of the procedure. Dissection through the right crux of the diaphragm often helps to facilitate access to the proximal abdominal aorta. It is important to start the dissection of the aorta in the correct avascular plane and to pay attention not to damage any aberrant branches from the left gastric artery that supply the left lobe of the liver, nor to damage any side branches supplying the diaphragm crura themselves. Of note, encircling the distal part of the oesophagus with a rubber traction sling and its left lateral mobilisation may facilitate dissection of this area. After the proximal abdominal aorta has been dissected free, a sling can be placed around it in order to allow its easy clamping, especially in the presence of multiple members of various organ procurement teams standing together around the same table.

Essential intra-abdominal dissection prior to cannulation of the aorta

The distal common bile duct is then isolated in the hepato-duodenal ligament and its anterior part incised to allow its extensive rinsing with normal saline at low pressure to evacuate the bile. Flushing of the bile duct is of paramount importance, because stagnating cold bile is toxic for the bile ducts and can cause biliary strictures. Flushing of the bile duct should be repeated at the back-table as well. A purse-string is placed on the gallbladder fundus. The bile is evacuated and the gallbladder is cleaned with normal saline. Although some centres routinely perform a cholecystectomy, it is avoided in our centre to leave the biliary anatomy untouched and to minimise bleeding from the gallbladder bed upon reperfusion. In case of doubt as to the grade of steatosis, a liver biopsy can be performed at the inferior border of the left liver lobe for immediate histological examination. A U-suture can then be placed for haemostasis. Generally, 'over'-manipulation of the liver and the abdominal organs should be avoided, as it activates Kupffer cells and increases the risk of damage to the organs and their blood supply. Consequently, extensive intra-abdominal dissection is avoided at our centre.

The greater omentum is divided at the inferior part of the stomach and the greater sac is opened. The gastro-pancreatic ligament is divided to expose the anterior surface of the pancreas. The greater curvature of the stomach is fully mobilised. Therefore, the short gastric vessels are clipped and cut, so that the stomach can be lifted up and the pancreas can be inspected. Care must be taken not to damage the left gastric artery and vein. The mesocolon transversum is partially incised and the vascular pedicle of the superior mesenteric vessels is evaluated at the inferior part of the head of the pancreas. The ligament at the angle of Treitz is cut and the inferior mesenteric vein is followed and dissected free up to the inferior border of the pancreas.

In situ cold perfusion; the start of the cold ischaemia

The most essential abdominal dissection is now completed and the major vessels are ready for cannulation and perfusion of the abdominal organs.

Hereafter, the cardiac and thoracic teams will prepare the thoracic organs for procurement by isolating the superior and inferior intrapericardial vena cava and placing a vascular purse string suture on both ascending aorta and pulmonary artery. Once all the other thoracic and abdominal organs have been prepared adequately, cold perfusion will take place following systemic administration of heparin to the donor (300–500 units/kg). The abdominal team will first ligate the distal abdominal aorta just above the iliac bifurcation. Alternatively, a vascular clamp can be placed to avoid damaging the aorta, so that it can be procured as a homograft. An 18 or 24 Fr gauge cannula is inserted into the distal abdominal aorta. In the case of pronounced atherosclerosis, care must be taken not to damage the back wall of the aorta, because a perforation or a dissection of the lumen could easily be made. Of note, a wide atraumatic umbilical tape-like ligature can be used for this purpose. Simultaneous venting of the venous outflow is made possible through insertion into the distal inferior vena cava of a 28/30 Fr gauge cannula. As mentioned above, cannulation of the inferior vena cava can be replaced by direct venting through the right atrium, when no thoracic organs are procured. Both cannulae are tightly fixed and secured. Needless to say, smaller sized cannulae will be used in the case of a paediatric donor. The bowel is replaced in its anatomical position and obstruction of the portal vein avoided, allowing recirculation of the preservation solution via the mesenteric vessels into the portal vein. Cannulation of the ascending aorta and pulmonary artery is now performed and the donor organs can be flushed. Facilitated by gentle traction on the sling placed earlier, the proximal abdominal aorta is cross-clamped with two vascular clamps, venous decompression is done and abdominal perfusion can be started. This is the start of cold ischaemia. Simultaneously, a vascular clamp can be placed on the thoracic inferior vena cava for cardiac inflow occlusion. In addition to aortic cooling with ice-cold preservation solution, some procurement teams perfuse the portal vein. In addition to the intravascular cold perfusion, topical cooling is essential, and abundant amounts of slushed ice saline should be poured into the abdominal cavity to complete the cooling process. The quality of perfusion of all organs is checked and topical cooling is continued for as long as needed.

Dissection and procurement of the organs according to urgency (heart, lungs, liver/pancreas and kidneys)

At the end of the cold flush (post-perfusion dissection), which normally takes about 15 minutes, procurement of the thoracic organs is performed first. Meanwhile topical cooling of the abdominal organs is assured. After the thoracic organs have been retrieved, procurement of the abdominal organs is started with an 'en-bloc' procurement of the liver and the pancreas. Our centre prefers en-bloc over *in situ* procurement because it avoids warming up of the organs after the cold flush and minimises 'over'-dissection in the abdominal cavity. The diaphragm is incised on the left side straight onto the oesophagus. The right diaphragm is incised until the right adrenal gland, taking care to avoid traction and tears to the liver capsule. The right gastric and gastroepiploic artery are clipped and divided, and the proximal duodenum is stapled immediately distal to the pylorus using a 55 mm GIA mechanical stapler. The left gastric artery and concomitant vein are ligated and cut close to the stomach. The completely detached stomach and distal oesophagus can be flipped over into the thorax to allow a better exposure. At the distal border of the pancreas the inferior mesenteric vein is clipped and cut. Close to the third part of the duodenum and the inferior border of the head of the pancreas, the superior mesenteric artery (or its branches) is (are) identified and ligated. The same is done for the superior mesenteric vein. Alternatively, some procurement surgeons prefer the placement of a GIA stapler across the whole mesenteric root (radix mesenterii). The third and fourth part of the duodenum are now dissected free and a GIA stapler can be placed distal to the angle of Treitz. A povidone iodine in water solution is injected into the isolated duodenum through separate punction. Alternatively, povidone iodine in water solution can be injected in the duodenum through the nasogastric tube prior to division of the stomach and after having placed this tube distal to the pylorus. The spleen is mobilised and used as a handle to lift up the pancreatic tail and to dissect and divide the splenocolic ligament and the left gastroepiploic artery. The dorsal side of the pancreas can be liberated with electrocautery in an avascular plane between the upper pole of the left kidney and the left adrenal gland. The dissection of the vascular pedicle for the 'en-bloc' procurement of the liver and pancreas is started at the aorta at the level of the origin of the superior mesenteric artery (previously dissected free and encircled during the preparation phase), just above the left renal vein. Care must be taken not to damage the left and right renal arteries, which must be clearly visualised before aortic transsection and creation of a superior mesenteric artery-patch. First, the aorta is incised obliquely in cephalic direction, immediately under the origin of the superior mesenteric artery (Fig. 6.1). After the aorta has been incised halfway, the scissors are turned obliquely upwards to the

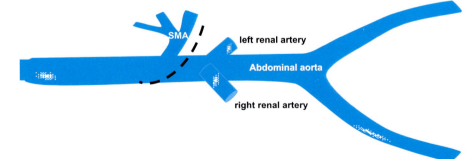

Figure 6.1 The abdominal aorta is transsected between the origin of the superior mesenteric artery (SMA) and the renal arteries. This is done in an oblique way (dotted line) to achieve a maximal and correct Carrel patch for both renal arteries (left and right renal artery, LRA and RRA), without compromising the aortic patch around the SMA.

aortic wall and transsection is completed. The inferior vena cava distal to the liver is dissected and the left and right renal veins are clearly identified. The inferior vena cava is isolated by blunt dissection and divided, just above the renal veins. With the division of the paravertrebral muscles and transsection of the right adrenal gland, the right side of the bloc is already detached. When the right adrenal gland is transsected, care must be taken not to damage either the upper pole of the right kidney or the liver. The left side of the aorta is now exposed by cutting through the paravertebral muscles and the left adrenal gland, so that the sling previously placed around the proximal aorta can be found and the descending thoracic aorta can be divided. The release of the liver–pancreas block can be completed by dissection of the loose prevertebral connective tissues.

Thereafter, both kidneys can be retrieved, and so we refer to the section on 'Kidney-only retrieval'.

Preparing the organ for cold-storage on the back-table

The liver–pancreas block (organ quality, anatomy, possible lesions, complete cold-flush . . .) is re-evaluated at the back-table while immersed in preservation solution. First, the spleen is removed by ligation of the splenic artery and vein. Care must be taken not to damage the tail of the pancreas. Alternatively splenectomy can be done at the pancreas recipient center. The division of the liver and pancreas is started in the hepatoduodenal ligament with the dissection of the common hepatic artery. The next step is the division of the gastroduodenal artery proximal to the superior border of the pancreatic head, paying attention to leave a short stump on the common hepatic artery (for possible later vascular reconstructions if needed and for arterial venting in the recipient). The origin of the splenic artery is dissected and divided exactly in the middle between its origin from the coeliac trunk and the first branches to the pancreas. A 5/0 Prolene™ stitch is used as a marker, because the splenic artery tends to retract and may become difficult to identify. The portal vein is transsected superior to the confluences of the splenic and superior mesenteric veins. Attention should be given not to accidently transsect an accessory right hepatic artery arising from the superior mesenteric artery and present dorsolateral to the portal vein. Priority is usually given to the liver and the superior mesenteric artery patch remains with the liver, although a reconstruction onto the gastroduodenal artery is also feasible whenever needed and the vessels have an appropriate size. The common bile duct is clipped just above the head of the pancreas and the second part of the duodenum. It is rinsed again with normal saline at low pressure to clean it from toxic cold bile. The separation of the liver and the pancreas ends with the preparation of an aortic patch from the celiac trunk and superior mesenteric artery for the liver and pancreas, respectively. After separation, the portal vein is perfused with 1 L of preservation solution. Anatomy is reviewed and the organs are packed. As mentioned, some centres separate the liver from the pancreas *in situ* before and after the start of cold perfusion. Anatomical landmarks are identical.

> ## Box 6.1 Tips for successful multiorgan procurement.
> **Twelve tips to remember for a successful multiorgan procurement**
>
> 1. Expect the unexpected.
> 2. Prepare cannulation first.
> 3. Identify (abnormal) anatomy.
> 4. Respect vascularisation.
> 5. Rinse gallbladder and common bile duct.
> 6. Cold ischaemia = intravascular and topical cooling.
> 7. En-bloc procurement (liver–pancreas and both kidneys).
> 8. Avoid traction; apply no-touch dissection.
> 9. Take your time.
> 10. Communicate with the local and remote procurement/recipient team.
> 11. Respect the donor and the donor family.
> 12. Fill in the organ report form.

The distal aorta and arterial iliac bifurcation are procured, serving as vascular toolkit for the recipient surgeons. One iliac axis (common, internal and external iliac artery) is given to the liver team and the contralateral one to the pancreas team, in order to provide vascular grafts in case vascular reconstruction is necessary in the recipients. The same is done for the venous iliacal bifurcation. A portion of spleen or mesenteric lymph nodes can be excised for tissue typing and crossmatching. At the end of the multiorgan retrieval, care must be taken to remove remaining preservation fluids and blood from the thoracic and abdominal cavity by suction. Meticulous closure of the body with a continuous suture is essential to prevent leakage and for aesthetic reasons. This closure should be done with maximal respect for the donor and his donor family. After the procedure, it is important to fill in a clear organ report form. In case of doubt, it is advisable to contact the recipient centre or transplant surgeon by phone (Box 6.1).

Kidney-only retrieval

Kidney retrieval en bloc
The retrieval of the kidneys most often takes place as the integral part of a multiorgan donor procedure and usually at the end of the procedure. Therefore, all preparatory steps described above for adequate intravascular and topical cooling are identical. Several techniques for removal of the kidneys have been described. In many institutions, including ours, the preferred technique is the so-called 'en-bloc' retrieval technique, in which both kidneys are procured en bloc and separated on the back-table. This is done following the division of the abdominal aorta, just distal to the origin of the superior mesenteric artery and just proximal to the left renal vein, which normally crosses the abdominal aorta anteriorly. This step should be done very carefully, to achieve the

maximal size of a correct aortic Carrel patch for both renal arteries. In our experience, this can be easily achieved by an oblique incision of the aorta from the origin of the superior mesenteric artery following a cranial and backwards direction (Fig. 6.1). After the division of the abdominal aorta, the inferior vena cava is also divided just proximal to the renal veins. Before the kidneys can be removed en bloc, the sigmoid colon is lifted up, the Toldt's fascia is incised and the left mesocolon is transsected to expose the retroperitoneum. At the lateral side, the ureters, together with as much peri-ureteral tissue as possible, are identified, encircled and dissected free as low as possible. Both ureters are transsected at the ureterovesical junction to supply sufficient length. After division they are clearly marked with small mosquito clamps, and under gentle retraction anteriorly kept out of the surgical planes. By gentle traction the left kidney is retracted medially and the peri-renal fat is incised and the left kidney completely mobilised. The right kidney is mobilised and freed in the same manner as the left kidney. Both the inferior vena cava and the aorta cannulae are then used for a safe en-bloc removal of both kidneys, and used as a handle to complete the posterior and lateral dissection by dividing the residual attachments between the left colon and the spine by dissection in the prevertebral space. The procurement is completed and both kidneys are extracted en bloc.

Back-table preparation

At the back-table, anatomy is reviewed and separation of the kidneys then proceeds in a standard manner. The division of the kidneys in our institution takes place as follows starting from an anatomical position. First, the left renal vein is dissected free with a rim of inferior vena cava, to allow for sufficient length (Fig. 6.2). The kidneys are then turned upside down, so that the posterior surface of the aorta is laying anteriorly. The exact middle at the posterior surface of the aorta can be identified safely and easily by the presence of the lumbar arteries and is opened by cutting between the stumps of the lumbar vessels in a caudal to cranial direction (Fig. 6.2). This allows a clear view of the exact vascular anatomy of the renal arteries and an easy and correct division of the aorta on the anterior surface can then be achieved. At this point, the kidneys are gently flushed again to ensure that all blood has been removed. By opening the Gerota's fascia, the peri-renal fat can be removed but remaining at distance from the hilum, which is left untouched. The whole surface of the kidneys is inspected, and this procedure should be done with care to avoid any traumatic decapsulation of the kidney and to identify any abnormality at the kidney surface (cyst, tumour, etc.; Fig. 6.3). As for all donor organs, the kidneys are then placed in individual plastic bags; the inner bag contains a sufficient amount of cold preservation fluid, the middle contains sufficient slushed ice and water, and the outer bag is dry. Eventually, the packed organ is marked 'left kidney' or 'right kidney' and is placed in a transport container completely surrounded by ice. Machine perfusion is an

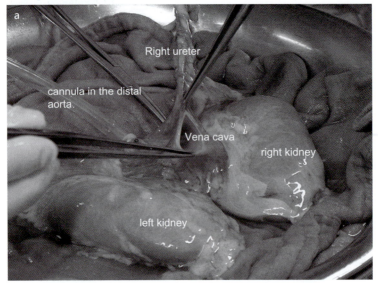

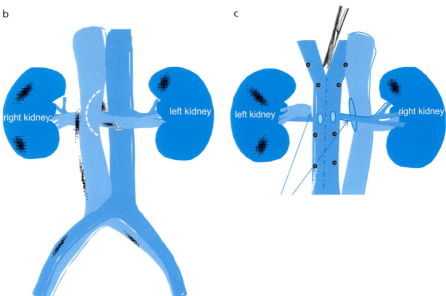

Figure 6.2 (a) Splitting of the en-bloc procured kidneys at the back table. Following en-bloc retrieval, the kidneys are first placed in a bowl in iced water in an anatomical position, and then both the ureters, the vena cava and the renal veins, as well as the aorta and the renal arteries, are identified. (b) After identification of all the renal vessels and structures, the left renal vein is first dissected free and divided (see dotted line) at the level of the vena cava, which remains with the right kidney (anterior view). (c) Following transection of the left renal vein from the vena cava (arrows), the kidney bloc is then turned upside down, so that the posterior surface of the aorta is laying anteriorly. The exact middle at the posterior surface of the aorta can be identified safely and easily by the presence of the lumbar arteries and is opened by cutting between the stumps of the lumbar vessels in a caudal to cranial direction. This allows a clear view of the exact vascular anatomy of the renal arteries and an easy and correct division of the aorta on the anterior surface can then be achieved (posterior view). (A full colour version of this figure appears in the colour plate section.)

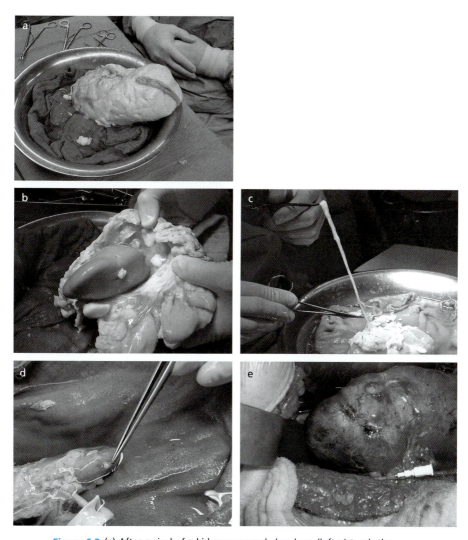

Figure 6.3 (a) After arrival of a kidney procured elsewhere (left picture), the redundant peri-renal fat is removed at the lower, middle and upper pole (but not around the pyelum, or pelvis) and between the lower pole and the upper ureter, revealing some unexpected and unreported lesions. Minimal defatting of the kidney immediately following the procurement will not only allow a better topical cooling but will also prevent unexpected findings to occur at the moment of unpacking the kidney at the recipient's centre; attention should be given not to devascularise the pyelum of the kidney. (b) During the removal of the fat, care must be taken not to cause any decapsulation that may render the renal graft no longer transplantable or compromise the transplantation. (c) One pitfall in the procurement of the ureter is to leave as much peri-ureteral tissue with the graft and not to dissect upon and to devascularise the ureter itself, resulting in the so-called 'spaghetti' ureter. (d) Image of a transected upper pole artery, which was responsible for a large zone of poorly vascularised renal parenchyma – this may be of particular importance for the lower pole, where the blood supply of the proximal ureter might be compromised. (e) A vascular reconstruction was done using the inferior epigastric artery. (A full colour version of this figure appears in the colour plate section.)

increasingly used method of preservation. In this case, the renal artery is connected to the perfusion system.

Non-heartbeating donation

Introduction

The terms 'non-heartbeating donation' (NHBD) or 'donation after circulatory death' (DCD) are generally used to define organ donation in a donor who succumbed to an irreversible absence of circulation and to differentiate this form of donation from the classical heartbeating donation. The main difference is the criteria used to diagnose death: in NHBD, conventional criteria of circulatory death are applied, whereas brainstem death criteria are used in heartbeating donors. Another distinction is that organs from NHBD are invariably exposed to a period of warm ischemia, which is deleterious for organ function and outcome. The first human kidney transplant by Voronoy involved a kidney procured in a NHBD [14]. Until 1968, all human kidneys were procured after cardiac arrest of the donor, because the concept of brain death was introduced later [15]. Of interest, before 1968, the first heartbeating organ procurement was performed by two Belgian surgeons, Professor Morelle and Professor Alexandre, who retrieved a kidney for transplantation [16]. The rationale for using NHBDs is that they represent a large pool of donors that could help to overcome the shortage of transplantable organs. The first international workshop on NHBD was organised in 1995 in Maastricht, The Netherlands. Since then, NHBDs have been classified into four categories, and a distinction is made between 'uncontrolled' and 'controlled' donors (Table 6.1) [17]. In controlled donors (category 3 of the Maastricht classification), a decision has been taken to withdraw support in a patient who is not brain dead, but where further treatment is felt to be futile with no realistic expectation of recovery. Of note, this decision is taken by the treating physician independently of the possibility of organ procurement. In these cases, cardiac arrest after withdrawal of therapy is awaited by the organ procurement team. Ischaemic times are kept short and lungs, liver,

Table 6.1 The classification of NHBDs as described during the First International Workshop on NHBD, Maastricht [17].

Category	Status of potential donor	Hospital department
Category I, uncontrolled	Dead upon arrival	Accident and emergency
Category II, uncontrolled	Resuscitation without success	Accident and emergency
Category III, controlled	Awaiting cardiac arrest	Intensive care
Category IV, controlled	Cardiac arrest while brain dead	Intensive care

pancreas and kidneys may be procured. Uncontrolled donors are declared dead after an accident or suicide outside the hospital (category 1) or suffer from a (witnessed) cardiac arrest (category 2) due to a major cardiac or cerebral event. In both categories, resuscitation will be commenced, but warm ischaemia times are usually longer or are not always known with certainty, compared with category 3 donors. Another issue in NHBD organ donation is the waiting time between cardiac arrest and the start of organ procurement. To make sure that cardiac arrest is irreversible, a 'no-touch' period is respected before procurement actually starts. The general consensus is to wait not less than 2 minutes and not more than 10 minutes between cardiac arrest and the start of the procurement [18]. A 'no-touch' period of 5 minutes is used in many centres.

The surgical procedure for NHBD organ procurement should be rapid. In NHBD organ retrieval, the procedure should be focused on the minimalisation of warm ischaemia, and early and effective establishment of *in situ* cold perfusion with abundant topical cooling and rapid venting of venous outflow.

Organ preservation and procurement in Maastricht category 1 and 2 NHBD

For uncontrolled donors (Maastricht categories 1 and 2), a double-balloon triple-lumen (DBTL) catheter is usually used for *in situ* preservation of kidneys, before the actual procurement takes place. This catheter can be introduced through the femoral artery into the aorta at the bedside, in the accident and emergency unit, in the intensive-care unit or in the operating room [19,20]. Additionally, peritoneal cooling can be done via catheters inserted into the peritoneal cavity [21]. Another option to provide normal tissue perfusion with oxygenated blood at body temperature is the use of extracorporeal membrane oxygenation (ECMO). Both femoral artery and vein should be cannulated either percutaneously or via cut down. In the opposite femoral artery, an aortic occlusion balloon may be advanced into the thoracic aorta under radiological guidance for selective perfusion of abdominal organs. This so-called ECMO-assisted NHBD technique was first developed and pioneered in Spain and is now also used in France and other countries, mostly in uncontrolled NHBD [22–24]. After adequate flushing and kidney preservation via the DBTL catheter or after a period of ECMO, standard and rapid procurement of the kidneys takes place in the operating theatre.

Organ preservation and procurement in Maastricht category 3 NHBD

In Maastricht category 3, if the family has agreed, the donor is transported to the operating theatre and will already be installed and draped. The ventilator switch-off (withdrawal of life support) will take place according to the local protocol. An experienced procurement surgeon who is familiar with rapid cannulation should perform the

NHBD procurement, which can be modified according to the technique described by the Pittsburgh group [25,26]. After cardiac death has been certified and after a 'no-touch' period has been respected, the procedure begins with a super-rapid midline sternotomy and laparotomy using a knife and a sternal saw. A rapid isolation and cannulation of the distal aorta is performed and can usually be achieved within 3 minutes. The aorta can be identified just above the iliac bifurcation on the left side of the vertebral column. The distal part of the aorta can be prepared for cannulation and the inferior mesenteric artery does not need to be tied off. The aorta is encircled once and an aortotomy is made to insert a cannula, which is fixed. A vascular clamp can be placed distally, to prevent backbleeding. Before perfusion starts, the inferior vena cava has to be drained, in order to prevent the ongoing congestion of the abdominal organs secondary to cardiac arrest. We recommend rapid drainage of the inferior vena cava at the level of the right atrium. It is also possible to cannulate and drain the infrarenal vena cava, but this usually takes longer than a sternotomy. Immediately thereafter, the descending aorta has to be cross-clamped just above the diaphragm, to allow for optimal and selective splanchnic perfusion. We recommend cross-clamping of the descending thoracic aorta instead of the supraceliac aorta, because it can easily be palpated just above the diaphragm in the left hemi-thorax and its access is less time-consuming. Topical cooling of the peritoneal cavity with saline ice slush is of paramount importance. In contrast to the earlier-described conventional procurement in DBD, the authors prefer a dual perfusion for a more rapid cooling of the organs. Dual perfusion can be obtained by identification and cannulation of the superior or inferior mesenteric vein, so that the liver is perfused via the hepatic artery and the portal vein. Due to the potential and increased risk for ischaemic bile duct injury and post-transplant intrahepatic biliary strictures in NHBD, it is very important to remove toxic bile during procurement. The gallbladder should be opened and the distal common bile duct should be identified and divided. Bile can be removed by extensive flushing of both gallbladder and common bile duct with saline at low pressure. After the flush, the actual organ procurement can start with particular attention to (arterial) anatomy. Vascular injuries to the graft can be made easily, as there is no blood flow. Because there is no pulsation, it might be more difficult to identify aberrant anatomy, such as left or right accessory hepatic arteries. For this reason, the authors prefer to procure pancreas and liver en bloc, without dissection in the hepatoduodenal ligament (Figs 6.4 and 6.5). The procedure continues with a Cattel-Braasch manoeuvre and release of hepatic ligaments. The greater and lesser sacs are opened and care must be taken not to damage an accessory left hepatic artery. The inferior vena cava is divided just above the origin of the left renal vein. The aorta is transsected between the origin of the superior mesenteric artery and the renal arteries to provide a sufficient patch if a right hepatic artery originates from the superior mesenteric artery. The suprahepatic inferior vena cava is divided intrapericardally, and the dissection ends by detaching the diaphragm. The left diaphragm is divided down towards the aorta and the right

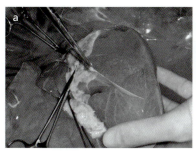
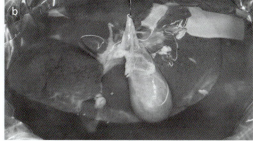

Figure 6.4 (a) All organs should always be handled with care. Here, an extensive capsular tear of the liver is shown. Although no longer considered a contraindiciaton, this may reflect the lack of gentle manipulation of the graft and its supplying blood vessels. (b) Example of an unflushed hepatic duct during procurement of the liver. Here, the common bile duct (CBD) was tied of instead of the cystic duct (CD). 'Over'-dissection of the hilum and surgery in the hepatoduodenal ligament should be avoided, apart from identification of the correct anatomy, adequate transection of the blood vessels between the pancreas and the liver, and redundant rinse of the common bile duct and the gallbladder. (A full colour version of this figure appears in the colour plate section.)

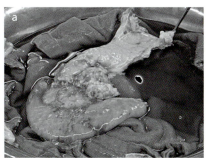
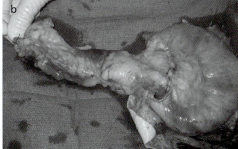

Figure 6.5 Representative image of a well-procured pancreas (a) and a pancreas that was discarded because of a large hematoma and capsular tear (b). (A full colour version of this figure appears in the colour plate section.)

diaphragm is divided down to the upper pole of the right kidney. The liver–pancreas block can be extracted and separated at the back-table as described earlier in this chapter in the multiorgan retrieval section. Subsequently, the kidneys are retrieved en bloc as described above. Both kidneys are divided on the back-table and in our centre routinely placed on machine perfusion, given the better preservation provided by machine perfusion versus cold storage, particularly in this type of kidney donor [27,28]. In some centres, cold flush in category 3 NHBD is obtained via the DBTL catheter (as described above for categories 1 and 2) and this is then followed by a standard procurement in the operating theatre. This strategy is used when therapy is withdrawn in the intensive-care unit. The aforementioned ECMO-assisted NHBD technique has also been used in controlled NHBD, prior to transportation to the theatre and organ procurement.

Acknowledgements

The authors thank Lydia Coolen for editorial assistance and Professor Benoit Barrou and Nicolas Terrier for the inspiration of the picture design (Figs 6.1 and 6.2).

References

1. Ackermann JR, Snell ME. (1968) Cadaveric renal transplantation: A technique for donor kidney removal. *Br J Urol* **40**, 515–521.
2. Alexandre GP. (1973) Organ procurement. *Proc Eur Dial Transplant Assoc* **10**, 31–56.
3. Veith FJ, Crane R, Hagstrom JW, *et al.* (1976) Preservation, transportation, and transplantation of the lung without functional impairment. *Trans Am Soc Artif Intern Organs* **22**, 216–222.
4. Shaw BW Jr, Rosenthal JT, Griffith BF, *et al.* (1983) Techniques for combined procurement of hearts and kidneys with satisfactory early function of renal allografts. *Surg Gynecol Obstet* **157**, 261–264.
5. Rosenthal JT, Shaw BW Jr, Hardesty RL, *et al.* (1983) Principles of multiple organ procurement from cadaver donors. *Ann Surg* **198**, 617–621.
6. Starzl TE, Hakala TR, Shaw BW Jr, *et al.* (1984) A flexible procedure for multiple cadaveric organ procurement. *Surg Gynecol Obstet* **158**, 223–230.
7. Starzl TE, Miller C, Broznick B, *et al.* (1987) An improved technique for multiple organ harvesting. *Surg Gynecol Obstet* **165**, 343–348.
8. Wright FH, Smith JL, Bowers VD, *et al.* (1989) Combined retrieval of liver and pancreas grafts: Alternatives for organ procurement. *Transplant Proc* **21**, 3522.
9. Margreiter R, Königsrainer A, Schmid T, *et al.* (1991) Multiple organ procurement–a simple and safe procedure. *Transplant Proc* **23**, 2307–2308.
10. Starzl TE, Shapiro R, Simmons RL. (1992) *Atlas of Organ Transplantation*. Gower Medical Publishing, New York.
11. Brockmann JG, Vaidya A, Reddy S, *et al.* (2006) Retrieval of abdominal organs for transplantation. *Br J Surg* **93**, 133–146.
12. Humar A, Matas A, Payne W. (2009) *Atlas of Organ Transplantation*. Springer-Verlag, London.
13. Baranski A. (2009) *Surgical Technique of Abdominal Organ Procurement. Step by Step*. Springer-Verlag, London.
14. Voronoy YY. (1936) Sobre el bloqueo del aparato reticulo-endothelial del hombre en algunas formas de intoxicacion por el sublimado y sobre la transplacacion del rinon cadaverico como metodo de tratamiento de la anuria consecutive a aquella intoxicacion. *El Siglo Med* **97**, 296.
15. Beecher H. (1968) A definition of irreversible coma. Report of the Ad Hoc Committee of the Harvard Medical School to examine the definition of brain death. *JAMA* **205**, 337–340.
16. Squifflet JP. (2003) The history of transplantation at the Catholic University of Louvain Belgium 1963–2003. *Acta Chir Belg* **103**(3 Spec No), 10–20.
17. Kootstra G, Daemen JH, Oomen AP. (1995) Categories of non-heart-beating donors. *Transplant Proc* **27**, 2893–2894.
18. Herdman R, Beauchamp TL, Potts JT. (1998) The Institute of Medicine's report on non-heart-beating organ transplantation. *Kennedy Inst Ethics J* **8**, 83–90.

19. Garcia-Rinaldi R, Lefrak EA, Defore WW, *et al.* (1975) In situ preservation of cadaver kidneys for transplantation: laboratory observations and clinical application. *Ann Surg* **182**, 576–584.
20. Kootstra G, van Heurn E. (2007) Non-heartbeating donation of kidneys for transplantation. *Nat Clin Pract Nephrol* **3**, 154–163.
21. Anaise D, Smith R, Ishimaru M, *et al.* (1990) An approach to organ salvage from non-heartbeating cadaver donors under existing legal and ethical requirements for transplantation. *Transplantation* **49**, 290–294.
22. Otero A, Gómez-Gutiérrez M, Suárez F, *et al.* (2003) Liver transplantation from Maastricht category 2 non-heart-beating donors. *Transplantation* **76**, 1068–1073.
23. Nuñez JR, Del Rio F, Lopez E, *et al.* (2005) Non-heart-beating donors: An excellent choice to increase the donor pool. *Transplant Proc* **37**, 3651–3654.
24. Fondevila C, Hessheimer AJ, Ruiz A, *et al.* (2007) Liver transplant using donors after unexpected cardiac death: Novel preservation protocol and acceptance criteria. *Am J Transplant* **7**, 1849–1855.
25. Heineman E, Daemen JH, Kootstra G. (1995) Non-heart-beating donors: Methods and techniques. *Transplant Proc* **27**, 2895–2896; Discussion 2896–2897.
26. Olson L, Davi R, Barnhart J, *et al.* (1999) Non-heart-beating cadaver donor hepatectomy 'the operative procedure'. *Clin Transplant* **13**, 98–103.
27. Moers C, Smits JM, Maathuis MH, *et al.* (2009) Machine perfusion or cold storage in deceased-donor kidney transplantation. *N Engl J Med* **360**, 7–19.
28. I Jochmans, C Moers, JM Smits, *et al.* (2010) Machine perfusion versus cold storage for the preservation of kidneys donated after cardiac death: A multicenter randomized controlled trial. *Ann Surg* **252**, 756–764.

7 Live donor nephrectomy

Jiří Froněk and Nicos Kessaris

Kidney transplantation is the ideal method of treatment for renal failure patients. Live donor kidney transplantation is one of the ways of having a kidney transplant. The first successful kidney transplant was performed from a live donor in 1954. After the legal acceptance of brainstem death, deceased donor renal transplantation became the most common method. Until the late 1990s, the number of deceased donor transplants was increasing in most countries around the world. By the end of the 20th century it became clearer that deceased donor transplantation (deceased donor and non-heart beating) could not serve the population on the waiting list. Because of the increasing gap between the number of kidneys available for transplant every year and number of patients in need of kidney transplants, other possible sources were explored: namely, donation after circulatory death kidney transplantation, live donor kidney transplantation and, more recently, HLA- and ABO-incompatible kidney transplantation, as well as paired donation. Such changes and the speed of progress in different kidney transplant programmes varied and still vary between countries, for religious, ethical and legal reasons.

Establishing or expanding a living donor transplant programme is one of the possible solutions for the growing lack of deceased donor grafts as well as for reducing the length of time on the waiting list. Moreover, such a programme is the preferred method of transplantation because it brings the best possible long-term outcomes for patients with end-stage kidney failure.

Live donor nephrectomy is a major surgical procedure, which is being performed in special circumstances. If we follow the basic classification of surgical procedures of amputation and reconstruction, live donor nephrectomy could be compared with amputation. Unlike standard amputation procedures, though, live donor nephrectomy together with other live donor procedures is unique because the excised organ must be in excellent condition once removed so that it is successfully transplanted to the recipient. In addition, live donation surgery is more challenging because there is no direct medical benefit to the donor. The live donor is a healthy person with no need for any surgery except the wish to help somebody else. The surgeon must therefore perform a major surgical procedure on a healthy person, which is followed by a smooth and quick recovery and ideally no complications. All these put enormous pressure on the performing surgeon.

Handbook of Renal and Pancreatic Transplantation, First Edition. Edited by Iain A. M. MacPhee and Jiří Froněk.
© 2012 John Wiley & Sons, Ltd. Published 2012 by John Wiley & Sons, Ltd.

A number of different nephrectomy techniques have been described and used for live donation. In principle, either open or endoscopic approaches can be used. Both can be performed either transperitoneally or extraperitoneally, and can be purely endoscopic or hand-assisted. Combinations of these give the full spectrum of surgical techniques.

The aim of this chapter is to explain and compare all the surgical techniques that may be used for live donor nephrectomy. **Colour versions of all figures used in this chapter appear on the website that accompanies this book, at www.wiley.com/go/macphee/transplantation.**

Pre-operative preparation

Living donor kidney transplantation, as well as live donor nephrectomy, are elective –and therefore planned – procedures. The potential donor and recipient are admitted to the hospital, usually on the day before surgery. It is important to place both donor and recipient on a ward where all staff are well trained and experienced in transplantation. The beds for the potential donor and recipient must be booked well in advance. It is unacceptable to cancel such surgery or place potential donors or recipients on an inexperienced ward because of bed shortage.

The first part of the pre-operative preparation includes the general principles that are applicable early on to any surgical procedure. Information must be given to the potential live donor to help him/her understand all the parts of the surgical process of donation and be willing to proceed. Without donor participation, the procedure cannot be successful. The psychological preparation starts at the time of first meeting with the clinical team. The donor must be fully informed and engaged in the process. Trust must be established to help the donor and allow active participation.

The second part of the preparation is specific for the procedure of live donor nephrectomy. The potential donor must be fully aware of the pre-operative work-up results and all possible risks after donation, including short- and long-term ones. In addition, the various nephrectomy techniques must be described to the potential donor. The technique that is going to be used in his/her case must be explained in great detail, including the conversion rate related to the endoscopic techniques and all possible complications and risks. One could discuss the worldwide experience as well as the national and local results. This discussion should include not only aspects related to donation, but transplantation as well.

The third part of the pre-operative preparation is the preparation of the operative field. Live donor nephrectomy is described as a clean procedure. The overall risk of infection is relatively small. Taking adequate intraoperative and postoperative measures, this risk can be further minimised. The day before surgery, the side of the nephrectomy is marked on the donor's abdomen. A permanent skin marker, which does not irritate skin, must be used for this. On the day of surgery this must be checked before the potential donor is moved from the ward to the

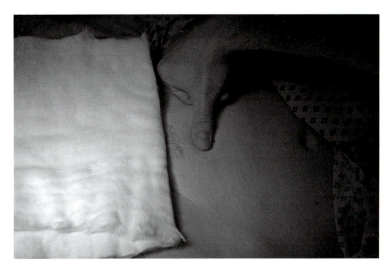

Figure 7.1 Hand assisted retroperitoneoscopic live donor nephrectomy – suprapubic incision is placed about one inch above symphisis pubis. Copyright © Jiří Froněk. All rights reserved.

operating theatre. Sometimes, after a shower, the mark may not be clearly visible and it may have to be remarked. The surgeon performing the nephrectomy is responsible for the correct marking. The anaesthetist should never start a case that is not clearly marked.

Once the donor is under general anaesthetic, a urinary catheter is inserted and the incision is marked after shaving. Shaving must be done carefully without any damage to the skin, otherwise the risk of infection may increase. Marking is important to perform before positioning to the lateral side, as that makes the abdominal wall move. Finally, the donor is positioned onto his/her side before the operative field is prepared (Figs 7.1–7.6). Positioning is essential for adequate access during the procedure and for preventing any harm to the donor. The operative field is cleaned using non-inflammable antiseptic, surrounded by drapes before covering with an adhesive sterile drape (e.g. 3MTM Steri-Drape; Fig 7.7).

Insertion of a central venous line and/or arterial line is generally not recommended. It is up to the individual centre to decide whether it includes such insertions of catheters in its protocol. Such decisions must be audited annually and of course justified.

Live donor nephrectomy techniques

- open live donor nephrectomy
  - lumbotomy (flank incision)
  - anterior subcostal extraperitoneal approach
  - open transperitoneal approach
  - mini-open or 'finger-assisted' approach
- endoscopic live donor nephrectomy
  - laparoscopic transperitoneal approach
  - hand-assisted laparoscopic transperitoneal approach

  ○ hand-assisted laparoscopic extraperitoneal (retroperitoneoscopic) approach
  ○ robotic hand-assisted laparoscopic donor nephrectomy
  ○ NOTES live donor nephrectomy.
• combined live donor nephrectomy techniques

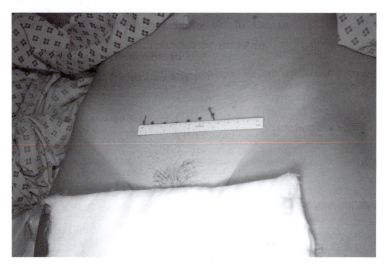

Figure 7.2 Hand assisted retroperitoneoscopic live donor nephrectomy – skin incision must be marked and measured before the patient is positioned to the lateral side. Copyright © Jiří Froněk. All rights reserved.

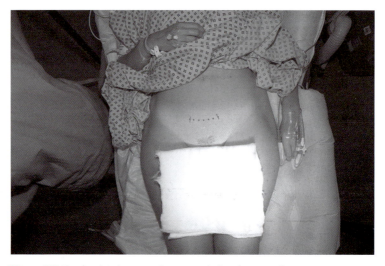

Figure 7.3 Hand assisted retroperitoneoscopic live donor nephrectomy – suprapubic incision must be correctly placed and curved. Copyright © Jiří Froněk. All rights reserved.

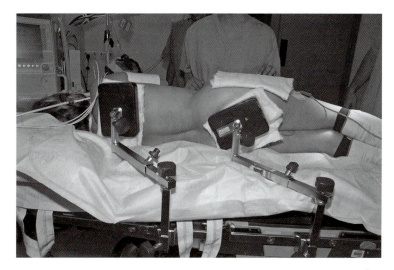

Figure 7.4 Hand assisted retroperitoneoscopic live donor nephrectomy – donor's position on the table – view from the back. Copyright © Jiří Froněk. All rights reserved.

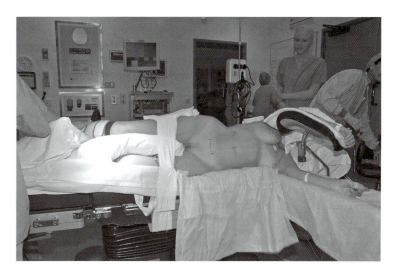

Figure 7.5 Hand assisted retroperitoneoscopic live donor nephrectomy – donor's position on the table – view from the front. Copyright © Jiří Froněk. All rights reserved.

Open live donor nephrectomy techniques

Open surgical techniques for live donor nephrectomy are generally safe, offering very good exposure to the kidney. Bleeding can be controlled by hand or vascular clamps. However, the incision is usually large and mostly muscle-cutting, requiring more pain relief. Recovery time is also

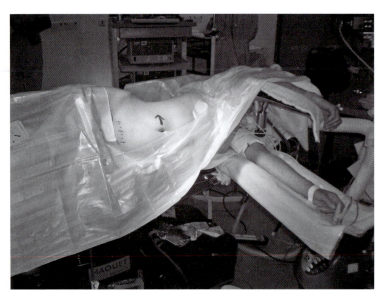

Figure 7.6 Hand assisted retroperitoneoscopic live donor nephrectomy – donor is covered with warming mat. Copyright © Jiří Froněk. All rights reserved.

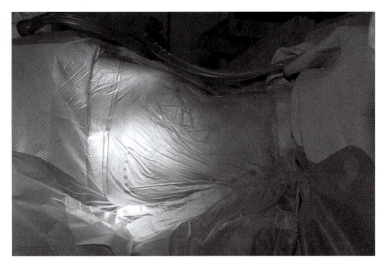

Figure 7.7 Hand assisted retroperitoneoscopic live donor nephrectomy – skin is covered with steri-drape. Copyright © Jiří Froněk. All rights reserved.

usually longer compared with the endoscopic techniques. Many centres still use open techniques as the method of choice in all cases and some only for right nephrectomy cases. In general, open techniques usually result in more pain, a higher rate of complications, longer recovery and worse cosmetic effect.

Advantages of open techniques
- very good exposure to the kidney (except mini-open 'finger-assisted')
- possible bleeding can be controlled by hand and vascular clamps.

Disadvantages of open techniques
- large incision (except mini-open 'finger-assisted')
- muscle-cutting approach with related possible complications include chronic pain and 'bulging' caused by denervation of the muscle
- more postoperative pain requiring more analgesia
- longer hospital stay
- higher morbidity rate

Lumbotomy approach (flank incision)

The traditional open 'flank incision' (also called 'loin incision') nephrectomy technique (Fig. 7.28) is derived from experience from the urology field. This has been modified for the purpose of live donation. This involves dissection around the whole kidney first, including the vessels and ureter, followed by clamping at the end of procedure. In urology, the dissection is done after clamping of the vessels. The flank incision technique is 'muscle cutting', and the size of the scar may vary from 10 to 20 cm, depending on the size of the donor. This technique can include excision of the rib if a wider approach to the kidney is required. This worsens postoperative pain and increases the chance for a pneumothorax. Insertion of an epidural anaesthetic catheter can help with the extra pain but adds an extra complexity to the operation.

Lumbotomy approach to live donor nephrectomy step by step
- The patient is placed in the lateral position; operation table is usually flexed.
- The size of the incision depends on size of the donor; usually 15–20 cm (Fig. 7.28). The incision is through skin, subcutaneous fat and muscle layers, between the 11th and 12th rib or below the 12th rib.
- The extraperitoneal fat is dissected and the peritoneum is mobilised medially. The Gerota's fascia is opened after palpating the convexity of the kidney in craniocaudal direction.
- The perinephric fat is dissected and the lateral aspect of the kidney cleared. Dissection progresses in circles from the medial part to the lower pole, the lateral part and the upper pole. Dissection of vessels comes last. When dissecting the lower pole it is important to preserve the ureter and its vessels. The ureter must be divided further down to the level where it crosses the iliac vessels. Once fully dissected the ureter can be either tied or clipped distally and divided. Some centres leave

the gonadal vein together with the ureter in order to make sure the ureteric vessels are preserved.

- During dissection of the upper pole special attention is given to the suprarenal gland. If this is damaged during surgery, it may bleed quite significantly and make the following dissection difficult.
- Before any irreversible step is taken, the whole kidney must be fully dissected with the vessels and ureter still intact. Once the artery, vein and ureter are visualised, red, blue and yellow slings, respectively, are passed around them. The renal vessels form the last part of dissection. This sequence of dissection is particularly important to prevent extended warm ischaemia. In case of bleeding, clamps can be applied on the vessels and, as the kidney is already free of all the surrounding attachments, it can be removed for perfusion immediately.
- First the ureter is tied or clipped distally before dividing. Then the artery followed by the vein are either clamped and tied or cut using an endovascular stapler. The arterial clamp is applied first to avoid the elevated intra-renal pressure with no outflow that occurs when the venous clamp is applied first. Venous clamping follows arterial clamping.
- Once the kidney is removed from the donor the perfusion is performed on the bench.
- After back-table kidney-graft preparation, the surgeon returns to the donor. The nephrectomy bed must be carefully reviewed. When the endovascular stapler is used for the vessels, no further haemostasis needs to be done. When vascular clamps are used, the renal artery and vein stumps must be sutured using Prolene™ 3/0 or 4/0 after removing the graft. Haemostatic powder can be applied to the kidney bed to prevent any haematoma formation especially when no drain is used.
- A drain can be used but in most cases is not needed. Muscle layers are usually closed with continuous loop polydioxanone (PDS) and the skin with absorbable continuous subcutaneous suture. To reduce pain, 0.25% bupivacaine can be given as local anaesthetic.
- The surgeon is responsible not only for positioning on the table but also for placing the donor back in the supine position on their bed.

Advantages of the technique
- very good exposure to the kidney
- possible bleeding can be controlled by hand and vascular clamps
- widely used, easy to learn

Disadvantages of the technique
- large incision
- muscle-cutting approach with related possible complications, including chronic pain
- risk of 'bulging' caused by denervation of the muscle

- painful procedure with long hospital stay and prolonged recovery time
- higher morbidity rate compared with endoscopic techniques

Anterior subcostal extraperitoneal approach

This approach has some advantages compared with the traditional lumbotomy. The incidence of hernia is lower and the incision can be quite small in slim cases. It is still an extaperitoneal approach that minimises the chance of intra-abdominal organ damage.

Anterior subcostal extraperitoneal approach step by step

- The patient is positioned in the supine position; the operation table can be a little flexed if required, and the lumbar part of the donor on the nephrectomy side can be supported using, for example, a 1 L bag of saline (Figs 7.29, 7.30).
- The size of incision depends on the size of the donor. This is usually a 5–15 cm horizontal incision that starts about 3 cm from the midline up to 3 cm above the umbilicus (see Fig. 7.31). After cutting through the skin, subcutaneous fat and the muscle layers, the extraperitoneal space is created.
- The extraperitoneal fat is dissected and the peritoneum is mobilised medially. The Gerota's fascia is opened after palpating the convexity of the kidney in craniocaudal direction.
- The rest of the dissection is the same as for the lumbotomy approach.

Advantages of the technique

- very good exposure to the kidney (but smaller than flank)
- possible bleeding can be controlled by hand and vascular clamps
- widely used, easy to learn

Disadvantages of the technique

- same as for lumbotomy

Open transperitoneal approach

This technique requires much more extensive dissection, so it is not commonly used. The risk of intra-abdominal organ damage, including splenic and small bowel injury, together with postoperative adhesions and related ileus is increased.

Transperitoneal approach step by step

- The donor is placed in the same position on the table as for the anterior subcostal extraperitoneal approach.
- The incision can be either horizontal, subcostal or paramedian. All the abdominal wall layers must be divided.

- On the left side, the descending colon must be mobilised to reveal the Gerota's fascia and the kidney. On the right side, the ascending colon must be mobilised. This phase of procedure is in principal the same as the transperitoneal laparoscopic live donor nephrectomy approach.
- Once the Gerota's fascia is reached and the convexity of the graft is palpable, dissection is the same as for the lumbotomy approach.

Advantages of the technique
- very good exposure to the kidney
- large operating field for dissection

Disadvantages of the technique
- possibility of intra-abdominal organ damage
- possibility of delayed intra-abdominal complications

Mini-open or 'finger-assisted' approach

This is a variation of the traditional lumbotomy loin incision first described by Nadey Hakim. The donor is placed in the same position as for the lumbotomy approach. What makes this technique different is the small size of the incision and the use of endovascular staplers for the ureter and the vessels. All three muscle layers are divided, but the rib is not resected. Retraction is accomplished using two 2.5 cm wide hand-held wound retractors and the surgeon's index and middle finger. The lead surgeon uses a headlight with 2.5× magnification loupes to enhance the view.

Mini-open or 'finger-assisted' approach step by step
- The donor is placed in the same position on the table as for the anterior subcostal extraperitoneal approach – the lateral decubitus position.
- Incision follows the line of the lower ribs and is 4 cm or more in size.
- Once Gerota's fascia is reached and convexity of the graft is palpable, dissection is the same as for the lumbotomy approach.
- The vessels as well as the ureter are divided using linear articulated stapling device (ETS-Flex 35 mm, Articulation, Endoscopic Linear Cutter, Ethicon Endo-surgery, Inc., Cincinnati, OH).

Advantages of the technique
- good cosmetic effect
- less pain compared with other open techniques

Disadvantages of the technique
- limited exposure to kidney and major vessels
- advantages may not apply to large donors

Endoscopic live donor nephrectomy techniques

The first laparoscopic live donor nephrectomy was performed by
Ratner in 1995 at the John Hopkins Medical Centre. Since then many
centres worldwide have adopted this technique instead of the open
approach.

The main benefits of the endoscopic techniques are: less pain, small
scar(s) and shorter hospital stay, as well as shorter recovery time and time
away from work. Since the introduction of such techniques, live kidney
donation has increased.

The endoscopic techniques are more expensive, and the operative
times seem to be longer. Warm ischaemic time (WIT) has been reported
to be longer as well. The length of WIT depends on the technique used.
Hand-assisted techniques offer shorter WIT. Some centres may be
reluctant to perform right-sided endoscopic nephrectomies as the right
renal vein is short.

There are some specific risks related to the use of endoscopic
techniques. These are CO_2 emphysema, pneumoperitoneum,
pneumothorax, pneumomediastinum, gas embolism, injury related
to trocar insertion, failure of endoscopic instruments (especially
stapler or endoclip failure) and limited access if there is major bleeding.
Some delayed complications may occur as well, such as bleeding and
peritonitis.

In general, endoscopic techniques have fewer complications in donors
but provide similar transplant outcomes to those of the open techniques.
When taking into consideration the early return to work and cost
implications of that, endoscopy is cheaper overall.

Laparoscopic transperitoneal approach step by step

- The donor is placed in the lateral decubitus position. The table can be
  flexed.
- Umbilicus port for camera and another two ports for dissection.
- Inspection of abdominal cavity follows.
- To access Gerota's fascia, the colon must be dissected. Gerota's facia is
  opened on convexity of the kidney in the craniocaudal direction.
- The perinephric fat is dissected and the lateral aspect of the kidney
  cleared. Dissection progresses in circles from the medial part to the
  lower pole, the lateral part and the upper pole. Dissection of vessels
  comes last. When dissecting the lower pole it is important to preserve
  the ureter and its vessels. The ureter must be divided further down
  to the level where it crosses the common iliac vessels. Once fully
  dissected the ureter can be either tied or clipped distally and divided.
  Some centres leave the gonadal vein together with the ureter in order
  to make sure the ureteric vessels are preserved.

- During dissection of the upper pole, special attention is given to the supra-renal gland. If this is damaged during surgery, it may bleed significantly and make the following dissection difficult.
- Before any irreversible step is taken, the whole kidney must be fully dissected with the vessels and ureter still intact. The ureter is clipped and divided distally. The artery and vein are divided separately using 35 mm vascular endostapler (e.g. ETS-Flex 35 mm, Endoscopic Linear cutter, Ethicon Endo-Surgery, Inc., Cincinnati OH). This may or may not be articulating. The arterial stapler is applied first to avoid the elevated intra-renal pressure due to loss of outflow if the venous clamp is used first. The venous stapler follows the arterial one.
- The renal vessels form the last part of dissection. This sequence of dissection is particularly important to prevent extended warm ischaemia. For example, in the case of bleeding, clamps can be applied on the vessels, and as the kidney is already free of all the surrounding attachments, it can be removed for perfusion immediately.
- After nephrectomy, the graft is placed into the endobag and removed from another incision. The graft removal incision can be placed either in the left lower quadrant or suprapubically. Performing the graft removal incision before clamping the vessels reduces the warm ischaemia time.
- Once the kidney is removed from the donor the perfusion is performed on the bench.
- After back-table kidney graft preparation, the surgeon returns to the donor. The nephrectomy bed must be carefully reviewed. Haemostatic powder can be applied to the kidney bed to prevent any haematoma formation, especially when no drain is used.
- A drain can be used but in most cases is not needed. The linea alba or anterior rectus sheath is usually closed with continuous loop PDS and the skin with absorbable continuous subcutaneous suture. To reduce pain, 0.25% bupivacaine can be given as local anaesthetic.
- As before, the surgeon is responsible not only for positioning on the table but also for placing the donor back in the supine position on their bed.

Advantages of the technique
- very good exposure to the kidney
- large space for dissection

Disadvantages of the technique
- Extensive dissection is needed to approach the kidney; similar to the open, transperitoneal nephrectomy. This may lead to intra-abdominal organ damage.
- The kidney is handled by metallic surgical instruments.
- Possible bleeding cannot be controlled by hand or vascular clamps.
- At the end of the procedure, the kidney is clamped but cannot be quickly removed until an adequate incision is made. This extends the warm ischaemic time.

Hand-assisted laparoscopic approach

Hand assistance was first described by Wolf in 1998. This approach has the additive effect of making the nephrectomy technique safer and quicker. Handling the kidney with the hand instead of laparoscopic instruments offers more accuracy and it is more gentle to the kidney tissue. Possible bleeding can be controlled easily by applying a finger over it. This gives the operating surgeon enough time to assess the severity of the bleeding and choose the best way of stopping it. Once the ureter and vessels are divided, the kidney graft is already in the surgeon's hand so can be removed straightaway for flushing with preservation solution. This aspect is essential for reducing the length of warm ischaemic time.

Hand-assisted laparoscopic approach step by step

- The donor is placed in the lateral decubitus position. The table can be flexed.
- Upper midline incision (for left-sided nephrectomy) or lower midline/horizontal incision (for right-sided nephrectomy) is performed for the hand port (size roughly 7 cm).
- Gelport (Applied Medical, CA, USA) is inserted.
- Two other 12 mm ports are placed in the lateral aspect (for camera and dissection).
- Inspection of the abdominal cavity follows.
- For dissection a Harmonic scalpel system (Ethicon Endo-Surgery, Inc., Cincinnati, OH, USA) or Ligasure (Valleylab, a division of Tyco Healthcare Group LP, Colorado, USA) is used.
- To access Gerota's fascia, the colon must be dissected. Gerota's fascia is opened on the convexity of the kidney in the craniocaudal direction.
- The perinephric fat is dissected and the lateral aspect of the kidney cleared. Dissection progresses in circles from the medial part to the lower pole, the lateral part and the upper pole. Dissection of vessels comes last. When dissecting the lower pole it is important to preserve the ureter and its vessels. The ureter must be divided further down to the level where it crosses the iliac vessels. Once fully dissected the ureter can be either tied or clipped distally and divided. Some centres leave the gonadal vein together with the ureter in order to make sure the ureteric vessels are preserved.
- During dissection of the upper pole special attention is given to the suprarenal gland. If this is damaged during surgery, it may bleed quite significantly and make the following dissection difficult.
- Before any irreversible step is taken, the whole kidney must be fully dissected with the vessels and ureter still intact. The ureter is clipped and divided distally. The artery and vein are divided separately using 35 mm vascular endostapler (e.g. ETS-Flex 35 mm, Endoscopic Linear cutter, Ethicon Endo-Surgery, Inc., Cincinnati OH). This may or may not be articulating. The arterial stapler is applied first to avoid the elevated intrarenal pressure due to loss of outflow if the venous clamp is used first. The venous stapler follows the arterial one.

- The renal vessels form the last part of dissection. Such a sequence of dissection is particularly important to prevent extended warm ischaemia. For example, in the case of bleeding, clamps can be applied on the vessels and as the kidney is already free of all the surrounding attachments, it can be removed for perfusion immediately.
- After nephrectomy, the graft is removed (it is already in surgeon's hand at the time of stapling) through the hand port incision for perfusion on the bench.
- After back-table kidney graft preparation, the surgeon returns to the donor. The nephrectomy bed must be carefully reviewed. Haemostatic powder can be applied to the kidney bed to prevent any haematoma formation, especially when no drain is used.
- A drain can be used but in most cases is not needed. The linea alba or anterior rectus sheath is usually closed with continuous loop PDS and the skin with absorbable continuous subcutaneous suture. To reduce pain, 0.25% bupivacaine can be given as local anaesthetic.
- As before, the surgeon is responsible not only for positioning on the table but also for placing the donor back in the supine position on their bed.

Advantages of the technique
- all the advantages applicable to laparoscopy when compared with open surgery
- plus comparing with pure laparoscopy:
  - better bleeding control if required
  - more gentle kidney graft handling
  - shorter warm ischaemic time (kidney in hand when clamping)

Disadvantages of the technique
- transperitoneal approach with possible intra-abdominal organ injury
- previous abdominal surgery might be a contraindication or cause a difficult procedure due to adhesions

Hand-assisted laparoscopic extraperitoneal (retroperitoneoscopic) approach

As explained above, hand assistance provides extra benefits to the laparoscopic procedure. The published rate of complications following either pure laparoscopic or hand-assisted laparoscopic nephrectomy varies in the literature. Some of the serious complications are related to intra-abdominal organ damage. Some live donor procedures were difficult or impossible to perform owing to adhesions following previous surgery. Because of these reasons other techniques have been developed. Jonas Wadström first published his experience with hand-assisted laparoscopic extraperitoneal nephrectomy in 2002. This technique, although delivering an ideal combination of benefits both from laparoscopy, hand assistance and an extraperitoneal approach, has not been widely adopted yet.

Hand-assisted laparoscopic extraperitoneal (retroperitoneoscopic) approach step by step

- The donor is placed in the lateral decubitus position with the table flat (Figs 7.1–7.6).
- For left-sided nephrectomy as well as for right-sided nephrectomy, a 7 cm suprapubic horizontal (Pfannenstiel-like) incision is performed. The linea alba is divided longitudinally in midline. The peritoneum is separated from the posterior aspect of the muscle using hand dissection. The wall is lifted using a deaver retractor. When enough space is created a Gelport (Applied Medical, CA, USA) is inserted (Figs 7.7–7.16).
- A 12 mm port is placed 2.5 cm medial and 2.5 cm inferior to the anterior superior iliac spine (for a camera at the beginning; later on for dissection; Figs 7.17, 7.18).
- The retroperitoneal space is created using hand dissection under vision.
- A 10 mm port is inserted under direct vision about 3 cm above the umbilicus in the mid-clavicular line. The camera is inserted here (Figs 7.19, 7.20).
- For dissection Harmonic scalpel system (Ethicon Endo-Surgery, Inc., Cincinnati, OH, USA) or Ligasure (Valleylab, a division of Tyco Healthcare Group LP, Colorado, USA) is used.
- To access Gerota's fascia the peritoneum is pushed medially. Gerota's fascia opened on convexity of the kidney in craniocaudal direction.
- The perinephric fat is dissected and the lateral aspect of the kidney cleared. Dissection progresses in circles from the medial part to the lower pole, the lateral part and the upper pole. An 11 mm port is used in most cases. This one is placed in the lateral aspect half way between the ribs and the iliac crest and it is used for retraction. Dissection of vessels comes last. When dissecting the lower pole it is important to preserve the ureter and its vessels. The ureter must be divided further down to the level where it crosses the iliac vessels. Once fully dissected the ureter can be either tied or clipped distally and divided. Some centres leave the gonadal vein together with the ureter in order to make sure the ureteric vessels are preserved.
- During dissection of the upper pole special attention is given to the suprarenal gland. If this is damaged during surgery, it may bleed quite significantly and make the following dissection difficult.
- Before any irreversible step is taken, the whole kidney must be fully dissected with the vessels and ureter still intact. The ureter is clipped and divided distally. The artery and vein are divided separately using 35 mm vascular endostapler (e.g. ETS-Flex 35 mm, Endoscopic Linear cutter, Ethicon Endo-Surgery, Inc., Cincinnati OH). This may or may not be articulating. The arterial stapler is applied first to avoid the elevated intra-renal pressure due to loss of outflow if the venous clamp is used first. The venous stapler follows the arterial one (Figs 7.21–7.27).
- The renal vessels form the last part of dissection. Such sequence of dissection is particularly important to prevent extended warm ischaemia. For example, in the case of bleeding, clamps can be applied

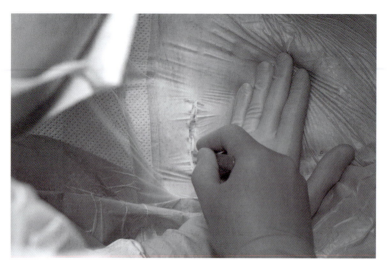

Figure 7.8 Hand assisted retroperitoneoscopic live donor nephrectomy – suprapubic incision. Copyright © Jiří Froněk. All rights reserved.

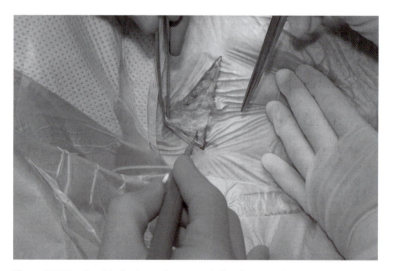

Figure 7.9 Hand assisted retroperitoneoscopic live donor nephrectomy – subcutaneous fat dissection. Copyright © Jiří Froněk. All rights reserved.

on the vessels and as the kidney is already free of all the surrounding attachments, it can be removed for perfusion immediately.

- After nephrectomy, the graft is removed (it is already in surgeon's hand at the time of stapling) through the hand port incision for perfusion on the bench.
- After back-table kidney graft preparation, the surgeon returns to the donor. The nephrectomy bed must be carefully reviewed. Haemostatic powder can be applied to the kidney bed to prevent any haematoma formation, especially when no drain is used.

- A drain can be utilised but in most cases is not needed. The linea alba or anterior rectus sheath is usually closed with continuous loop PDS and the skin with absorbable continuous subcutaneous suture. To reduce pain, 0.25% bupivacaine can be given as local anaesthetic.
- As before, the surgeon is responsible not only for positioning on the table but also for placing the donor back in supine position on his bed.

Advantages of the technique

Combines all three benefits of:

- endoscopy
- hand assistance
- extraperitoneal approach.
   This combination offers:
- reduced pain
- short hospital stay
- quick recovery
- good control of possible bleeding
- gentle kidney handling
- short warm ischaemic time.

Disadvantages of the technique

- relatively unusual approach for surgery
- used in a few centres worldwide only
- so far, unknown length of learning curve

 A video demonstration of this technique (one left- and one right-sided case) appears on the website that accompanies this book at www.wiley.com/go/macphee/transplantation.

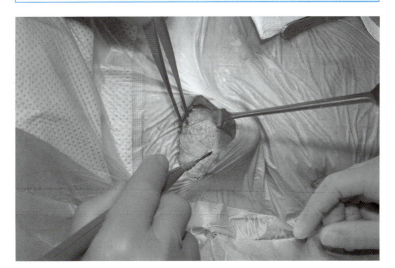

Figure 7.10 Hand assisted retroperitoneoscopic live donor nephrectomy – fascia dissection. Copyright © Jiří Froněk. All rights reserved.

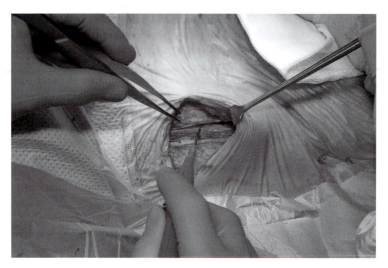

Figure 7.11 Hand assisted retroperitoneoscopic live donor nephrectomy – Dissection underneath the rectus muscle. Copyright © Jiří Froněk. All rights reserved.

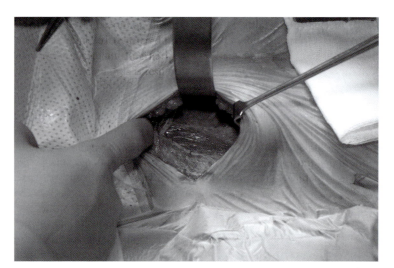

Figure 7.12 Hand assisted retroperitoneoscopic live donor nephrectomy – access to the retroperitoneum space for further dissection. Copyright © Jiří Froněk. All rights reserved.

Combined laparoscopic/open techniques

Some centres adopted techniques that combine open and endoscopic methods. One such technique includes a small pararectal incision as well as laparoscopic ports. Dissection is made without gas insufflation but under laparoscopic camera vision. There is very little evidence to support this technique.

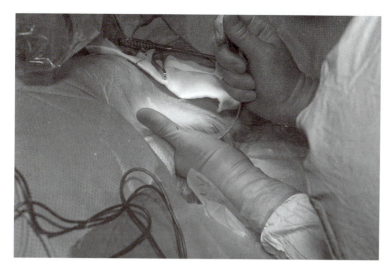

Figure 7.13 Hand assisted retroperitoneoscopic live donor nephrectomy – hand insertion into retorperitoneum space I. Copyright © Jiří Froněk. All rights reserved.

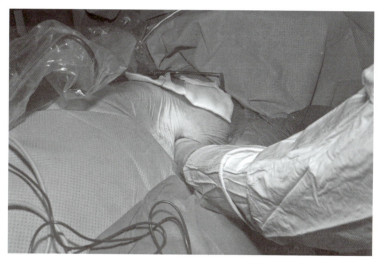

Figure 7.14 Hand assisted retroperitoneoscopic live donor nephrectomy – hand insertion into retorperitoneum space II. Copyright © Jiří Froněk. All rights reserved.

Robotic-assisted laparoscopic live donor nephrectomy

Robotic-assisted live donor nephrectomy can be performed either as pure laparoscopic or as hand assisted. In case of hand assistance, an assisting surgeon is scrubbed with one hand through a hand port similarly to the laparoscopic approaches described above. This technique, even though popular in some centres in the USA, has not been widely accepted, most probably because of the high cost.

Advantages of the technique
- restores the 3D vision lost in the laparoscopic approach
- enhances the ability to perform complex tasks in a laparoscopic environment

Disadvantages of the technique
- expensive
- operating surgeon not scrubbed
- transperitoneal
- prolonged setup of robot
- learning curve of about 80 cases

Natural orifice translumenal endoscopic surgery live donor nephrectomy

The first natural orifice translumenal endoscopic surgery live donor nephrectomy (NOTES) live donor nephrectomy was performed in 2008. In 2010 vaginal graft extraction techniques were described.

Advantages of the technique
- absence of scars

Disadvantages of the technique
- prolonged warm ischaemic time
- possible graft contamination
- difficult control of possible bleeding
- intraperitoneal technique with related complications
- indications not clear yet
- further development of instruments required

As some of the techniques described above offer small scars as well, it is not clear how NOTES can offer a big advantage without compromising safety at the moment. Over the next few years we may see NOTES live donor nephrectomy established as an alternative technique.

Comparison of approaches and relevant points for decision-making

Open versus endoscopic

Some centres still use the traditional flank incision nephrectomy technique, either for right-sided cases or for all the cases. This technique offers the worst results of all. Some centres use the anterior subcostal extraperitoneal approach. This technique is less invasive but still an open approach. Few centres use the mini-open approach.

Endoscopic techniques in general offer less pain, shorter hospital stay, quicker recovery for donor and the same transplant outcomes for recipient when compared to the open technique. More and more

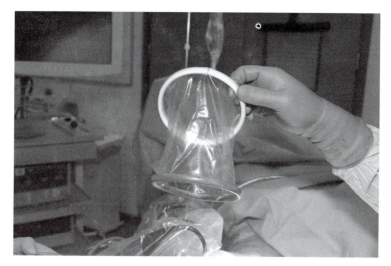

Figure 7.15 Hand assisted retroperitoneoscopic live donor nephrectomy – handport placement I. Copyright © Jiří Froněk. All rights reserved.

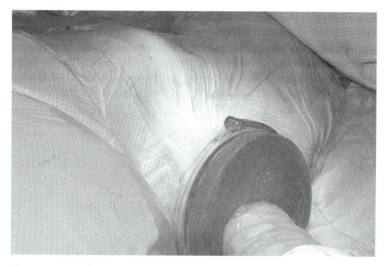

Figure 7.16 Hand assisted retroperitoneoscopic live donor nephrectomy – handport placement II. Copyright © Jiří Froněk. All rights reserved.

units worldwide offer an endoscopic approach for live donor nephrectomy.

Pure endoscopic versus hand assisted

Pure endoscopic techniques came first followed by hand-assisted approaches. Hand assistance offers gentle handling of the graft during dissection, better control of possible large bleeding and shorter warm ischaemia.

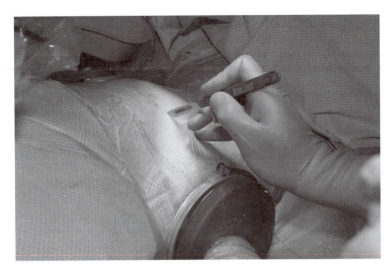

Figure 7.17 Hand assisted retroperitoneoscopic live donor nephrectomy – first trocar placement I. Copyright © Jiří Froněk. All rights reserved.

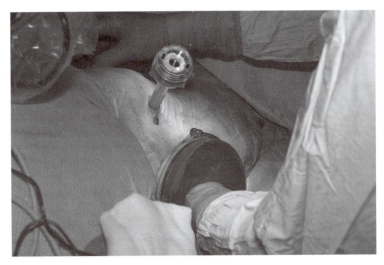

Figure 7.18 Hand assisted retroperitoneoscopic live donor nephrectomy – first trocar placement II. Copyright © Jiří Froněk. All rights reserved.

Intraperitoneal versus extraperitoneal

Transperitoneal laparoscopic nephrectomy (pure laparoscopic or hand assisted) offers very good exposure during surgery but requires extensive mobilisation of the colon. Extraperitoneal techniques (both open and hand-assisted laparoscopic) require much less dissection. Previous surgery, scarring and adhesions do not affect the procedure.

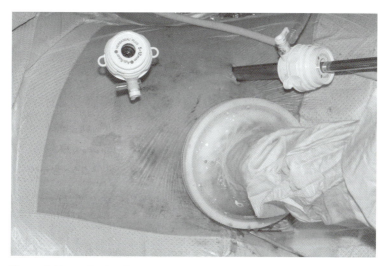

Figure 7.19 Hand assisted retroperitoneoscopic live donor nephrectomy – all trocars in place I. Copyright © Jiří Froněk. All rights reserved.

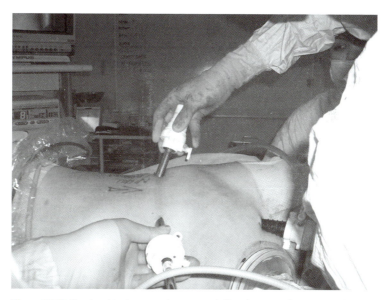

Figure 7.20 Hand assisted retroperitoneoscopic live donor nephrectomy – all trocars in place II. Copyright © Jiří Froněk. All rights reserved.

As there is less dissection and no exposure to intra-abdominal organs, it is nearly impossible do get complications such as bowel/colon/spleen injury or postoperative adhesions. Also the incidence of postoperative paralytic ileus is lower and if present, the donor recovers quickly.

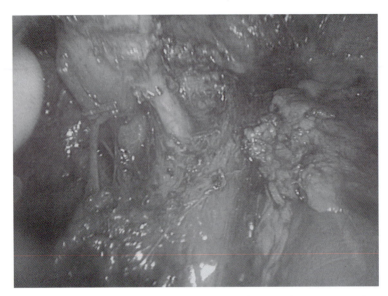

Figure 7.21 Hand assisted retroperitoneoscopic live donor nephrectomy – renal pedicle. Copyright © Jiří Froněk. All rights reserved.

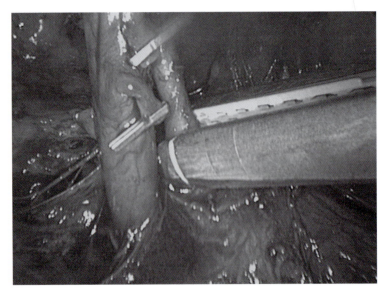

Figure 7.22 Hand assisted retroperitoneoscopic live donor nephrectomy – renal vein and artery ready for stapling. Copyright © Jiří Froněk. All rights reserved.

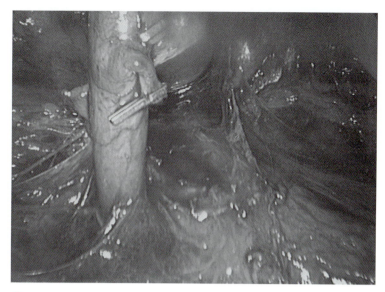

Figure 7.23 Hand assisted retroperitoneoscopic live donor nephrectomy – renal artery stapled. Copyright © Jiří Froněk. All rights reserved.

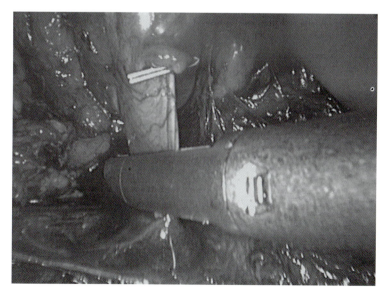

Figure 7.24 Hand assisted retroperitoneoscopic live donor nephrectomy – renal vein stapling. Copyright © Jiří Froněk. All rights reserved.

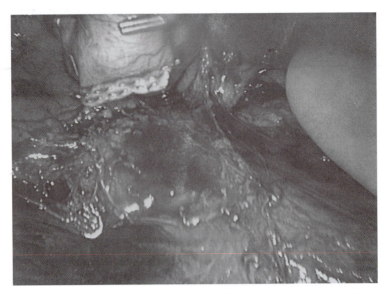

Figure 7.25 Hand assisted retroperitoneoscopic live donor nephrectomy – graft extraction. Copyright © Jiří Froněk.

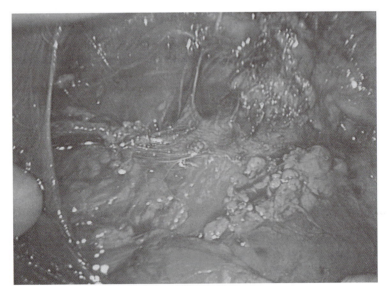

Figure 7.26 Hand assisted retroperitoneoscopic live donor nephrectomy – operation field review I. Copyright © Jiří Froněk.

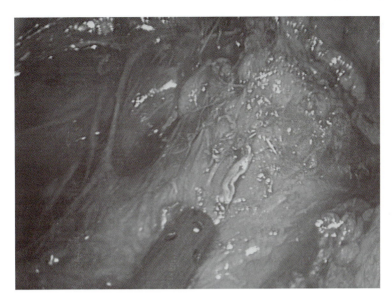

Figure 7.27 Hand assisted retroperitoneoscopic live donor nephrectomy – operation field review II. Copyright © Jiří Froněk. All rights reserved.

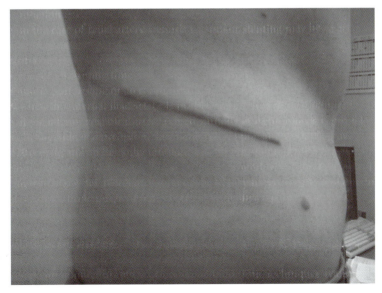

Figure 7.28 Live donor nephrectomy via Flank incision – scar (right sided nephrectomy). Copyright © Jiří Froněk. All rights reserved.

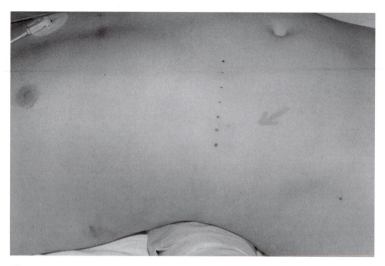

Figure 7.29 Live donor nephrectomy via anterior subcostal extraperitoneal approach – positioning on the table (right sided nephrectomy). Copyright © Jiří Froněk. All rights reserved.

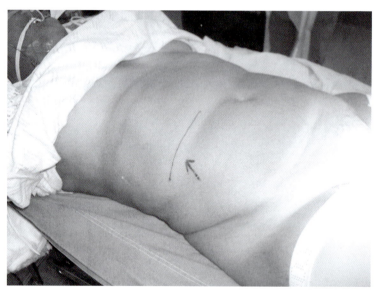

Figure 7.30 Live donor nephrectomy via anterior subcostal extraperitoneal approach – incision marking (right sided nephrectomy). Copyright © Jiří Froněk. All rights reserved.

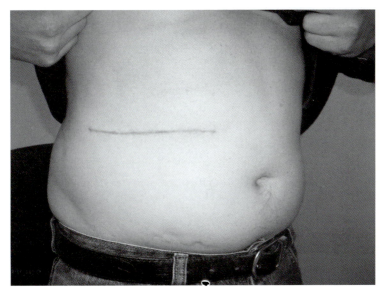

Figure 7.31 Live donor nephrectomy via anterior subcostal extraperitoneal approach – scar (right sided nephrectomy). Copyright © Jiří Froněk. All rights reserved.

Handling of ureter and renal vessels

The quality of both ureter and renal vessels is crucial for successful transplantation. During live donor nephrectomy, the ureter should be divided down to the level where it crosses the iliac vessels. During deceased donor retrieval, the ureter is usually cut below this point and is therefore much longer. For transplantation, the ureter should be long enough to create a tension-free anastomosis and short enough to prevent ischaemic complications (stenosis/necrosis/leak). The upper two-thirds of the ureter are supplied with blood from the renal pelvis, whereas the lower third is supplied from the bladder. If the ureter is left too long, ischaemia with its related complications may occur. Renal vessels must be long enough to create a secured anastomosis and aid positioning of the kidney graft before closing. If the vessels are too long, a kink may occur, which may be followed by stenosis/thrombosis. If vessels are too short, positioning may be difficult and thrombosis may occur again. Grafts with multiple vessels must be treated with special care. All arteries must be anastomosed (except small capsular arteries supplying small superficial area of the graft). In the case of two equal veins, both must be anastomosed. If one or more veins are small compared with the main one, they can be tied off. This is because a collateral venous system is present in the kidney.

Right-sided nephrectomy

Right-sided nephrectomy is indicated when the quality of that kidney is inferior (the better kidney being left in the donor), or when simple anatomy is present, compared with the left side. The right renal vein is always shorter than the left one. However, the right vein is unlikely to have an associated lumbar or other tributary. Early branching of the right renal artery behind the inferior vena cava should always be taken into consideration, as it may result in multiple arteries. Occasionally, dissection might be difficult because of the liver. Most units prefer to perform a left-sided nephrectomy because of renal vein length and easier dissection. Right-sided nephrectomy should not be a problem for the experienced team, and if indicated, this must offer the same outcomes for both donor and recipient.

Warm ischaemic time and kidney graft cold perfusion

During the live donor nephrectomy procedure all the kidney structures e.g. artery, vein and ureter are stapled/clipped and divided. Once the kidney is completely separated from the donor's body, it should be called 'kidney graft'. After removing the graft from the donor, it is perfused via renal the artery/arteries on the back-table using preservation solution. At the time the arterial clamp is applied, the warm ischaemic time starts. Warm ischaemic time ends once cold perfusion flow starts. This period of time must be as short as possible to minimise damage to the graft. Usually this lasts 2–3 minutes.

Morbidity and mortality

According to the published data, donor mortality is approximately 1/3000 and morbidity between 2 and 20%. The use of laparoscopic techniques for living donor nephrectomy results in less postoperative pain, a short hospital stay and a quick return to normal life and work. It is necessary to offer and maintain regular follow-up to all donors for life. This may prevent the development of complications following the nephrectomy and detect any new pathologies at an early stage. One study from Sweden showed that donors live longer than the rest of the population, which is probably explained partly by the fact that at time of the nephrectomy, they were 'healthy individuals' and partially by the early detection and treatment of other pathologies, during postoperative monitoring.

Risks and possible complications in general

All surgical procedures are associated with some risks. The same is true for live donor nephrectomy. It is useful to divide these risks into early and late complications. The group of early complications involves all those related to major surgery: bleeding, wound infection, chest infection, deep vein thrombosis and pulmonary embolism. Every potential live donor must be fully informed and aware of all these potential complications. According to the literature, the incidence of the above-mentioned risks vary and rate of those depends on the technique used for nephrectomy as well as on the technique/device used for handling vessels (stapler/clip/suture). The risk of thrombophilia must be assessed pre-operatively on an individual basis. Based on this assessment adequate prophylaxis is decided. This approach is particularly important in cases of living donation. In 1992 Najarian published 17 deaths following live donor nephrectomy and concluded that the risk of death is around 1/3000. This was also shown to be true in the 2010 by Montgomery. Long-term risks are the same irrespective of the surgical techniques. Risk of hypertension, diabetes, proteinuria and renal failure are described in detail in Chapter 24.

Comparing the techniques – which approach might be ideal?

Based on techniques and their pros and cons described above, the combination of laparoscopy, hand assistance and extraperitoneal approaches seems to offer most of the benefits. For this reason, the hand-assisted retroperitoneoscopic live donor nephrectomy technique may be the method of choice. In general, if the operating surgeon and team are experienced, the short-term results may be similar after any of the techniques; nevertheless, we should try to combine the benefits of each approach to minimise the risks.

Key references

1. Chandak P, Kessaris N, Challacombe B, *et al.* (2009) How safe is hand-assisted laparoscopic donor nephrectomy? Results of 200 live donor nephrectomies by two different techniques. *Nephrol Dial Transplant* **24**, 293–297.
2. Cooper M, Al-Qudah HS, Jacobs SC, *et al.* (2006) Laparoscopic donor nephrectomy for transplantation: 10 years and 1000 consecutive cases. *Am J Transplant* **6**, 286.
3. Dols LF, Kok NF, Terkivatan T, *et al.* (2010) Optimizing left-sided live kidney donation: Hand-assisted retroperitoneoscopic as alternative to standard laparoscopic donor nephrectomy. *Transpl Int* **23**, 358–363.
4. Dosani T, Olsburgh J, Mustafa N, *et al.* (2007) Key-hole mini-open donor nephrectomy: A single institution experience. *Am J Transplant* **7**,489.
5. Fehrman-Ekholm I, Möller S, Steinwall J, *et al.* (2009) Single or double arteries in the remnant kidney after donation: Influence on the long-term outcome of the donor. *Transplant Proc* **41**, 764–765.
6. Fronek JP, Morsy MA, Singh U, *et al.* (2006) Retroperitoneoscopic live donor nephrectomy in a patient with a double inferior vena cava. *J Laparoendosc Adv Surg Tech* **16**, 378–380.
7. Giessing M, Turk I, Roigas J, *et al.* (2005) Laparoscopy for living donor nephrectomy – particularities of the currently applied techniques. *Transpl Int* **18**, 1019–1027.
8. Gorodner V, Horgan S, Galvani C, *et al.* (2006) Routine left robotic-assisted laparoscopic donor nephrectomy is safe and effective regardless of the presence of vascular anomalies. *Transpl Int* **19**, 636–640.
9. Hadjianastassioua VG, Johnson RJ, Rudge CJ, *et al.* (2007) 2509 Living donor nephrectomies, morbidity and mortality, including the UK introduction of laparoscopic donor surgery. *Am J Transplant* **7**, 2532–2537.
10. Halgrimson WR, Campsen J, Mandell MS, *et al.* (2010) Donor complications following laparoscopic compared to hand-assisted living donor nephrectomy: An analysis of the literature. *J Transplant* **2010**, 825689.

11. Kessaris N, Fronek J. (2008) Hand-assisted retroperitoneoscopic living-donor nephrectomy: 106 consecutive left and right sided cases. *Transplantation* **86**, 394.

12. Kohei N, Kazuya O, Hirai T, *et al.* (2010) Retroperitoneoscopic living donor nephrectomy: Experience of 425 cases at a single center. *J Endourol* **24**, 1783–1787.

13. Kokkinos C, Nanidis T, Antcliffe D, *et al.* (2007) Comparison of laparoscopic versus hand-assisted live donor nephrectomy. *Transplantation* **83**, 41–47.

14. Laca L, Daniel–Lacková K, Daniela-Nyulassy, Š, *et al.* (1998) *Orgánove transplantácie. Transplantácia obličiek.* DALI, Banská Bystrica.

15. Laca L, Grandtnerova B. (2003) *Transpantácie obličiek od žijúcich darcov.* Enterprise, Banská Bystrica.

16. Leventhal JR, Paunescu S, Baker TB, *et al.* (2010) A decade of minimally invasive donation: Experience with more than 1200 laparoscopic donor nephrectomies at a single institution. *Clin Transplant* **24**, 169–174.

17. Ma L, Ye J, Huang Y, *et al.* (2010) Retroperitoneoscopic live-donor nephrectomy: 5-year single-center experience in China. *Int J Urol* **17**, 158–162.

18. Modi P, Kadam G, Devra A. (2007) Obtaining cuff of inferior vena cava by use of the Endo-TA stapler in retroperitoneoscopic right-side donor nephrectomy. *Urology* **69**, 832–834.

19. Najarian JS, Chavers BM, McHugh LE, *et al.* (1992) 20 years or more of follow-up of living kidney donors. *Lancet* **340**, 807–810.

20. Nanidis TG, Antcliffe D, Kokkinos C, *et al.* (2008) Laparoscopic versus open live donor nephrectomy in renal transplantation: A meta-analysis. *Ann Surg* **247**, 58–70.

21. Treska V. (2002) *Transplantologie pro mediky.* Karolinum, Prague.

22. Troppmann C, Perez RV, McBride M. (2008) Similar long-term outcomes for laparoscopic versus open live-donor nephrectomy kidney grafts: An OPTN database analysis of 5532 adult recipients. *Transplantation* **27**, 916–919.

23. British Transplantation Society. (2011) *UK Guidelines for Living Donor kidney Transplantation.* Available online from: http://www.bts.org.uk/transplantation/standards-and-guidelines/.

24. Viklický O, Janoušek L, Baláž P. (2008) *Transplantace ledviny v klinické praxi.* Grada, Prague.

25. Wadstrom J, Biglarnia A, Gjertsen H, *et al.* (2011) Introducing Hand-Assisted Retroperitoneoscopic live donor nephrectomy. Learning curves and development based on 413 consecutive cases in four centres. *Transplantation* **91**, 462–469.

26. Wadström J, Lindström P. (2002) Hand-assisted retroperitoneoscopic living-donor nephrectomy: Initial 10 cases. *Transplantation* **73**, 1839–1841.

27. Yashi M, Yagisawa T, Ishikawa N, *et al.* (2007) Retroperitoneoscopic hand-assisted live-donor nephrectomy according to the basic principle of transplantation in donor kidney selection. *J Endourol* **21**, 589–594.

28. Segev DL, Muzaale AD, Caffo BS, *et al.* (2010) Perioperative mortality and long-term survival following live kidney donation. *JAMA* **303**, 959–966.

8 Organisation of transplant services, organ sharing and organ allocation: A perspective from the UK and Eurotransplant

James Neuberger and Axel Rahmel

Introduction

Transplantation of kidneys and other solid organs is now a well-established procedure for patients with end-stage disease but remains an expensive procedure, both in financial terms and in the extent of the multidisciplinary team of clinicians, scientists and others required to assess, transplant and follow-up patients. The coordination of donor (whether living or deceased) and recipient matching to ensure optimal outcome depends on the availability of a central structure or structures that will be responsible for the transplant process, from identification of potential donors, maintaining good clinical governance, commissioning the service, developing the processes for organ allocation and agreeing and monitoring clinical standards. Achieving a successful outcome requires close coordination between a number of agencies. In this chapter, we will outline the approaches taken in two health-care administrations: in the UK and in the Eurotransplant zone.

The situation in the UK and the Eurotransplant countries

In the UK, the responsibility for organ transplantation lies with several groups:
- the Departments of Health of the four UK nations (England, Scotland, Wales and Northern Ireland) determine overall policy
- local National Health Service (NHS) groups commission the renal transplant services from Hospital

Handbook of Renal and Pancreatic Transplantation, First Edition. Edited by Iain A. M. MacPhee and Jiří Froněk.
© 2012 John Wiley & Sons, Ltd. Published 2012 by John Wiley & Sons, Ltd.

- the Human Tissue Authorities (HTAs) have responsibility for ensuring the integrity of living donation
- NHS Blood and Transplant (NHSBT) is responsible for commissioning the National Organ Retrieval Service, employing donor transplant coordinators, facilitating organ donation through funding the Clinical Leads for Organ Donation in every acute Hospital, setting selection and allocation policies and ensuring equity of access and outcomes, maintaining the national transplant waiting list, maintaining the UK Transplant Registry and maintaining and promoting the Organ Donor Register. Clinical input is provided by Organ Advisory Groups. The Kidney Advisory Group includes representatives from all designated transplant units, scientists, coordinators as well as relevant professional organisations. There is an annual meeting with patients and patient groups and one open meeting for all stakeholders.

The UK has a population of about 60 million people. Currently, deceased donor rates per million population (pmp) are just above 15. In the financial year from 1 April 2010 to 12 December 2010 there were 707 deceased organ donors (449 donations after brain death and 258 donations after circulatory death) and 698 living kidney donations. In that period of time, there were a total of 1057 kidney deceased donor kidney transplants and 683 living donor kidney transplants. There were 6779 patients registered on the UK National Transplant List for kidney transplants and 261 registered for kidney–pancreas transplants [1].

The Eurotransplant International Foundation (ET), with its office in Leiden, the Netherlands is responsible for the allocation of organs from deceased donors in the Eurotransplant regions. Currently seven countries – Austria, Belgium, Croatia, Germany, Luxembourg, the Netherlands and Slovenia – are cooperating within the Eurotransplant framework, representing a total population of 124.5 million inhabitants.

Eurotransplant is not only responsible for the organisation of organ allocation, it also supports the development of new allocation algorithms. For this purpose several organ specific advisory committees (ACs) were established, in which transplant experts from the different ET member countries are represented. Proposals of these ACs are developed based on close monitoring of waiting list dynamics (including access to transplantation and mortality on the waiting list), transplant activities and outcome after transplantation. To gather the necessary information, Eurotransplant maintains a registry department.

In 2010 there were 2109 utilised deceased donors reported in the Eurotransplant countries (a utilised donor is a donor of whom at least one organ was transplanted). From these donors 6985 organs were procured, resulting in 6683 transplants – among them 3702 kidney transplants. In addition, 1399 living donor transplants were performed (1262 kidney and 137 liver transplants). For all non-renal organs the number of patients waiting for a transplant has been increasing over recent years: at the time of writing (1 January 2011) 15,605 patients are on the Eurotransplant waiting list. However, the number of patients awaiting kidney transplantation has been slightly but steadily decreasing over the past 9 years, from 12,653 in 2002 to 10,768 in 2011 (1 January of each year). This decline in the kidney transplant waiting list size is due to several factors, among them the increased use of elderly kidney donors boosted by the introduction of the Eurotransplant Senior Program (for details, see below) and the steady rise in living donor kidney transplantation (129 in 1991, 1262 in 2010; Fig. 8.1).

Organ retrieval

Since April 2010, the UK has had a National Organ Retrieval Service, commissioned by NHSBT. There are seven abdominal retrieval teams that cover the entire UK. These are based primarily in the seven designated liver transplant centres, but there are partnership arrangements. The potential donor is identified in the intensive-care units (ICUs), emergency departments and other areas of the hospital. NHSBT employs about 250 specialist nurses in organ donation (SN-ODs) across the UK who work very closely with clinicians, especially in ICUs. In addition, there are just under 200 clinical leads in organ donation who are usually intensivists working in those ICUs where there is a high probability of donation. The family of the potential donor will be approached either by the SN-OD or a member of the clinical team, to seek consent for organ (and tissue) donation. If granted, the donor details are sent electronically to NHSBT, who will contact transplant teams to identify suitable recipients. The local retrieval team will be contacted and retrieval arranged. If the nearest retrieval team is already retrieving, then the next nearest team will be alerted. Teams must gather within 1 hour and the aim is that the team will arrive at the donor hospital anywhere within the UK within 3 hours in 95% cases. The European Union has issued a Directive about the safety of organs for transplantation. This will be implemented in 2012 in the member states of the European Union. This will provide an additional layer of control and regulation. In the UK, the Competent Authority (CA) is the Human Tissue Authority and the NHS Blood and Transplant has been asked to assist in several functions including reporting and investigation of serious adverse and unexpected reactions (SAR).

In each of the ET countries CA's will be appointed. The role of ET in this regard will probably vary from country to country. Due to fact that ET facilitates the international exchange of organs it will continue to guarantee traceability and will assist in reporting SAR, especially in case of transborder exchange of organs.

Organ retrieval falls under the responsibility of the organ procurement organisations of the different ET member countries and therefore varies both with regard to the legal framework and the organisation structure. For example, donation after circulatory death and transplantation of kidneys from these donors is currently not allowed in Croatia and Germany. Another major difference is the type of consent to donation from deceased donors laid down in the legislation of the different ET member countries. Most countries (Austria, Belgium, Croatia, Luxembourg, Slovenia) use the principle of presumed consent, or

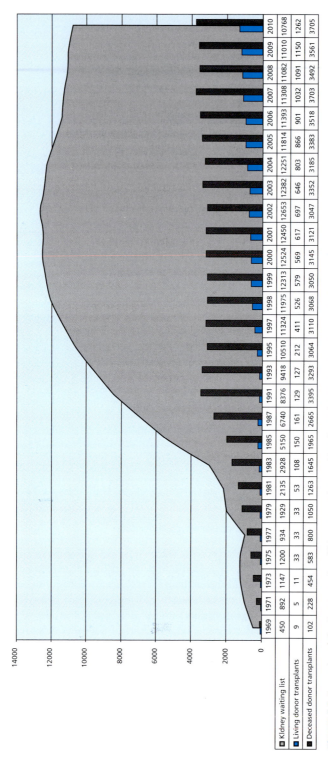

	1969	1971	1973	1975	1977	1979	1981	1983	1985	1987	1991	1993	1995	1997	1998	1999	2000	2001	2002	2003	2004	2005	2006	2007	2008	2009	2010
☐ Kidney waiting list	450	892	1147	1200	934	1929	2135	2928	5150	6740	8376	9418	10510	11324	11975	12313	12524	12450	12653	12382	12251	11814	11393	11308	11082	11010	10768
■ Living donor transplants	9	5	11	33	33	33	53	108	150	161	129	127	212	411	526	579	569	617	697	646	803	866	901	1032	1091	1150	1262
■ Deceased donor transplants	102	228	454	583	800	1050	1263	1645	1965	2665	3395	3293	3064	3110	3068	3050	3145	3121	3047	3352	3185	3383	3518	3703	3492	3561	3705

Figure 8.1 Dynamics of the Eurotransplant kidney transplant waiting list and transplants between 1969 and 2010.

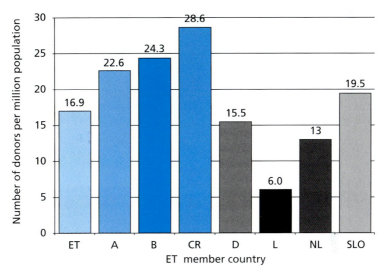

Figure 8.2 Deceased organ donation rates (utilised donors per million population) in the Eurotransplant member countries 2010 (ET, average all Eurotransplant countries; A, Austria; B, Belgium; CR, Croatia; D, Germany; L, Luxembourg; NL, The Netherlands; SLO, Slovenia). Reproduced with permission from Eurotransplant International Foundation Annual Report 2010.

'opting-out'; Germany and the Netherlands, by contrast, use explicit consent (the 'opting-in' system) [2]. These differences are probably one of the reasons for the substantial variety in organ donation rates between the ET member countries (Fig. 8.2).

Selection and allocation

In virtually all health-care administrations, there is a shortfall between the number of people who would benefit from kidney transplantation and the availability of kidneys. As a consequence, there needs to be rationing of resources. Rationing can be achieved either at the time of selection (that is when the patient is placed on the national transplant waiting list) or else at allocation (when the recipient of a donated organ is determined).

Rationing at the time of selection will, depending on the aims of the selection policy, ensure that for those on the waiting list, there is a reasonable expectation that the listed patient will receive a graft in a timely fashion. However, such an approach will significantly understate the numbers of patients who might benefit from a transplant and so give misleading reassurance about the extent of the need for more grafts. Rationing at the time of allocation is harder to achieve, as there will be more people to be considered and allocation models may struggle to differentiate between and rank fairly a large number of potential recipients.

The basis of rationing and therefore development of the selection and allocation policies must be overt and transparent, developed after full discussion with all interested parties and evidence-based where possible. There needs to be a clear understanding of the aims of the allocation policy. There are several possible, and sometimes competing aims, of any allocation policy. The need to consider and balance utility, benefit, equity, and fairness will be sometimes in conflict. Furthermore, public perceptions may be counter to legal requirements: for instance, several studies have shown that the public in general, donor families, health-care professionals and even some recipients are supportive of priority being given to children, and this can be supported by the ethical 'good innings' argument, yet such an approach runs counter to legislation on age discrimination. Of course, younger age may be a surrogate marker for other, legitimate factors, such as correction of growth retardation or considerations about lack of vascular access.

The term 'equity' is used widely and often without further definition. The term could apply to age, so that people of all ages would have the same probability of being allocated a transplant and the very elderly would be treated in the same way as a child. The term could also apply to geographical equity, so that a recipient in the north of the country, for example, would have the same probability of receiving a graft as someone in the far south. Equity of access may mean that all patients who meet the criteria for eligibility would have the same chance of getting a graft or that all patients with the same characteristics would have the same probability. Does equity mean that all patients would have the same probability of receiving a graft or dying on the list? If so, is it important to consider waiting time? There are no simple answers to these questions; however, it is essential that the aims of the selection and allocation policies are defined before policies are developed, modelled and tested and finally implemented, modelled and, if needed, revised.

Whichever approach is taken to allocation of donated kidneys (and indeed other organs and tissues), the aims should be clear and outcomes closely monitored to show that the aims are being achieved. With the changing patterns of disease and of organ donation, changes in medical practice and advances in surgical techniques and improvements in therapy, such policies need continued review and often frequent revision.

In this chapter, we will outline the policies adopted in the UK and the countries served by ET. We recognise that there are other effective and efficient transplant organisations both within and without Europe but a full review of all administrations would, we feel, add little more knowledge for the reader.

UK kidney allocation scheme

Allocation of kidneys from donors after brain death

The UK allocation scheme was introduced in 1998 and was known as the National Kidney Allocation Scheme (NKAS); it was a national scheme for the allocation of kidneys from deceased donors after brain death (DBDs)

[3]. The model was based on an analysis of factors that affect graft outcome. UK data [4] show that 1-year graft survival is affected by donor age, donor type, donor cause of death, recipient age, waiting time to transplant, primary renal disease, HLA mismatch group, cold ischaemic time, recipient ethnicity and 1-year patient survival. At 5 years, graft survival is related to graft year, donor age, donor type, donor cause of death, recipient age, waiting time to transplant, primary renal disease, HLA mismatch group, recipient ethnicity and patient. One of the major aims of the scheme was to improve HLA matching. There were three tiers, according to the degree of HLA matching. The scheme was not truly national, as only about half the donated kidneys were allocated nationally and the others were allocated according to local policy; thus it was a centre-based approach, often without full transparency.

A review in 2004 [5] suggested that, although the 1998 scheme had partially achieved its aims, there were still inequities in the system, so a task force was set up to define the requirements for allocation and develop an algorithm that could be modelled, make simulations and then introduce them. The task force identified several objectives: the most important factor was to ensure equity of access, which was defined as access to transplantation for kidneys from DBDs regardless of geographical location, ethnicity, rarity of HLA or blood group and, where biologically possible, regardless of blood group and degree of sensitisation to HLA. Further aims were: reducing the number of patients waiting more than 5 years; ensuring that paediatric, young adult and highly sensitised candidates are allocated suitable kidneys; matching graft with recipient life expectancy; and avoiding prolonged cold ischaemia times.

One of the major concerns lay with the HLA matching. Those with rare HLA types had waited longer than those with more common types: this discrepancy affected especially those from ethnic minority groups, in which the demand for transplantation was greater and the donation rates lower. This was partly overcome by replacing the then current method of matching based on broad specificities with matching those antigens that are rare in the donor population with the nearest specificity as assessed by serological cross-reactions and sequence analysis. There were concerns that defaulting rare antigens could result in increased sensitisation rates, but it was felt that the potential consequences of sensitisation would be outweighed by the benefits of shorter waiting times and better access.

2006 National Allocation Scheme

In the 2006 National Allocation Scheme, five tiers were agreed (shown in Box 8.1). Paediatric patients (aged below 18 years) in tiers A and B are prioritised according to waiting time, as defined below. Others are prioritised according to several factors, as shown in Box 8.2. The waiting time is determined from date of first active listing for a graft. Each day on the list accrues 1 point, including all days of temporary suspension from the list. For the majority of patients, waiting time starts at zero on the day they are registered as active on the kidney transplant list. However, any patient whose previous graft failed within the first 180 days after a

> ## Box 8.1 Tiers for the UK National Kidney Allocation Policy.
> - Tier A: 000 mismatched paediatric patients – highly sensitised* or HLA-DR homozygous
> - Tier B: 000 mismatched paediatric patients – others
> - Tier C: 000 mismatched adult patients – highly sensitised* or HLA-DR homozygous
> - Tier D: 000 mismatched adult patients – others and favourably matched paediatric patients (100, 010, 110 mismatches)
> - Tier E: all other eligible patients
>
> *≥85% calculated reaction frequency (based on comparison with pool of 10,000 donor HLA types on national database).

> ## Box 8.2 Factors affecting prioritisation in the UK National Allocation Policy.
> - Waiting time
> - HLA match and age combined
> - Donor–recipient age difference
> - Location of patient relative to donor
> - HLA-DR homozygosity
> - HLA-B homozygosity
> - Blood group match

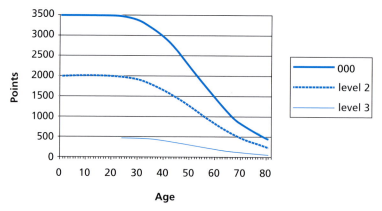

Figure 8.3 Point scores for HLA and age.

transplant, starts with a waiting time as it was on the day of the failed transplant. Waiting time is transferable when a patient transfers from one transplant centre to another. HLA match and age points combined are defined as: level 1, mismatch points: $3500/(1+(age/55)5)$; level 2 mismatch, $2000/(1+(age/55)5)$; and level 3 mismatch $500/(1+(age/55)5)$. This is shown in Fig. 8.3. Priority is given to HLA-DR homozygous patients are these are associated with better outcomes. The age difference points are calculated as Age difference points = –½(donor–recipient age difference)[2]. Location points: 900 for patients at the same centre as the donor and 750 for patients at another centre within the local area, as defined geographically. HLA-DR homozygous points: 500 for all HLA-DR homozygous patients (where HLA level >1). HLA-B homozygous points = 100 for all HLA-B homozygous patients (where HLA level >1). Blood group points = −1000 for blood group B patients when the donor is group O (tiers D and E only). The defaulting of HLA antigens is described in more detail elsewhere.

In addition for patients in Tier E, additional points are allocated for paediatric patients who have a waiting time in excess of 2 years; additional points will be allocated in tiers D and E to improve the chance of being allocated a kidney. It is preferable for paediatric patients to receive a well-matched kidney, but in some cases this is not possible and if a patient has not been transplanted within 2 years they will be prioritised for any compatible kidney. For patients waiting 2–3 years, 2500 extra points will be awarded and for patients waiting in excess of 3 years, 5000 additional points will be awarded. Patients on the transplant list under 18 years old are classed as paediatric patients for the purposes of the kidney allocation scheme. However, since 15 July 2009, patients registered active on the list before their 18th birthday but still waiting for a kidney after they reach 18 years retain their paediatric status and the associated benefits until such time as they are removed from the list for whatever reason (e.g. transplant). Periods of suspension from the list do not affect this entitlement.

If a kidney needs to be reallocated because the patient for whom the kidney has been accepted cannot subsequently receive the transplant, then allocation will depend on the following agreement: if the kidney has not been dispatched to the transplant centre it will continue to be offered for prioritised patients in the usual way. If the kidney has been dispatched to the transplant centre, it will be offered back to any patients in tiers A to D. If there are no suitable patients in tiers A to D, the kidney can be kept by the centre to which the kidney has been dispatched. The centre will select the most appropriate patient from their local list. In all cases, offering kidneys will only continue as specified until 20 hours of cold ischaemia time has elapsed, when the centre holding the kidney (or the centre to which the kidney has been dispatched) can use the kidney in a patient of their choice. In either of these cases, the kidney will be offered back to the designated local transplant centre if not required for local use as permitted. When selecting a patient of their own choice, a centre may, in exceptional circumstances, select a patient with a level 4 HLA match or a patient who is blood group compatible but falls outside of the blood-group-matching criteria specified.

Highly sensitised patients (HSPs) (>=85% calculated reaction frequency) will be considered for offers of kidneys: Level 1 HLA match (000 mismatches) – all HSPs. Level 2 HLA match (100, 010, 110, 200 or 210 mismatches) – all local centre HSPs and all other HSPs where all antibody specificities have been identified (i.e. residual sensitisation level = 0). Levels 3 and 4 (all other mismatches) – no kidneys will be offered to HSPs. Note that the HLA match is that based on defaulting of rare antigens.

Kidneys from donors over 50 years of age will not be offered for paediatric patients (i.e. those <18 years at time of offer). Patients requiring a kidney/pancreas transplant are prioritised after tier A–C kidney-only patients. Kidneys from donors aged 4 years and under will be retrieved and offered en bloc (but may be split if appropriate), whereas kidneys from donors aged 5 years and over will be retrieved and transplanted singly wherever possible. En-bloc kidneys will be offered on a centre rather than patient basis to any centre wishing to receive offers of such kidneys.

The policy for donor–recipient blood-group matching is that O donors may donate to O, A, B and AB recipients, A donors to A and AB recipients, B donors to B and AB recipients, and AB donors to AB recipients only.

Paediatric patients: the current system defines a paediatric patient as one aged less than 18 years. There are concerns about the validity of giving priority to any group on the basis of age. The reasons for this priority are several: firstly, transplantation will allow catch-up of growth, retarded by renal disease. Secondly, younger people are more likely to develop problems with venous access over time. Although the general public do indicate they would give children priority over adults, this approach must be considered in the light of current legislation.

Declined kidney scheme: if a donated kidney donated from a deceased donor after brain death is declined by five centres for the same donor- or graft-related reason, the kidney is then offered though the declined kidney scheme. This was designed to allow those centres that were able and willing to take those offered organs in a timely fashion. The kidney is then offered to the participating centres according to the kidney run; however, the centre is allowed to use that kidney for a recipient other than that identified by the matching run, using other clinical criteria that are deemed relevant. This scheme is monitored regularly and works well. If the kidney is declined by all centres, then the organ is disposed of appropriately or sent for research, according to the wishes of the donor and their family. The allocation scheme was reviewed and revised slightly in 2010.

Allocation of kidneys from donors after circulatory death

At present, kidneys from donors after circulatory death are retrieved either by the National Organ Retrieval Service or, for kidney-only donors, by the local team. At present, such kidneys are allocated locally. However, with increasing experience and greater numbers of DCDs, this policy is being reviewed. It is agreed that donated organs, whether from DCDs or DBDs, are a national and not a local resource and therefore there must be transparency and equity in how these organs are allocated. Although many of the same principles will apply to the allocation of DCD and DBD kidneys, there are significant differences (for example, the impact of cold ischaemia time may be more important). The policy is currently being discussed.

The National Pancreas Allocation Scheme

In 2010, NHSBT adopted a new approach to allocation of pancreases from deceased donors (DBDs and DCDs). Those that are transplanted as part of a multi-visceral organ transplant are excluded from the scheme and will take priority over pancreas-only and pancreas-and-kidney transplants.

Prioritising kidneys between kidney-only and simultaneous kidney–pancreas (SPK) transplants: kidneys are allocated through the National Kidney Allocation Scheme as indicated above. Those listed for kidney only in tiers A, B and C will receive priority over those listed for SPK. If there is one suitable kidney recipient in tiers A–C, then one kidney will be allocated to the kidney-only recipient and the kidney–pancreas to the kidney-pancreas recipient. If there is no suitable kidney recipient, then the kidney will be allocated to a recipient in tier D or E and the pancreas offered as a pancreas-only graft. If both kidneys are allocated to tier A–C recipients, the pancreas will be offered as a single organ.

There is a fast-track scheme where the pancreas needs to be placed rapidly, such as where the pancreas is retrieved before allocation or when the intended recipient is found to be unsuitable because of, for example, infection or unexpected HLA crossmatched positivity. Then the pancreas is offered simultaneously to all centres.

The points system for pancreas allocation was developed using factors that were considered to be clinically relevant, objective and verifiable and associated with outcome. There was an exhaustive modelling exercise and validation process to develop a points system to prioritise recipients. Only after validation and support from the clinical and patient community was the system introduced.

The factors in the model are:

- HLA mismatch
- waiting time
- sensitisation
- travel time from retrieval to implantation hospital
- donor body mass index (BMI)
- dialysis status
- donor–recipient age match.

Those with 0–4 HLA-A, -B and -DR mismatches are allocated 730 points and with five or six mismatches 0 points in order to minimise the number of mismatched transplants. The waiting time points are calculated on the formulae for all vascularised and first islet graft points are (waiting time (days))2/365. To prioritise those listed for a second islet graft, the points are calculated as (waiting time (days))2/44.4, as there is evidence that there should be short interval between the first and second islet graft. Sensitisation points are calculated to discourage transplantation in the presence of appropriate anti-HLA antibodies and are calculated as sensitisation as calculated reaction frequency (%)3/1000. 180 points are given to those on dialysis or other forms of renal support. The travel time points are calculated to minimise the cold ischemia time between retrieval and implantation. For pancreases retrieved after brain death, the patients registered at the three centres closest to the retrieving hospital are given 365 points and the routine islet patient also gets 365 points. For pancreas retrieved after circulatory death, the recipients at the closest centres get 10,000 points and at the next three closest centres 5000 points, and islet recipients will get 10,000 points if registered at a centre with 150 miles of he isolation laboratory. BMI points are given to encourage allocation of a pancreas from low-BMI donors as vascularised graft and from a heavier donor, as islet. Thus for BMI of ≤ 22, 23–25, 26–28, 29–31 and $\geq 32\,kg/m^2$ are +730, +365, 0, −365 and −730, respectively, for a vascularised graft candidate and the reverse for islet recipient. Finally, the points allocated for donor and recipient age matching according to the formula (age difference(years))2/13.9.

It should be noted that the formula appears complex but is, in practice, simple to calculate. Recipients are ranked in order and the pancreas offered in sequence.

Pancreases are also allocated according to blood-group match: donor O to O or B recipient, A to A or AB recipient, B to B recipient and AB to AB recipient, unless there is no suitable matched recipient.

The scheme has been in operation for nearly 1 year and appears to be working effectively.

ET Kidney Allocation System (ETKAS)

The Eurotransplant International Foundation started in 1967 as a scientific cooperation between several transplant centres in Belgium, Germany and the Netherlands based on the initiative of Professor Jon van Rood, who believed that the results of kidney transplantation could be improved by improving HLA matching between donors and recipients. Kidney transplantation is still the cornerstone of ET allocation activities. Since the early days, the kidney allocation rules have been continuously monitored and adapted when necessary. The ETKAS is based on a point-scoring system, with specific modifications for high urgent patients and children. For highly immunised patients and for the allocation of kidneys from elderly donors to elderly recipients special allocation programmes were established (Fig. 8.4).

ETKAS point scoring system
The ranking of the recipients is based on several scoring factors – HLA-matching, mismatch probability, waiting time, expected ischaemic time and organ exchange balance. The recipient with the highest point score is ranked highest and receives the first offer.

HLA typing
Because HLA matching between donor and recipient directly influences the acute and long-term outcome of kidney allocation and has an impact on the probability of immunisation of the recipient, it is one of the major factors in the ETKAS. Only HLA-A, -B and -DR loci are considered in the match and are currently weighted equally. Using the HLA typing of the

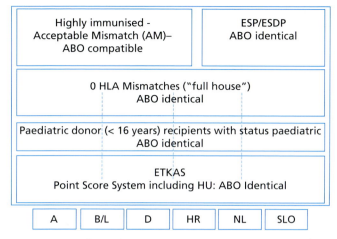

Figure 8.4 Eurotransplant Kidney Allocation Scheme.

donor and the recipient, the number of HLA mismatches is determined. For HLA-A and -B the broad antigens, and for the HLA-DR the split HLA antigens, are taken into account. The point score is calculated according to the following formula:

$$= 400 \times (1 - (\text{number of mismatches}/6))$$

Mismatch probability
Recipients with a rare combination of HLA typing, ABO blood group and panel reactive antibody (PRA) screening would have a disadvantage in the HLA-based scoring system. To compensate for this, the mismatch probability (MMP) is calculated. The MMP reflects the chance of receiving a kidney offer with no or only one mismatch, taking the above-mentioned factors into account. The higher the MMP, the more points are given – up to a maximum of 100 points.

Waiting time
Waiting time starts with the onset of maintenance dialysis; for every year of waiting time 33.3 points are assigned (i.e. 0.091 points per day of waiting). There is no upper limit for the number of waiting time points that can be accrued. Patients listed for pre-emptive deceased donor transplantation do not receive waiting time points.

Expected ischaemic time
A short ischaemic time positively influences the outcome of kidney transplantation. Because the ischaemic time for an individual transplant depends on a number of different factors and is therefore difficult to estimate, the distance between donor and recipient hospital are used as a surrogate parameter for this factor. With some national modifications the following rules apply:
• local donor (recipient in the same centre as the donor): 300 points
• regional donor (recipient centre in the same region as the donor centre): 200 points

- national donor (recipient centre in the same country as the donor centre): 100 points
- international donor (recipient centre outside the country of the donor centre): 0 points.

National kidney exchange balance

Donation rates between countries vary substantially, as explained earlier. Therefore it is necessary to introduce a balancing system between the ET member countries in order to prevent a substantial net export of donor kidneys from a country with a high donation rate to a country with a low donation rate. A balanced organ exchange between the ET member states reflects the underlying ethical principle of national self-sufficiency. In order to balance the organ exchange between the countries without using a simple payback system that would not be in line with the other allocation principles described so far, national balance points are included in the ETKAS. The difference between the number of kidneys procured (and later transplanted) in a country and the number of kidneys transplanted in that country is calculated on a daily basis for the proceeding 365 days. If there are more kidneys procured than transplanted in a country, a negative balance ('net export') results. If more kidneys are transplanted than procured, a positive balance ('net import') results. The higher the export of kidneys from a country, the more national balance points the recipients from this country receive in the kidney match.

Modifications of the ETKAS point score system

High urgent patients

A patient on the kidney waiting list can receive a high urgency (HU) status if at least one of the following criteria is fulfilled:
- no conventional access to haemodialysis and peritoneal dialysis not possible
- severe (uraemic) polyneuropathy
- inability to cope with dialysis with a high risk for suicide
- severe bladder problems (haematuria, cystitis, etc.) due to kidney graft failure after SPK transplantation, provided that the pancreas graft is bladder drained and functioning adequately.

If an external kidney transplant expert audit group has accepted the HU status for a recipient, this patient receives 500 bonus points in the allocation.

Paediatric and adolescent patients

Children and adolescents with end-stage renal disease are threatened by irreversible disturbances of somatic and mental development. In addition, the mortality of paediatric patients on chronic dialysis therapy is four- to fivefold higher than after successful renal transplantation. Several mechanisms are implemented in the ETKAS to address these disadvantages of paediatric recipients:

- paediatric patients receive 100 bonus points
- kidneys from donors <16 years of age are preferentially allocated to paediatric patients
- for paediatric transplant candidates the points for HLA typing (see above) are doubled.

In the past ET assigned the paediatric status to a patient, if dialysis treatment started prior to the 16th birthday. As this definition does not cover all patients who are in special need for a transplantation to overcome the threats mentioned above, the definition of a paediatric patient was recently extended and does now include those adolescent patients >16 years of age who still have existing growth potential. For evaluation, an X-ray of the left hand has to be made, and if epiphysical closure has not yet taken place, the paediatric status can be assigned by an external audit group.

Kidney after liver transplant

The allocation of donor organs in case of a combined transplantation, in general, takes place according to the organ specific allocation rules of the non-renal organ. Liver allocation is in most ET countries performed based on the Model for End-stage Liver Disease (MELD) score. Performing a simultaneous liver and kidney transplantation is not always the optimal solution. In some cases the kidney function might recover after transplantation (hepatorenal syndrome). In patients with a very high MELD, however, mortality after liver transplantation is increased and the risk of losing a functioning kidney due to the death of the patient might therefore be high. Therefore, it was decided to open the option for a sequential kidney-after-liver transplantation. In the case of a patient registered for liver and kidney transplantation, the transplant centre can decide to perform a liver-only transplantation first. If the recipient has a creatinine clearance <15 mL/min) he/she will receive 500 bonus points between 87 and 360 days after liver transplantation.

Special allocation programmes

Acceptable Mismatch programme

Highly sensitised patients have a reduced chance to receive a crossmatch-negative donor kidney. Therefore ET has introduced a special programme that gives the highest priority to highly sensitised (PRA >85%) patients as soon as a donor becomes available, which is compatible with the patient's antibody profile: the Acceptable Mismatch (AM) programme. For highly immunised patients, those HLA antigens towards which the patient never formed antibodies are identified (acceptable mismatches). If a kidney donor has an HLA phenotype, which consists only of the patients' own HLA and one or more AMs, a negative crossmatch is assumed and the kidney is allocated to the highly immunised patient. Upon arrival at the recipient centre a crossmatch is performed prior to the transplant [6].

Zero-mismatch allocation

If there is no AM-programme recipient, a donor kidney is allocated to a fully HLA-matched (HLA-A, -B, -DR) kidney recipient (zero mismatch). Only if there is no zero-mismatch recipient, the kidneys are allocated according to the ETKAS point scoring system.

Eurotransplant Senior Program

The poorer graft survival of elderly kidneys is in part due to a greater susceptibility to increased ischaemia-reperfusion injury and delayed graft function, which in turn makes the allograft more susceptible to acute rejection and graft failure. Therefore a shorter ischaemic time is considered advantageous in the transplantation of kidneys from elderly donors. In elderly recipients HLA matching might be less important, because immunisation – if it occurs due to poor matching – will be less relevant as retransplantation will be uncommon. Taking these aspects into account, the ET Senior Program (ESP) was introduced in 1999. ESP allocates kidneys from donors aged >65 to recipients aged >65 locally or regionally to minimise cold ischaemic time. Allocation is driven by blood group and waiting time; HLA-matching, by contrast, is not taken into account. After introduction of ESP the usage of kidney from elderly donors increased substantially and the waiting time of elderly recipients dropped significantly [7].

General allocation principles

Blood group rules

Kidneys are primarily allocated to blood-group-identical recipients; only if no blood-group-identical recipient can be identified, blood-group-compatible recipients may be transplanted, see Table 8.1 for the blood-group rules that apply.

Donation after cardiac death

As described earlier, donation after cardiac death and transplantation of DCD organs is not allowed in Croatia and Germany. In the other ET countries allocation of DCD kidneys follows the same general rules as described above.

Rescue allocation

If a donor kidney has been rejected at least five times by different transplant centres for donor-related medical reasons, or if the donor's condition becomes unstable so that the donor kidneys might get lost, ET

Table 8.1 Blood-group rules.

Donor blood group	Eligible recipients
A	A and AB
B	B and AB
AB	AB
O	O, A, B and AB

can switch to the so-called rescue allocation. Whereas kidney allocation as described so far is strictly patient-oriented, in the case of rescue allocation organs offers are centre-oriented. As a consequence the physicians in the transplant centre can select the best-suited recipient on their local waiting list. The aim of the rescue allocation is to reduce the risk of losing a donor kidney. Currently less than 5% of all donor kidneys are allocated via this alternative allocation scheme; nevertheless, this policy increases the usage of available donor kidneys without hampering short- and long-term outcome of the transplants [8].

ET pancreas allocation system

Pancreas allocation within Eurotransplant takes place in a two-step process: first suitable recipients are identified based on blood-group rules and recipient-specific donor profiles taking into account donor age, donor BMI and certain other donor characteristics (hepatitis serology, history of tumour disease, sepsis, meningitis, drug abuse). Among the suitable recipients the allocation sequence is determined in a second step, with a straightforward point-scoring system taking into account waiting time, distance between donor and recipient (as surrogate marker for ischemic time) and international organ exchange balance.

Pancreas–kidney allocation follows the rules of pancreas-only transplants. All other combined organ transplants involving a pancreas are allocated based on the rules for the other organs.

Preference is given to special urgent and highly immunised patients.

Special urgency for vascularised pancreas transplantation

Indications for special urgency (SU) status of patients on the waiting list for pancreas transplantation are:
- pancreas graft failure within 2 weeks after vascularised pancreas transplantation due to graft thrombosis
- patient suffering from hypoglycaemia unawareness at least twice in one year requiring hospitalization.

SU status can be assigned via an audit procedure involving independent transplant experts from different Eurotransplant countries on request of the transplant centre. If SU status is assigned, the recipient gets priority over all elective patients; in the case of there being more than one eligible SU patient, allocation is based on the general pancreas point score described above.

Highly immunised patients in need of a combined kidney pancreas transplant

In the case that HLA typing is already available at the time of starting the pancreas match, an immunised patient (PRA >85%) waiting for a combined pancreas–kidney transplant will get priority in allocation over all other pancreas (and kidney) recipients, in case the donor organs seem to be suitable according to the rules and procedures of the kidney AM programme as described above.

Blood group rules

For the allocation of SU or HU recipients blood-group compatibility between donor and recipient is sufficient; for all other transplants ABO blood-group-identical recipients have priority over ABO blood-group-compatible recipients.

Conclusions

The allocation of organs retrieved from deceased donors is complex, and different jurisdictions have adopted slightly different approaches. The broad principles, however, remain the same, focused on providing a transparent process that balances equity and utility in proportions that are supported by the public, the donors and their families, the recipients and the health-care professionals and are consistent with current legislation. The resulting process is complex and will not be perfect and cannot account for all possible clinical situations, so these rules must be implemented with common sense. Furthermore, with advances in clinical practices and changes in social and other factors, these processes will need monitoring, regular review and modification as required.

Acknowledgement

The NHSBT schemes were developed by members of the Directorate of Statistics and Clinical Audit, NHSBT.

References

1. NHS Blood and Transplant. *Statistical Methodology*. Available online from: http://www.organdonation.nhs.uk/ukt/statistics/centre-specific_reports/statistical_methodology.jsp.
2. Roels L, Rahmel A. (2011) Strategies to meet organ shortage – The European experience. *Transpl Int* **4**, 350–367.
3. Johnson R, Fuggle SC, Mumford L, *et al.* (2010) A new UK 2006 kidney allocation scheme for deceased heart-beating donor kidneys. *Transplantation* **89**, 387–394.
4. Johnson RJ, Fuggle SV, O'Neill J, *et al.* (2010) Factors influencing outcome after deceased heart-beating donor kidney transplantation in the United Kingdom: An evidence base for a new national kidney allocation policy. *Transplantation* **89**, 379–386.
5. Fuggle SV, Johnson RJ, Bradley JA, *et al.* (2010) Impact of the 1998 UK National Allocation Scheme for deceased heartbeating donor kidneys. *Transplantation* **89**, 372–278.
6. Claas FHJ, Rahmel A, Doxiadis IN. (2009) Enhanced kidney allocation to highly sensitized patients by the acceptable mismatch program. *Transplantation* **88**, 447–452.
7. Frei U, Noeldeke J, Machold-Fabrizii V, *et al.* (2008) Prospective age-matching in elderly kidney transplant recipients – A 5-year analysis of the Eurotransplant Senior Program. *Am J Transplant* **8**, 50–57.
8. Vinkers MT, Smits JM, Tieken IC, *et al.* (2009) Kidney donation and transplantation in Eurotransplant 2006–2007: Minimizing discard rates by using a rescue allocation policy. *Prog Transplant* **19**, 365–370.

9 Deceased donor kidney transplantation

Luisa Berardinelli

Terminology

Deceased donation remains the main source of kidneys for transplantation in many countries. Deceased donors (DDs) can be classified as following:
- donor after brainstem death (DBD), which used to be known as a heartbeating donor (HBD)
- donor after circulatory death (DCD), which used to be known as a non-heartbeating donor (NHBD).

DBDs are those who have died from brain trauma, cerebrovascular accident or primary brain tumours. The ongoing shortage of available organs, with wide variations observed around the world, has led to increasing use of suboptimal donors with increased risk of graft failure and recipient morbidity. These expanded criteria donors (ECDs) are characterised by donor age over 60 years, or aged 50 to 59 years with two additional risk factors: brain death due to a cerebrovascular accident, history of hypertension/diabetes or elevated terminal serum creatinine, which may influence the choice of surgical strategy either for kidney retrieval or for transplantation. DCD donors are those in whom the heart stopped beating after withdrawal of medical support; hence the terminology 'non-heartbeating deceased donors'. Comparable long-term graft survival is achieved across these donor groups but with a higher incidence of delayed graft function for DCD and ECD kidneys. Retrieval techniques are discussed in detail in Chapter 6.

The technique of transplantation

Preparation of recipient

Kidney transplantation should be an 'elective' surgical procedure for uraemic patients who have been previously submitted to careful assessment of the cardiovascular status, liver function, clotting disorders

Handbook of Renal and Pancreatic Transplantation, First Edition. Edited by Iain A. M. MacPhee and Jiří Froněk.
© 2012 John Wiley & Sons, Ltd. Published 2012 by John Wiley & Sons, Ltd.

and lower urinary system and to exclude malignancies or infections that would contraindicate transplantation and immunosuppression (see Chapter 2).

However, the recipient must be admitted to the hospital on an urgent basis. An accurate history, particularly for vascular problems, must be taken to assess the risk of surgery. The site of vascular access or cutaneous exit of peritoneal catheter must be protected, as well as other sites of potential infections. On admission to the hospital, a chest radiograph, electrocardiogram, complete blood count, electrolyte panel, prothrombin, partial thromboplastin times and crossmatch tests between donor and recipient are required urgently. Systemic anticoagulation, with warfarin for example, should be reversed by the administration of vitamin K and clotting factors. For patients on aspirin with an absolute indication, such as coronary artery or stroke disease, treatment should probably be continued but heparin should only be used if absolutely necessary in this instance owing to increased risk of haemorrhage. Clopidogrel is a more difficult issue. Patients with drug-eluting coronary stents who have an absolute indication for clopidogrel for 6 months should be excluded from the transplant list, as the risk of coronary thrombosis on stopping clopidogrel is high. When anticoagulation is needed in the immediate post-transplant period, one should keep in mind that platelet dysfunction due to aspirin or clopidogrel use can persist for several days after stopping treatment.

The patient with a haemoglobin level higher than 8 g/dL does not have an absolute requirement for transfusion, but many surgeons would regard a haemoglobin of at least 10 g/dL to be safer. If the patient has received dialysis within the last 24 hours or is on peritoneal dialysis, and serum potassium is <5.5 mmol/L and bicarbonate concentration >15 mmol/L, no pre-operative dialysis is necessary. The patient should be maintained at 1–2 kg above their usual dry weight to ensure optimal renal perfusion and reduce the risk of postoperative acute tubular necrosis.

Beta-blockers should not be discontinued, but these patients may need low doses of dopamine (1–4 μg/kg/min) to control hypotension during anaesthesia. Patients who had received alpha sympathetic and/or calcium channel blockade must receive more intra-operative volume expansion, owing to decreased peripheral resistance induced by vasodilators. A single dose of antibiotic, administered at the time of induction and given as short-term prophylaxis, is sufficient for patients who have undergone careful pre-operative assessment, who do not present skin infection or potential infections in other sites and who receive the kidney from a standard criteria deceased donor.

After induction of general anaesthesia, a central venous catheter may be inserted, preferably through the internal jugular vein, to support an adequate filling pressure, monitor central venous pressure (CVP) and derive blood samples. However, adequate fluid management can be achieved through careful clinical assessment without CVP monitoring, and some centres have now abandoned routine insertion of central venous cannulae to reduce the potential for complications. Functional vascular access must be carefully protected during surgery, as well as the superficial veins of the forearm. Non-invasive measurement of arterial pressure should be preferred to avoid damage to the recipient superficial vessels, which can be possibly used in the future for vascular access construction. Constant vigilance over the anaesthetised patient's cardiovascular system is a joint responsibility of the surgeon and the anaesthetist: the minimum CVP must remain at values of over 12 mmHg under mechanical respiration, and the systolic arterial blood pressure above 120 mmHg to ensure adequate intravascular volume, promote diuresis from the new kidney and prevent postoperative anuria.

A urethral catheter, large enough to prevent the possibility of obstruction from blood clots from the cystotomy, is inserted into the bladder aseptically and any urine is sent for culture. The catheter is connected to a closed drainage system, and the bladder is cleaned and may be filled with antibiotic solution. A nasogastric tube may be inserted to remove secretions and vomitus from the airway during and after the operation. Extremity wrapping should be preoperatively applied to prevent pulmonary embolism, particularly in anaemic, malnourished or obese patients.

Before the general anaesthesia, a pad of one to two folded towels are placed underneath the gluteus on the side of operation to elevate the pelvis and allow improved access to the bladder.

Strict asepsis, rigorous haemostasis, gentleness to tissues, meticulous reconstruction of wound layers and attention to detail are imperative to avoid complications and minimise infection risks in a patient who will receive immunosuppressive treatment, with consequent diminished host resistance and impaired wound healing. Moreover, the uraemic state itself engenders enhanced susceptibility to infection due to hypercatabolism, inhibition of natural immunity, occult inflammation and tendency to bleeding.

At the end of the transplant procedure, before wound closure, local infiltration of subcutaneous tissue with local analgesic drugs is useful to reduce postoperative pain and excessive need of opioids.

Preparation of the graft

The operation should be planned well in advance, with a clear pre-operative assessment and treatment plan depending either on the recipient characteristics, such as presence of obesity, small size, atherosclerosis, thrombosis of the external iliac vein, or the anatomical properties of the kidney.

The cold-preserved kidney must always be inspected and excess fat removed, taking care not to damage the 'golden triangle' that contains the ureteral blood supply. All vessel branches that will not be reconstructed are ligated and the aorta/vena-cava patches are prepared.

The most frequent bench reconstruction is the elongation of the right renal vein, as inadequate length of vein or implantation in an obese patient may be a potential cause of graft failure, thrombosis or kinking of the longer renal artery. The DD-procurement team should always retrieve

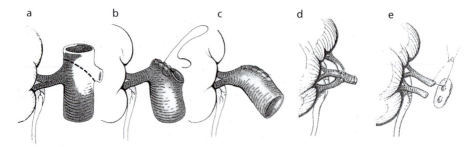

Figure 9.1 (a) The deceased donor vena cava is used to elongate a right renal vein. (b) The proximal opening of the donor vena cava is sutured. (c) The right renal vein is elongated. (d) Two renal arteries are anastomosed at bench, end-to-side to the main renal artery. (e) End-to-side anastomosis of two renal arteries to a biological patch. Reproduced from Vegeto A, Berardinelli L. (1999) *Il Trapianto di Rene*, with permission from UTET, Periodici Scientifici, Torino.

the right kidney with the vena cava attached, to perform an extension if required. The donor vena cava may be easily used to elongate the right venal vein (Fig. 9.1a,b,c), suturing its proximal opening [1]. Insufficient renal vessel length may also be addressed by placing a bypass graft in an end-to-end fashion to extend the artery or the vein. Biological/semi-biological materials may be employed as patch or vascular substitute, if any vessel segment coming from the same donor is not available. Synthetic grafts should be avoided, because of risk of infection.

As there is no collateral arterial supply in the kidney, every ligation of even the smallest arterial branch results in an ischaemic parenchymal area after revascularisation. Although tiny vessels of the upper pole can be ligated if the parenchymal tributary area is smaller than 1–2 cm in diameter, all lower polar arteries must be reconstructed, owing to the high risk of ureteral necrosis. The use of diluted supravital dyes, as methylene blue, may be useful to identify the parenchymal area of arterial supply.

Arterial injuries or polar arteries damaged at retrieval, intrinsic diseases or anatomic variations may require reconstruction 'at bench' using cold perfusion liquid before the patient is anaesthetised. Bench reconstruction must be performed in order to minimise the anastomosis time, the so-called 'second warm ischaemia period'. This minimises the risk of postoperative acute tubular necrosis, and optimises the results of microvascular anastomoses. Optical magnification systems are essential for best results and a fibre-optic headlamp may be useful to illuminate the critical area of the operating field.

The kidney is placed in a shallow basin of cold perfusion liquid and ice. If a Carrel patch is not available, one or two renal arteries may be anastomosed end-to-side to the larger one (Fig. 9.1d), using running or interrupted monofilament sutures of 8/0 or 9/0 polypropylene, according to the diameter of the vessels [2]. Depending on anatomical considerations or the presence of arterial disease, a biological or semi-biological patch can be employed for an end-to-side anastomosis of one or multiple arteries (Fig. 9.1e), using simple devices as vascular shields [3].

In the case of two renal arteries of equal diameter originating close together on the donor aorta, a less satisfactory option consists in suturing them together to obtain a common trunk.

Standard transplant procedure

The kidney transplant should be made in a surgical room with laminar airflow ventilation with high-efficiency particulate air-filtered air to reduce risk of infection.

The kidney transplant is placed heterotopically and extraperitoneally in the lower abdomen. The side of transplantation is pre-operatively selected on the basis of a previously failed transplant, dampened femoral/ peripheral pulses or according to the Doppler ultrasonography findings. The right iliac fossa is generally preferred, as in such location the right iliac vein is generally more superficial. However, some surgeons continue to use the side contralateral to the donor kidney, in order to have the renal pelvis always anterior, so making it easily accessible in case of urologic re-operations. For second transplants, the opposite side to the first one is generally adopted. In the case of further transplants, an intraperitoneal approach may be necessary.

A transparent sterile plastic drape, placed on the operative field after skin preparation with an iodine-containing solution, prevents contamination.

Two cutaneous incisions may be used in the lower quadrant of the abdomen for placing the new kidney into the recipient iliac fossa: the 'hockey-stick' approach in the lower abdomen, which is parallel to the lateral border of the rectus muscle and allows minimal muscle splitting, and the Gibson-like approach in the pelvis, which extends from 1 cm above the symphysis pubis to about 2 cm medial to the anterior superior iliac spine and allows a better exposure of the iliac vessels, facilitates the location of a big graft and moreover enables implantation of very short ureter to the bladder, maintaining a good ureteric blood supply.

The external oblique muscle and fascia are cut in line with the skin incision, the internal oblique, transversus abdominis muscles and transversalis fascia are divided simultaneously on the rectus sheath with electrocautery, and the peritoneum is reflected cephalad and medially. The iliac vessels are exposed in the retroperitoneum.

It is seldom necessary to remove a non-functioning kidney to make room for the new organ or to eliminate a potential source of infection, as nephrectomy is generally made as elective surgical procedure at least 1 month before transplantation to minimise the stress of transplant operation, to prevent intraoperative hypotension with risk of delayed graft function and to eliminate infections before immunosuppression begins. However, occasionally during the waiting time a polycystic kidney may become so large as to occupy the lower abdominal quadrant: in this case, a nephrectomy may be performed at the time of transplant operation using the same iliac incision to prevent compression of the new kidney. Less invasive approach to create space, such as draining cysts, are now practically abandoned, because of potential risk of infection.

The iliac vessels are wrapped by lymphatics, which must be ligated using non-absorbable fine stitches before dividing them to prevent the development of lymphoceles. Another surgical skill useful to minimise the incidence of lymphocele consists in dissecting the external iliac vessels as little as possible and never above the lymph nodes that underlie the inguinal ligament.

The inferior epigastric vessels are ligated and divided. An exception to this is when the inferior epigastric artery is used to perfuse a lower polar artery that was harvested without an aortic patch. In females, the round ligament is ligated and interrupted to prevent potential compression of the transplanted ureter, as well as the spermatic cord in males, if it crosses the operative field, otherwise the spermatic cord may be retracted medially.

The key surgical risk is incurred in the dissection of the external iliac vein and ligature of its tiny tributary veins or internal iliac vein.

Placement of mechanical auto-retractors should avoid traction or compression of lateral femoral cutaneous and femoral nerves to prevent neuropraxias.

Vascular anastomoses

During the vascular anastomoses, the kidney must be completely wrapped in gauze, kept wet by continuous irrigation of cold solution to minimise the effect of second warm ischaemia time. Vascular anastomoses are made easier by maintaining the kidney hung with a tape.

Renal vein–iliac vein anastomosis

The deeper venous anastomosis is usually performed first, in order to avoid traction on the kidney and tearing of the vein wall, taking care that the adventitia does not intrude into the vessel lumen to avoid vascular thrombosis. The external iliac vein is generally adopted, exposing it according to the principle of traction and counter traction; a silicone vessel loop can be passed around and used for retraction during dissection.

The division of the posterior tributaries and hypogastric vein allows a maximum mobility with superficialisation of the iliac vein, makes the venous anastomosis easier and prevents tearing of the renal vein wall, particularly in the presence of a short right vein.

Proximal and distal soft jaw vascular clamps are applied to the external iliac vein and a linear venotomy of the approximate size of the renal vein is made using a No. 15 scalpel blade and the lumen is flushed with 1% heparin solution. The venotomy is extended to the appropriate length using Pott vascular scissors and the venous anastomosis is constructed, passing two double-needle 6/0 polypropylene sutures at each of the corners of the donor renal vein and the external recipient iliac vein. A third temporary stitch is applied at the back row of the anastomosis before tying the two corner sutures by the so-called 'triangulation

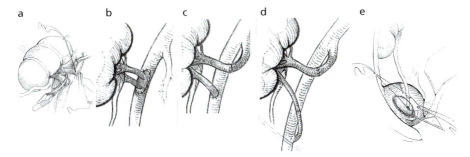

Figure 9.2 (a) A delicate vascular clamp is applied to the renal vein cephalad to the anastomosis to allow the removal of venous clamps from the external iliac vein, during the anastomosis of the donor renal artery to recipient arterial iliac vessels. (b) End-to-side anastomosis of a Carrel patch with two renal arteries to the external iliac artery. (c) End-to-side anastomosis of a renal artery to external iliac artery, and end-to-end anastomosis of a second renal artery to hypogastric artery. (d) End-to-end-anastomosis of a tiny lower polar artery to the recipient inferior epigastric artery. (e) Extravesical uretero-cystoneostomy with a small opening on the bladder dome. Reproduced from Vegeto A, Berardinelli L. (1999) *Il Trapianto di Rene*, with permission from UTET, Periodici Scientifici, Torino.

technique' to prevent inadvertent injury to the back wall. A running over-and-over stitch is then used, beginning from the two corners of the suture and tying the everting sutures at the midpoint. The kidney is then rotated to the other side, the temporary retraction stitch is removed and the suture is completed in the same fashion from both angles.

At this point, a delicate Fogarty clamp may be applied to the renal vein, cephalad the anastomosis (Fig. 9.2a) to allow the removing of venous clamps from the external iliac vein, in order to restore the venous flow of the lower limb during the arterial anastomosis, reducing the risk of formation of clots in the lower limb, potentially leading to pulmonary embolism. This also avoids the arterial hypotension that can occur with simultaneous, sudden reflow to arterial and venous beds. Moreover, the manoeuvres for the arterial anastomosis are made easier.

Alternative techniques for venous anastomosis

In some patients, insufficient venous outflow or external iliac vein thrombosis is observed at operation, owing to previous venous catheterisations for urgent dialysis through the great veins of the leg. In these cases, no attempt must be made to restore the blood flux into the external iliac vein and the venous outflow is searched for cephalad, using the recipient common iliac vein or inferior vena cava. In this case, a partial occlusion with a Satinski, Glover or Lambert-Kay clamp is advocated during the venous anastomosis, to prevent formation of distal clots, pulmonary embolism and acidosis. A bench elongation of the renal vein is particularly useful in these cases.

In the presence of two renal veins of similar diameter, a patch of deceased donor vena cava with multiple veins may be employed for a single anastomosis. Two separate venous anastomoses are also possible, whenever a bench reconstruction has not been made previously. A less satisfactory option consists in a side-to-side suture of the two veins to obtain a single trunk for anastomosis. If the diameter of the multiple veins is quite different, the smaller ones can be, in general, safely ligated, as the venous drainage of the kidney is widely interconnecting, unlike the arterial vascular supply. However, if the graft after reperfusion becomes tight and darkish, and excessive bleeding from renal capsular/hilar vessels is observed, venous hypertension may be suspected. In this case, the smaller vein(s) may be anastomosed to the iliac vein or on the first one, after its partial clamping, to avoid risk of thrombosis or graft rupture.

Renal artery anastomosis

The arterial site for anastomosis depends on the vascular anatomy of the graft and of the recipient, as well as on the preference of the surgeon. In the early transplant experience, the DD renal artery was anastomosed end-to-end to the recipient internal iliac (or hypogastric) artery, using the triangulation technique (Fig. 9.2a). This one remains as an optional technique when the donor source is a living donor or in case the kidney had been harvested from the DD without an aortic patch. A vascular clamp is placed on the proximal origin of the hypogastric artery and its distal end is double-ligated, placing a transfixing non-absorbable vascular stitch above the bifurcation of the superior gluteal artery. The dissection of the hypogastric artery must be extended to the distal common iliac artery and to the proximal external iliac artery to mobilise it sufficiently and avoid kinking of the hypogastric artery. The 6/0 double-needle polypropylene stitches are typically placed from the outside to the inside so that the needle may pass through the intimal surface of the host vessel, pressing the host intima against the media to prevent atheromatous plaque disruption or dislocation. However, the use of the hypogastric artery is now discouraged, as its transaction may contribute to erectile dysfunction in males after transplantation, especially in the presence of occlusive atherosclerotic disease or bilateral section should a re-transplantation be needed.

Today, the choice option for arterial anastomosis is the use of the external (or common) iliac artery for an end-to-side anastomosis of the aorta Carrel patch with one or more (Fig. 9.2b) renal arteries, using a procedure identical to the one used for the venous anastomosis, thus minimising the dissection of the lymphatic vessels, shortening the operating time, preventing stenosis and providing a common patch for multiple arteries.

Alternative techniques for anastomosing multiple or diseased arteries

Uraemic patients are prone to atherosclerotic disease, and kidneys coming from older DDs may present heavy atherosclerosis. The presence of atherosclerosis and multiple or diseased arteries may require alternative techniques and the use of common iliac artery or the distal aorta.

Atherosclerotic plaques producing stenosis and ulceration of the intima must be treated by endarterectomy. The atheromatous plaque is dissected away from the iliac artery by establishing a plane in the layer between media and adventitia using a Freer septum elevator. Optical magnification provides an accurate view. The atherosclerotic plaque is divided at its proximal end and divided in such a way that it remains proximally tightly attached to the arterial wall. Sharp scissors may be used to remove the plaque. Care should be taken to ensure that the remaining intima distally is tightly adherent to the arterial wall. When required, tacking Kunlin stitches may be used to prevent intimal flap elevation and arterial thrombosis.

Sometimes, especially in small children, the renal parenchyma becomes mottled after revascularisation, owing to arterial spasm, which can generally be solved by topical application of warm saline, 2% xylocaine solution and intravenous administration of dopamine (2–4 mg/kg/min).

Approximately 25% of all kidneys present multiple arteries that should be anastomosed, because the arterial system of the kidney is not interconnected. Failure to recognise and/or revascularise multiple renal arteries may cause ureteric necrosis, parenchymal infarction or calyceal-cutaneous fistula, resulting in urological complications, infection and hypertension.

Upper polar renal arteries can be ligated if they feed less than 10% of the renal parenchyma.

A variety of 'direct revascularisation techniques' may be adopted to anastomose multiple arteries using one or more patches of aorta for end-to-side anastomosis to the external/common iliac artery and/or end-to-end to hypogastric artery, adopting various combinations (Fig. 9.2c). Sometimes, serious urological complications due to a lower polar artery that had not been noted at donor nephrectomy and at pre-operative inspection of the graft can be prevented by anastomosing it end-to-end to the recipient inferior epigastric artery (Fig. 9.2d).

However, in case the renal arteries have been harvested individually without aortic patches, the best option, as already mentioned, remains the reconstruction at bench prior to transplantation with microsurgical techniques.

Reperfusion of the kidney graft

Before restoring renal perfusion with the recipient's blood, systolic arterial pressure should be over 120 mmHg and CVP over 12 mmHg. The renal vein and distal artery clamps are sequentially removed to avoid air embolus in the transplanted kidney and check for leakage. In case of blood leakage, oxidised cellulose may be useful to control haemostasis. If major leakage is expected, owing to recipient vascular atherosclerosis/calcifications or coagulation disorders, PEG should be applied before the clamps are removed or fibrin glue after revascularisation.

Adequate intravascular volume and stable haemodynamics allow the new kidney to become firm and pink immediately, with urine output in the first few minutes. Transient compression of the renal vein and of the distal external iliac artery may be useful in the case of poor perfusion of the kidney.

Reconstruction of the lower urinary tract

The preferred method for restoring urinary tract continuity is the ureteroneocystostomy and its modifications. However, several other methods are available for restoring urinary tract continuity, such as uretero-ureterostomy, pyelo-ureterostomy, pyelo-pyelostomy and other techniques for restoring the urinary drainage of the abnormal urinary tract.

Extravesical uretero-cystoneostomy

The extravesical approach originally described by Gregoir [4] and Lich for the correction of vesicoureteral reflux has become very popular, initially described for renal transplantation by MacKinnon in 1968 [5]. It is now the preferred technique, as a smaller cystotomy is made (Fig. 9.2e), reducing the risk of wide opening of the bladder, urinary fistula and bladder bleeding. Moreover, this approach is quicker and simpler than the Politano-Leadbetter technique [6,7] and, most importantly, requires the shortest length of ureter, with the advantage of avoiding distal ureteral ischaemia with consequent ureteral fistulae and stenoses. The only disadvantage is that reflux is perhaps more common in the case of a defunctionalised bladder, where a shorter submucosal ureteral tunnel is undertaken.

Then the bladder is closed and a prevesical drain with a closed system is left for 4–5 days.

The intravesical ureteroneocystostomy prevents reflux, but this approach is unsuitable for very small or scarred bladders, and increases the risks of wound infection due to contamination, cystotomy breakdown, postoperative haematuria and urinary fistulae.

Ureter-ureter, pyelo-ureter, pyelo-pyelo anastomoses

These alternative techniques are generally used as a second option whenever the ureteroneocystotomy cannot be employed owing to damage of the donor ureter at nephrectomy or if it is absolutely impossible to use a minimal capacity/very frail or scarred bladder. However, in patients who have been anuric for several years, it is advisable to confirm satisfactory drainage of the recipient ureter by injection of diluted (1:1000) methylene blue into the lumen. The recipient ureter (or pelvis) may be used to re-establish the urinary tract continuity, when it is healthy and non-refluxing, for an end-to-end anastomosis to the remnant donor ureter (or pelvis), using a 7/0 polydioxanone two running sutures after having introduced a double J stent.

The ipsilateral kidney can either be removed or left in place after ligation of the proximal recipient ureter, if the patient has been anuric for long and there is no other indication for nephrectomy [8].

More frequent ureteral complications associated with these techniques, and risk of arteritis due to contiguity to vascular anastomosis, outweigh the potential advantages, which include a sufficient blood supply to proximal donor and distal recipient ureter, limited dissection for isolation of the bladder and no contamination from the bladder opening.

Particular problems in re-establishment of abnormal urinary tract continuity

Double ureter

Two separate collecting systems are generally fed by the same blood supply that flows between the double ureters, and care must be taken to avoid damage at nephrectomy. Two separate ureteroneocystostomies with a single submucosal tunnel represents the best technique to follow, taking care to avoid damage to ureteral blood supply, rather than anastomosing one of the two ureters to the side of the other ureter.

Lower urinary tract dysfunctions and neurogenic bladder

Even a very small, scarred bladder can recover its compliance and normal function after transplantation, and urologic evaluation is not necessary in a transplant candidate who is continent without obstructive symptoms and has sterile urine cultures. However, characterisation of bladder dysfunction is a key element in considering the patient as candidate for transplantation. A voiding cystourethrogram, cystoscopy and urodynamic testing may be required to predict the results of pre-transplant surgical correction and the impact on graft outcome. The urodynamic results refer to the four Cs: capacity of the bladder reservoir, compliance of the bladder, contractility of the detrusor muscles and sphincter, and continence. Lower urinary tract sensation and evacuation with possible presence of post-void residual are also investigated.

The most difficult lower urinary tract problems are found in neurogenic bladder disease, owing to neurospinal dysraphisms or other acquired neurological conditions, that should be corrected at least 3 months before transplantation with a strict, coordinated interaction of transplant surgeon and urologist.

Implantation of the transplant ureter into the native bladder, even though enlarged is always preferred; however, patients whose lower urinary tract has been diverted into an ileal conduit can also be considered candidates for transplantation, without reversal of the urinary tract diversion if the urinary abnormalities cannot be corrected with other techniques.

Bladder augmentation

The urologic treatments of neurologic bladder dysfunction aim to obtain a continent, low-pressure storage container. Bladder enlargement using various techniques is a reliable means of increasing bladder capacity and reducing intravesical pressure [9]. Preserved detrusor elasticity and satisfactory management of bladder emptying are prerequisites for success.

Bladder augmentation can be obtained by the use of intestinal segments [10], such as ileum or colon; long-term complications of these enterocystoplasties include bacterial colonisation, increased incidence of urinary tract infections, metabolic acidosis, mucus production, vitamin B_{12} deficiency and somatic growth retardation. The stomach may also be adopted as an alternative [11], especially in children, owing to lower mucus production, reduced bacterial colonisation and reduced incidence of urinary tract infections. Typical complications are metabolic alkalosis and haematuria-dysuria syndrome [12]. After operation many surgical complications may arise [13]. Bladder augmentation may also be made using techniques that preserve the urothelium, such as ureterocystoplasty using a megaureter in the presence of non-functioning kidney [14] and seromuscular colocystoplasty: the advantages of these procedures, which in addition can be employed using a lower morbidity retroperitoneal approach, consist in avoiding electrolyte imbalances and mucus production. However, whichever technique is used, bladder emptying is generally impaired and most patients require clean self-intermittent catheterisation after enterocystoplasty, through the native urethra or through a Mitrofanoff procedure with a flap-valve mechanism. In the latter case, the catheterising stoma must be placed in the lower quadrant of the abdomen through the rectus muscle and below the 'bikini line' for a better quality of life.

Ileal conduit

The enteric bladder, generally obtained using the standard Bricker loop of terminal ileum with an external ileostomy and previously used for native ureter diversion, can be adopted for anastomosis of the transplant ureter too. The ileal conduit is also useful in patients with neurogenic bladder dysfunction who are unwilling or unable to perform self-catheterisation. Before transplantation takes place, the patency of the loop should be ensured with a radiopaque 'loopgram'.

After revascularisation of the kidney, using the usual retroperitoneal approach, a 22–24 Fr Foley catheter is passed into the catheterising stoma to reach the proximal end of the loop, the transplant ureter is spatulated and anastomosed to the loop proximal end, creating a watertight mucosa-to-mucosa apposition with interrupted fine (6/0) delayed absorbable sutures. An antireflux tunnel may be constructed on the ileum and an ureteral single J stent may be left in place.

Cutaneous ureterostomy

Is some cases where the bladder is missing or cannot be used, the ureterostoma can be performed. Sometimes, this technique requires kidney graft to be upside-down, and the ureter is tunnelled through muscle layers and anastomosed to the skin as a stoma, and a JJ stent is used to prevent stoma strictures.

Dual kidney transplantation

The surgical techniques of transplant procedures may vary for kidneys coming from ECDs, which are at higher risk for delayed graft function, owing to older donor age, higher donor serum creatinine at organ retrieval, history of hypertension in the donor and cerebrovascular accident as the cause of brain death. The cold ischaemia time should be in these cases as short as possible to reduce the risk of delayed graft function. Nevertheless, many kidneys from older ECDs are discarded, fearing inadequate function in the recipients. In these cases, the two-for-one-approach using dual kidney transplantation has been advocated, in order to overcome the reduced nephron mass of a single marginal kidney, using as decisive criteria the donor creatinine clearance (less than 65 mL/min), age over 60 years, presence of renal disease such as diabetes or significant histologic damage on the biopsy specimen taken at the time of organ retrieval (>20% glomerulosclerosis of both kidneys as determined by frozen-section biopsy).

One kidney may be placed in each iliac fossa using the standard technique through the conventional iliac incision, or through unique single midline incision.

Alternatively, both kidneys may be placed into the same iliac fossa, according to Masson's technique [15], implanting first the right kidney to the recipient vena cava and common iliac artery and then, after revascularisation of the right kidney, the left kidney by standard technique. However, some risks are increased in the recipient of dual transplantation, owing to an increase in preservation time that influences the immediate recovery of the graft, prolonged anaesthesia time in a recipient who is often old and technical complications that may double compared with a single kidney transplant. Against dual kidney transplantation are the better results obtained with single transplants from older donors, when compared with dual transplants, reported in large series and the uncertain role of the renal biopsy/glomerular filtration values for predicting the future outcome of the graft [16]. Moreover, an incorrect policy of dual kidney transplantation may halve, rather than increase, the number of available kidneys. This controversy remains to be resolved.

Transplantation of paediatric kidneys 'en bloc'

Paediatric kidneys should not be transplanted separately but en bloc. They should be retrieved together with a segment of aorta and inferior vena cava. Such a graft should be preferably transplanted to an adult recipient. The upper end of the aorta and inferior vena cava is closed, and the lower end is anatomosed to iliac vessels end-to side. Common complications after such a transplant can be kinking of the graft vessels or rupture of the kidney(s) because of hypertension.

Horseshoe kidneys

In this rare renal abnormality, the lower poles of the two kidneys are joined, forming an isthmus, and the axis of the kidneys is shifted towards the lumbosacral vertebrae.

The horseshoe kidney often has vascular and urological anomalies; therefore it is rarely used for transplantation, because of a fear of increased complications. Nevertheless, organ shortage has driven the use of horseshoe kidneys for transplantation, either for en-bloc transplantation in a single recipient or, after isthmectomy, for transplantation into two recipients, with good outcomes.

References

1. Benedetti E, Fryer J, Matas AJ, *et al.* (1994) Kidney transplantation outcome with and without right renal vein extension. *Clin Transplant* **8**, 416.
2. Vegeto A, Berardinelli L. (1999) *Il Trapianto di Rene*. UTET, Periodici Scientifici, Torino.
3. Berardinelli L, Vegeto A. (1978) A simple vascular shield for microanastomoses. *Am J Surg* **134**, 127.
4. Gregoir W, van Regemorter G. (1968) Le reflux vescicoureteral congenital. *Urol Int* **18**, 122.
5. MacKinnon KJ, Oliver JA, Morehouse DD, *et al.* (1968) Cadaver renal transplantation: Emphasis on urological aspects. *J Urol* **99**, 486.
6. Politano VA, Leadbetter WF. (1958) An operative technique for the correction of vescico-ureteral reflux. *J Urol* **79**, 932.
7. Leadbetter GW, Monaco AP, Russell PS. (1966) A technique for reconstruction of the urinary tract in renal transplantation. *Surg Ginecol Obstet* **123**, 839.
8. Jaffers GJ, Cosimi AB, Delmonico FL, *et al.* (1982) Experience with pyeloureterostomy in renal transplantation. *Ann Surg* **196**, 588.
9. Duel BP, Gonzalez R, Barthold JS. (1999) Alternative techniques for augmentation cystoplasty. *J Urol* **159**, 998.
10. Gough DCS. (2001) Enterocystoplasty. *BJU Int* **88**, 739.
11. Close CE. (2001) Autoaugmentation gastrocystoplasty. *BJU Int* **88**,757.
12. Nguyen DH, Bain MA, Salmonson KL, *et al.* (1993) The syndrome of dysuria and hematuria in pediatric urinary reconstruction with stomach. *J Urol* **150**, 707.
13. Shekarriz B, Upadhyay J, Demirbilek S, *et al.* (2000) Surgical complications of bladder augmentation: Comparison between various enterocystoplasties in 133 patients. *Urology* **55**, 123.
14. Bellinger MF. (1993) Ureterocystoplasty: A unique method for vescical augmentation in children. *J Urol* **149**, 811.
15. Masson D, Hefty T. (1998) A technique for the transplantation of two adult cadaver kidney grafts into one recipient. *J Urol* **160**, 1779.
16. Dahmane D, Audrad V, Hiesse C, *et al.* (2006) Retrospective follow-up of transplantation of kidneys from marginal donors. *Kidney Int* **69**, 546.

10 Living donor kidney transplantation

Jiří Froněk and Nicos Kessaris

Introduction

The first successful kidney transplantation was carried out in 1954 in Boston by Joseph Murray. This was a live donor transplant between identical twins. Currently, more than 1000 live donor transplants occur in the UK annually. The surgical technique of live donor kidney transplantation differs little from that for deceased donors, but there are some important differences. The main difference is absence of a patch for the arterial anastomosis. This is especially important when multiple arteries are present on the kidney graft, as multiple anastomoses are required. **Colour versions of all figures used in this chapter appear on the website that accompanies this book, at www.wiley.com/go/macphee/transplantation.**

Bench-table kidney-graft preparation

After the graft has been removed from the donor it must be immediately flushed via the renal artery/arteries using cold preservation solution (Figs 10.1 and 10.2). If there is any residual fat on the surface of the kidney, this must be removed to fully assess the surface of the kidney. The ureter should be kept long enough for the anastomosis but not too long, as this may cause ischaemic ureteric stricture. This is because the blood supply to the distal ureter is derived from the bladder. Both artery/arteries and vein/veins must be dissected long enough to enable the creation of the anastomoses and the placement of clamps for testing the anastomosis before reperfusion. The hilum and pelvis should not be touched. Some fat is always left there, as dissection in the hilum may cause vascular or pelvic damage. In the case of multiple arteries, some centres prefer to join these together on the bench and perform fewer arterial anastomoses. In the case of multiple veins, the smaller one/ones can be tied off safely. If there are two equal veins, both should be anastomosed. After flushing with preservation solution, the whole graft must change its colour from purple to light yellow. Finally, the quality of the renal vessels is assessed and the length measured and documented (Figs 10.3 and 10.4).

Handbook of Renal and Pancreatic Transplantation, First Edition. Edited by Iain A. M. MacPhee and Jiří Froněk.

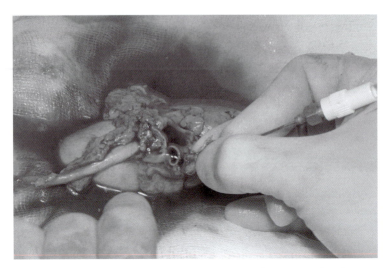

Figure 10.1 Live donor nephrectomy – kidney graft perfusion on the bench via renal artery.

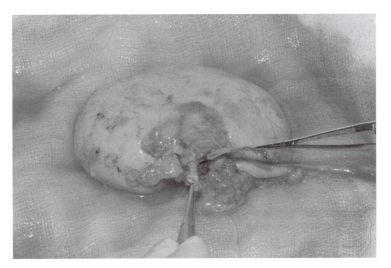

Figure 10.2 Live donor nephrectomy – kidney graft perfusion on the bench via renal artery: performed.

Incision and dissection of blood vessels

An incision, typically oblique or curvilinear, is made in the right or left lower abdominal quadrant (Fig. 10.5). This starts at the level or above the iliac crest and ends in the midline adjacent to the pubic symphysis. Most centres prefer a right-sided incision for the first transplant, as the iliac vessels lie more superficially. The external oblique muscle and fascia are divided as well as the internal oblique and transversus abdominis muscle.

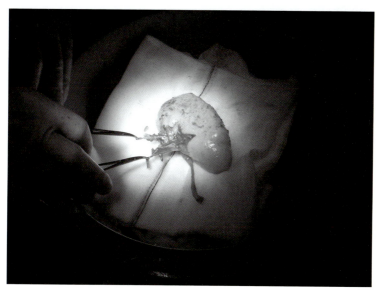

Figure 10.3 Live donor nephrectomy – graft vessels defined.

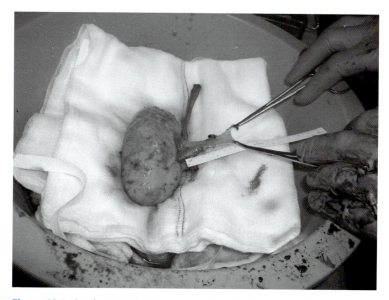

Figure 10.4 Live donor nephrectomy – renal vein length measured.

The peritoneum is pushed towards the midline and up to reveal the iliac vessels (Fig. 10.6). The spermatic cord is preserved, but the round ligament can be divided. Patient consent must be obtained for sacrificing the spermatic cord in cases where the surgeon expects difficult dissection that may cause damage to the cord. The inferior epigastric artery can be preserved for use in some cases of multiple vessels, where it can be

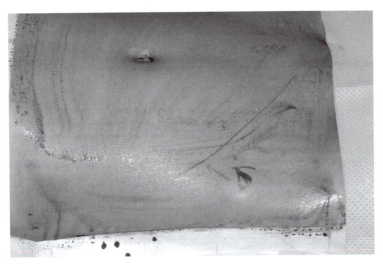

Figure 10.5 Living donor kidney transplantation – recipient's incision marked.

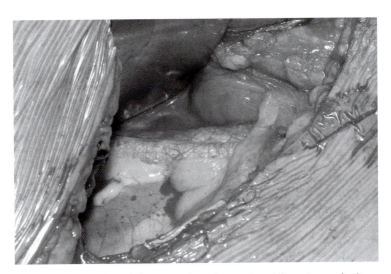

Figure 10.6 Living donor kidney transplantation – external iliac artery and vein identified.

utilised for one of the arterial anastomoses. The main renal vessels are anastomosed to external iliac vessels. Excessive dissection is unnecessary – there should be enough to allow clamping and for performing the anastomosis. During dissection all the lymphatics must be tied to prevent lymphatic leakage and creation of lymphocoele after transplantation (Fig. 10.7). After freeing a segment of roughly 5 cm of external iliac artery and vein, vascular slings are placed behind them (Figs 10.8 and 10.9). The length of the dissected segment depends on the number of graft vessels as well as the quality of the recipient's vessels. The external iliac artery

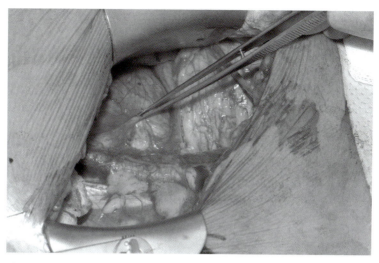

Figure 10.7 Living donor kidney transplantation – lymphatic vessels surrounding iliac vessels.

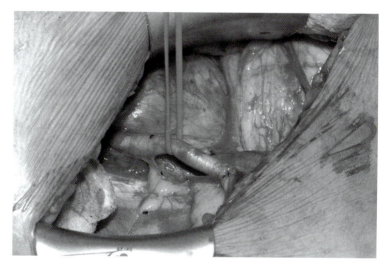

Figure 10.8 Living donor kidney transplantation – external iliac artery dissected.

should always be palpated for calcification. The vascular slings are kept in place until the end of the operation. They can be of help in cases of severe bleeding where the vessel can be lifted and easily found.

Revascularisation – venous anastomosis

The renal vein is anastomosed end-to-side to external iliac vein using 5/0 monofilament non-absorbable suture (Prolene™). On some occasions 6/0

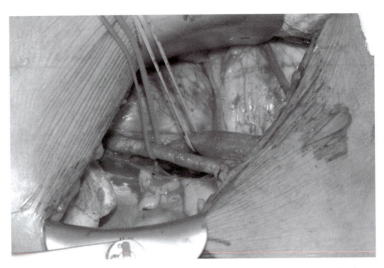

Figure 10.9 Living donor kidney transplantation – external iliac artery and vein dissected.

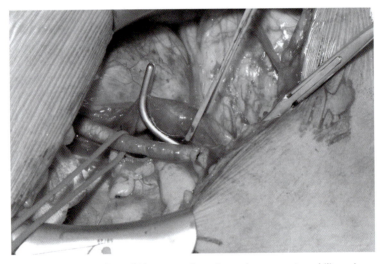

Figure 10.10 Living donor kidney transplantation – clamp on external iliac vein before venotomy.

can also be used. The dissected external iliac vein is lifted on the vascular sling to aid positioning of a Satinski clamp (Fig. 10.10). A venotomy is then performed. This should match the size of the renal vein. Either a two- or a four-corner technique is used for the anastomosis (Figs 10.11 and 10.12). Once this is finished, a baby Debakey clamp is placed on the renal vein above the anastomosis and the Satinski released (Fig. 10.13). This tests the integrity of the anastomosis while preventing blood flow to the kidney at this stage.

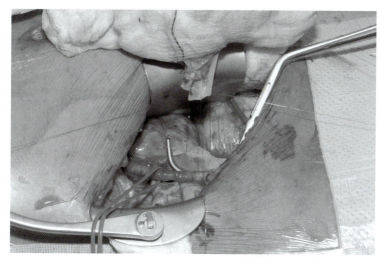

Figure 10.11 Living donor kidney transplantation – creation of renal vein to external iliac vein end-to-side anastomosis – four-corner technique.

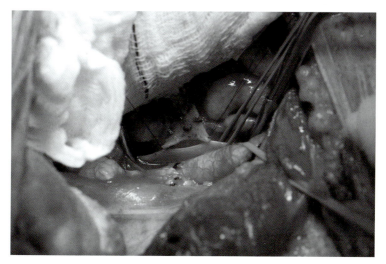

Figure 10.12 Living donor kidney transplantation – creation of renal vein to external iliac vein end-to-side anastomosis – two-corner technique.

Revascularisation – arterial anastomosis

The renal artery is usually anastomosed end-to-side to external iliac artery using 6/0 monofilament non-absorbable suture (Prolene™). The technique of end-to-end anastomosis on the internal iliac artery can be also used. This technique might be useful in multiple artery cases or in cases where for some reason the external iliac artery can not be used. The dissected external iliac artery is gently lifted on the vascular sling, the

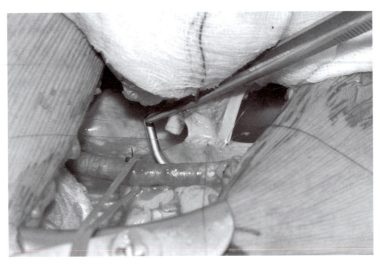

Figure 10.13 Living donor kidney transplantation – renal vein to external iliac vein end-to-side anastomosis created.

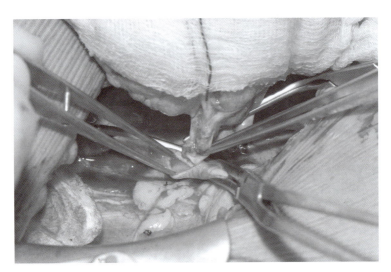

Figure 10.14 Living donor kidney transplantation – arteriotomy of external iliac artery.

Satinski clamp positioned and the arteriotomy performed using a size 11 blade. The size of arteriotomy should match the size of the renal artery. A 2 or 4 mm punch can be used to create a smooth, round ostium (Figs 10.14 and 10.15). Either a two- or four-corner technique is used for the anastomosis. Some centres prefer the parachuting technique using one suture only. Once the arterial anastomosis is finished, a baby Debakey or a bulldog clamp is placed on the renal artery above the anastomosis and the Satinski is released. This tests the integrity of the anastomosis and allows time for extra sutures to control bleeding without the need for

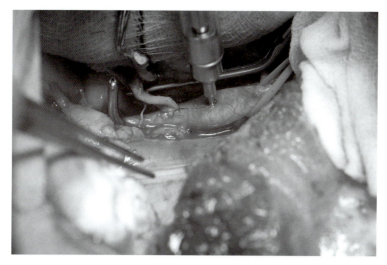

Figure 10.15 Living donor kidney transplantation – arteriotomy and punch ostium creation for renal artery anastomosis.

re-clamping and the risk of warm ischaemia after reperfusion. In the case of multiple arteries, an attempt to anastomose all vessels must be made to prevent loss of kidney parenchyma. These can be either joined together on the bench or anastomosed separately. Joining the arteries together on the bench makes the graft–recipient anastomosis simpler. However, if there is a thrombus, all joint vessels will be lost. The pros and cons of the two different approaches are summarised below.

Multiple artery bench reconstruction

Pros
- fewer graft–recipient anastomoses
- shorter rewarming time

Cons
- possible damage to the wall of the renal artery/arteries
- in the case of thrombosis of a single artery, the whole graft may be lost
- in the case of renal artery stenosis, treatment/stenting may be difficult or impossible

Multiple artery in-vivo reconstruction (Fig. 10.16)

Pros
- each artery can be cut to the right length
- good quality/level for anastomosis can be found
- end-to-end to inferior epigastric artery anastomosis of upper/lower polar artery can be performed (Figs 10.17 and 10.18)
- end-to-end to branches of internal iliac artery can be performed

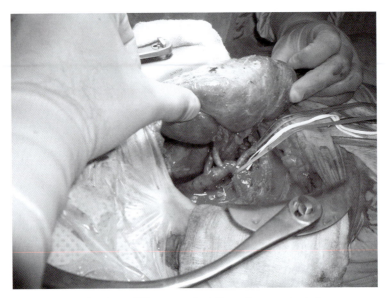

Figure 10.16 Living donor kidney transplantation – three renal arteries anastomosed separately to the external iliac artery in an end-to-side fashion.

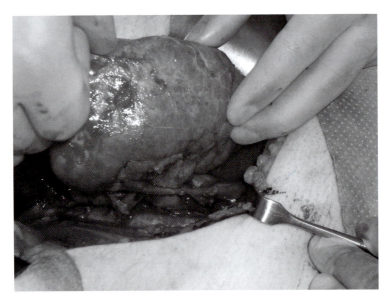

Figure 10.17 Living donor kidney transplantation – upper polar renal artery anastomosed end-to-end to the inferior epigastric artery.

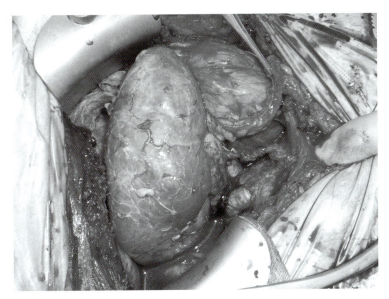

Figure 10.18 Living donor kidney transplantation – lower renal artery anastomosed end-to-end to the inferior epigastric artery.

- in the case of one branch thrombosis the rest of the kidney may still function
- in the case of renal artery stenosis treatment/stenting may be easier

Cons
- longer rewarming time
- more graft–recipient anastomoses
- when the internal iliac artery is utilised, more dissection is required
- if the inferior epigastric artery is used, atrophy of rectus muscle is possible

Before kidney reperfusion, the systolic blood pressure must be above 120 mmHg and all the induction immunosuppression must have been given. After reperfusion, it is useful to fill the wound with reasonably warm saline to allow the microcirculation of the kidney to recover from spasm. In most cases, urine production is observed soon after reperfusion.

Ureteric anastomosis

There are number of different ureteric anastomotic techniques available. These are summarised below. All the described techniques can be used for both live donor as well as deceased donor kidney transplantation.

Uretero-cysto anastomosis – simple, one layer
With this technique the incidence of ureteric complications is 0.5%. The technique is simple and involves anastomosing longitudinally the cut,

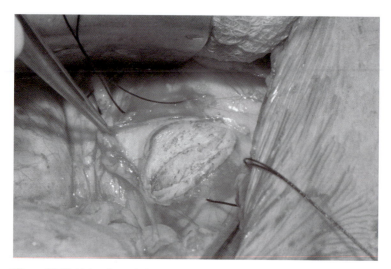

Figure 10.19 Living donor kidney transplantation – bladder wall cut using diathermy; mucosa still intact.

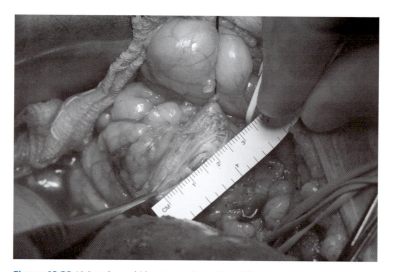

Figure 10.20 Living donor kidney transplantation – bladder wall cut using diathermy and measured; mucosa still intact.

distal end of the ureter down to the top of the bladder using one layer of monofilament absorbable 4/0 suture (PDS) (Figs 10.19–10.27). The anastomosis is usually 3–4 cm in length and involves taking the ureter together with the bladder mucosa and muscle with each suture.

Uretero–cysto anastomosis – antireflux mucosal tunnel

This technique is more difficult and has a higher rate of complications. It involves taking the ureter together with the bladder mucosa with each

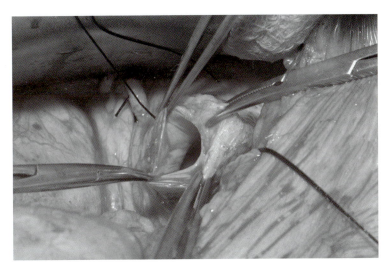

Figure 10.21 Living donor kidney transplantation – bladder opened wide for ureterocystoanastomosis.

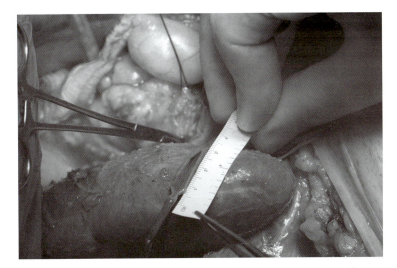

Figure 10.22 Living donor kidney transplantation – graft ureter cut short plus longitudinally.

suture and then creating a muscular tunnel at the top as an antireflux mechanism.

Uretero–uretero anastomosis

Can be used in cases where simple uretero–cysto anastomosis cannot be performed. Using recipient's native ureter is usually simple, with the added advantage of using healthy, unscarred tissue with a good blood supply. This technique may cause unilateral native kidney hydronephrosis

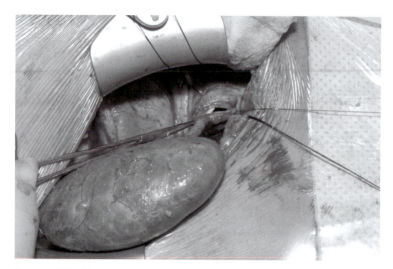

Figure 10.23 Living donor kidney transplantation – ureterocystoanastomosis creation using simple technique I.

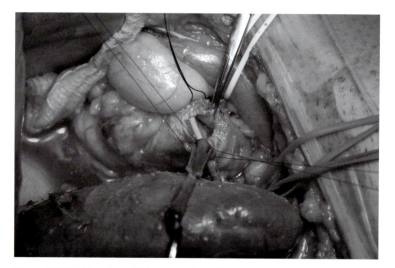

Figure 10.24 Living donor kidney transplantation – ureterocystoanastomosis creation using simple technique II.

in cases where there is still production of native urine. Embolisation of that kidney may be necessary in complicated cases.

Ileal conduit

This technique can be used in cases where the bladder has previously been excised or is damaged. Either a previously performed ileal conduit can be used or new one created using a segment of small bowel. If an old

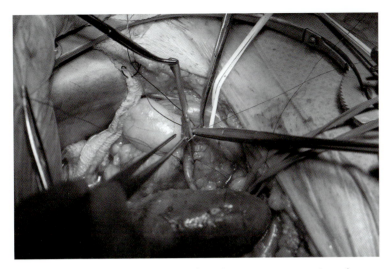

Figure 10.25 Living donor kidney transplantation – ureterocystoanastomosis creation using simple technique III.

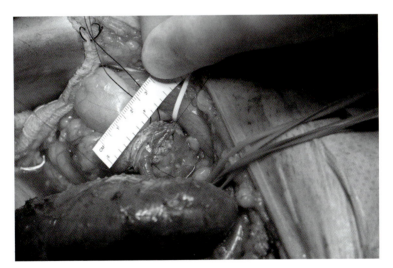

Figure 10.26 Living donor kidney transplantation – ureterocystoanastomosis creation using simple technique IV.

one is used, complications related to the quality of the small bowel may occur. The kidney must be placed upside down to allow for the ureter to be anastomosed to the conduit.

Ureter to skin anastomosis

In some cases where the above options are not possible, a ureterostoma can be performed. This technique requires the kidney graft to be placed

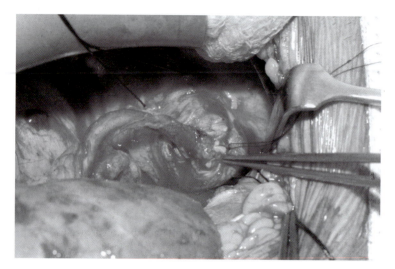

Figure 10.27 Living donor kidney transplantation – ureterocystoanastomosis completed.

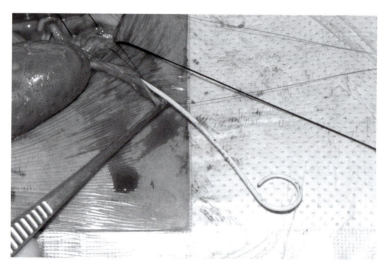

Figure 10.28 Living donor kidney transplantation – JJ stent insertion into the graft ureter.

upside down. The ureter is then tunnelled through the muscle layers and anastomosed to the skin as a stoma. A JJ stent is used to prevent stoma strictures.

Over the years, the techniques have been simplified. Such approaches offer a lower rate of complications. Some centres use double a JJ stent to prevent ureteric complications (Fig. 10.28). The stent is placed intraoperatively during the creation of the ureteric anastomosis and is usually removed 6 weeks after transplantation using cystoscopy.

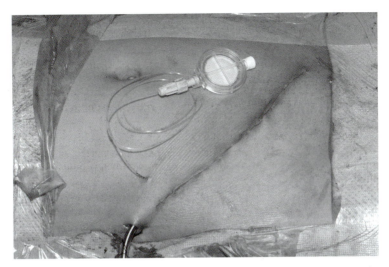

Figure 10.29 Living donor kidney transplantation – renal transplantation wound closed with epidural catheter for local anaesthetic infusion and drain in situ.

Biopsy, drainage and wound closure

After reperfusion the whole kidney must look pink. If part of the graft looks dark/blue, this indicates poor or no arterial blood supply and must be taken seriously and corrected. Unless there is a known clotting abnormality, the whole operation field should be dry with no bleeding. All possible bleeding sources must be stopped using diathermy, tie or clip. A wedge or needle 'time zero' biopsy should be taken and the defect closed with monofilament 5/0 non-absorbable suture. In the majority of cases a suction drain is placed. If the operation field is absolutely dry, a drain may not be necessary. Usually, the drain stays in for 48 hours after surgery. Muscle and fascia layers can be closed using various techniques. One simple way, with good results, is to perform a continuous two-layer monofilament absorbable (PDS loop 1) suture technique with an epidural local anaesthetic catheter placed between the two layers. Subcutaneous fat is apposed with interrupted or continues absorbable suture. The skin is closed using continuous absorbable subcutaneous suture (Fig. 10.29). The wound is covered with semipermeable adhesive dressing, such as tegaderm. This should not be disturbed on the ward, to reduce the risk of infection, unless necessary.

Postoperative care

Postoperatively, the patient is placed in the recovery unit for several hours for monitoring. Most of the patients can return to the ward but some high-risk patients may need more intensive care. In recovery, an ultrasound Doppler scan is performed to make sure there is no problem with blood flow throughout the graft after wound closure. Using this policy, we have detected and salvaged five grafts with perfusion problems after wound closure over a 6-year period. In the case of no flow, reduced flow, non-homogenous flow or a high resistance index, patients must be taken back to theatre for a second look operation. On the ward, urine output and vital signs must be monitored on a regular basis. Fluid replacement should be adjusted to urine output. At St George's Hospital in London, we use the protocol of urine output + 50 mL/hour replacement for patients over 75 kg. For patients below 75 kg we replace urine output + 25 mL/hour.

Two days after surgery, the urinary catheter, drain and local anaesthetic catheter can be removed and the intravenous fluids can be stopped. The usual hospital stay is 4 days after surgery. Following discharge, patients come to clinic three times a week.

Living donor kidney transplantation is elective surgery. All the attempts must be made to get the recipient fit for surgery. Kidney transplantation is not a life-saving procedure; it offers better quality of life to the patients. Any potential cause of morbidity or mortality must be disclosed to the recipient during the work-up. Only a high success rate after live donation as well as live donor transplantation can promote further donation and help the renal patient population.

Key References

1. Merrill LP, Murray JE, Harrison JH, *et al.* (1956) Successful homotransplantations of a human kidney between identical twins. *JAMA* **160**, 277.
2. Lee HM. (1994) Surgical technique of renal transplantation. In: Morris PJ. *Kidney Transplantation: Principles and practice*, 4th edn. WB Saunders, Philadelphia.
3. Odland MD. (1998) Surgical technique/post-transplant surgical complications. *Surg Clin North Am* **78**, 55–58.
4. Morris PJ. (1994) *Kidney Transplantation: Principles and practice*, 4th edn. WB Saunders, Philadelphia.
5. Danovitch GM. (2009) *Handbook of Kidney Transplantation*, 5th edn. Lippincott Williams & Wilkins, Philadelphia.
6. Kessaris N, Papalois V, Canelo R, *et al.* (2010) Live kidney transplantation. In: Hakim N, Canelo R, Papalois V (eds), *Living Related Transplantation*. Imperial College Press, London.
7. Gaston RS, Wadström J. (2005) *Living Donor Kidney Transplantation: Current practices, emerging trends and evolving challenges.* Taylor & Francis, London.
8. Ozremir FN, Ibis A, Altunoglu A, *et al.* (2007) Pretransplantation systolic blood pressure and the risk of delayed graft function in young living-related allograft recipients. *Transplant Proc* **39**, 842–845.
9. Berardinelli L. (2006) Best results in living donor transplantation using and aggressive policy in microsurgical bench reconstruction of nonoptimal arterial supply. *Transplant Proc* **38**, 991–993.

11 Pancreas transplantation

Guido Woeste and Wolf O. Bechstein

Simultaneous pancreas kidney (SPK) transplantation is considered to be a life-saving therapy for type 1 diabetics with concomitant end-stage kidney disease [1,2]. Pancreas after kidney (PAK) transplantation is performed in lower numbers. Regarding the excellent results of living donor kidney (LDK) transplantation, pancreas transplantation after LDK (PALK) offers the advantages of a living donor kidney with shorter duration of dialysis and a functional pancreas. An analysis of data from the United Network for Organ Sharing (UNOS) showed that PALK was associated with better kidney graft and patient survival compared with SPK, but the pancreas graft survival was inferior (80% versus 86% pancreas graft survival after 1 year). Despite worse pancreas survival, no significant difference in mortality rates was noted. Patients with type 1 diabetes with a potential living donor can be considered for living donor kidney followed by pancreas transplant. Pancreas transplantation alone, prior to presence of diabetic nephropathy, is performed very rarely and is indicated only for patients with severe problems in managing their diabetes (e.g. hypoglycaemic unawareness).

From 16 December 1966 to 31 December 2008 more than 30,000 pancreas transplants have been reported to the International Pancreas Transplant Registry, including more than 22,000 from the USA and more than 9000 from outside the USA [3]. After a constant increase in the number of pancreas transplants, the overall number started to decrease in 2002. Although pancreas transplantation has even been performed sporadically in patients with type 2 diabetes, this disease is not yet accepted to be a proven indication for pancreas transplantation [4].

Indication and diagnostics

Definition

Diabetes mellitus type 1 is an autoimmune disease with antibodies against islet cell antigens GAD, ICA and IA-2. Onset is usually in childhood and youth. Owing to destruction of all islet cells of the pancreas, there is no insulin secretion. By contrast, type 2 diabetics show

Handbook of Renal and Pancreatic Transplantation, First Edition. Edited by Iain A. M. MacPhee and Jiří Froněk.
© 2012 John Wiley & Sons, Ltd. Published 2012 by John Wiley & Sons, Ltd.

preserved or even increased insulin secretion with underlying peripheral insulin resistance.

Diagnosis

Diagnosis of diabetes
The verification of type 1 diabetes can be performed by measuring the islet cell antibodies Anti-GAD, -ICA and -IA-2. In the case of negative antibodies with typical clinical appearance of juvenile onset diabetes, the absence of secretion of c-peptide after stimulation of the pancreas can prove the loss of insulin secretion.

Assessment before transplantation
For identifying possible contraindications, clinical history, physical examination and investigations are required to identify diabetic long-term complications such as arteriosclerosis (carotid artery, coronary artery disease (CAD) and peripheral artery disease), polyneuropathy and retinopathy. The examinations required for evaluation of a pancreas transplant candidate are listed in Table 11.1.

The major cause of death after SPK is cardiac death due to CAD caused by myocardial infarction or arrhythmia [3]. The assessment of CAD is therefore the major concern in pre-transplant evaluation. Some centres require a coronary angiogram for all patients before entering the waiting list for SPK. As some patients are evaluated pre-emptively before the onset of dialysis, there are concerns about impairment of renal function by giving contrast media, precipitating the need for dialysis. In our algorithm we perform a cardiac stress test (echocardiography or myocardial scintigram with medical stress) for assessment of myocardial ischaemia.

Advanced arteriosclerosis with circular calcification, especially in diabetic patients, may cause severe problems during the transplant and should be ruled out in advance. Remarkably, an angiogram of the iliac

Table 11.1 The examinations required for evaluation of a pancreas transplant candidate.

Organ	Exam
Heart	ECG, echocardiography, cardiac stress test (in case of pathologic findings: coronary angiography)
Vascular	Doppler ultrasound of carotid artery, iliac artery and lower limb
Lung	Function test (lung capacity, FEV1)
Blood	Blood type, coagulation (screening for prothrombotic disorders)
Immune system	Viral test (HBV, HCV, CMV, EBV, VZV, HSV) HLA-typing, definition of HLA antibody specificities

CMV, cytomegalovirus; EBV, Epstein–Barr virus; ECG, electrocardiogram; FEV1, forced expiratory volume in the first second; HBV, hepatitis B virus; HCV, hepatitis C virus; HSV, herpes simplex virus; VZV, varicella roster virus.

vessels can show normal vascular lumen without relevant stenosis even in the presence of severe calcification. Calcification of the pelvic vessels is better demonstrated by plain radiography of the pelvis. In the case of calcification, a computerised tomography (CT) scan of the pelvis without contrast media with three-dimensional reconstruction can be very helpful to get an impression of the vessels.

One of the main reasons for pancreas graft failure is venous thrombosis. During the first visit the patient's history should be checked for a possible thrombotic disorder (history of deep vein thrombosis, thrombosis of dialysis access). In the case of a positive history, hypercoagulability screening should be performed, including protein S, protein C, activated protein C (APC) resistance, factor V Leiden and antiphospholipid syndrome [5].

Indication

Simultaneous pancreas kidney transplantation
The indication for SPK is mostly for type 1 diabetics with end-stage renal failure. Pre-emptive transplantation before the need for dialysis results in the best outcomes. There is no consensus about the right time for listing for transplantation. Admitting a patient to a waiting list below a creatinine clearance of 20 mL/min is undisputed. However, some centres have a threshold below 40 mL/min for registration for SPK.

In the following text, we refer to type 1 diabetic patients with advanced renal failure, if not otherwise specified. The advanced renal failure is just one of many characteristics of the late diabetic syndrome. Further diabetic complications such as retinopathy, peripheral and autonomic polyneuropathy, and macro- and microangiopathy occur frequently in diverse sites. An improvement of these complications (except neuropathy) cannot be expected, but with restoration of normal glucose metabolism after pancreas transplantation with physiologic euglycemia the progression of these complications can be slowed down or even stopped [6]. Patients younger than 50 years of age show the greatest benefit from SPK. Therefore, older age is considered a contraindication.

Further contraindications for both pancreas and kidney transplantation are:
- severe cardiopulmonary disease such as advanced CAD with reduced left ventricular function and chronic obstructive lung disease with reduced pulmonary capacity
- untreated or metastatic malignant disease
- active or untreated chronic infections; with the use of highly active antiretroviral therapy (HAART), HIV infection no longer constitutes a contraindication to transplantation when patients show undetectable HIV RNA for 3 months and CD4+ T-cell count of more than 200 cells/µL [7]).

Pancreas after kidney transplantation
PAK requires good renal allograft function. A creatinine clearance above 80 mL/min is mandatory, and SPK instead of PAK should be considered

where creatinine clearance is below 40 mL/min. The range of 40 to 80 mL/min requires careful consideration on a case-by-case basis.

Pancreas transplantation alone

Pancreas transplantation alone is performed rarely. Possible indications are life-threatening, recurrent hypoglycemic episodes not recognised by the patient due to hypoglycemic unawareness or rapid progression of non-renal diabetic complications (neuropathy, retinopathy). The decision for PTA is even more demanding, as lifelong immunosuppressive therapy with potential nephrotoxicity has to be initiated in contrast to SPK and PAK where the immunosuppression is required to maintain kidney graft function.

Surgical therapy in general

Today pancreas transplantation is always performed using the whole organ with a concomitant duodenal patch. Transplantation of a segmental pancreas or the gland with only a small peripapillar duodenal fragment is of historical interest and no longer used.

The following technical options are common today:
- arterial anastomosis
  - vascular reconstruction with donor iliac Y-graft (splenic artery – internal iliac artery, superior mesenteric artery – external iliac artery)
  - aortic patch of celiac trunk and superior mesenteric artery
- portal venous anastomosis
  - systemic – venous (vena cava)
  - portal – venous (branch of mesenteric vein)
- exocrine drainage
  - enteric (small bowel or duodenum)
  - bladder.

The different techniques can be mixed with one exclusion: bladder drainage cannot be performed with portal-venous drainage owing to technical factors. Furthermore, the placement of the pancreas graft can be variable: head-down/tail-up or head-up/tail-down. The pancreas graft can be placed intraperitoneally or retroperitoneally behind the right colon [8].

Pancreas transplantation with systemic-venous and enteric drainage

This is the most frequently used technique worldwide (85% enteric drainage, 79% systemic venous) [3]. The systemic-venous anastomosis is usually performed between the portal vein of the graft and the vena cava or the external iliac vein of the recipient.

Enteric anastomosis typically involves the proximal jejunum and is usually performed by a side-to-side anastomosis. The use of direct anastomosis is currently prevalent over Roux-en-Y loop [8]. Duodenoduodenostomy is a further option when the pancreas is placed in the right retrocolic space [8]. This technique allows endoscopic surveillance but entails challenging repair of the recipient's duodenum in the case of allograft pancreatectomy.

Pancreas transplantation with portal-venous and enteric drainage

Portal venous drainage has become popular since the mid-1990s when the technique was described by Gaber *et al.* and the development of further modifications [9]. As these methods place the pancreas graft in a mid-abdominal position, arterial anastomosis may be difficult. Boggi *et al.* described placement of the pancreas behind the right colon to overcome most of these difficulties. Even percutaneous access to the graft is good, as there are no overlapping bowel loops [8].

The more physiological secretion of the insulin with a first-pass through the liver (in contrast to a permanent hyperinsulinaemia of the systemic-venous drainage) is assumed to be beneficial. However, there is no proof of a beneficial metabolic effect of the portal-venous drainage compared with systemic-venous drainage.

A reduced rejection rate with the portal-venous technique has been described repeatedly but has not been proven in randomised controlled studies.

Pancreas transplantation with systemic-venous and bladder drainage

Bladder drainage helped make pancreas transplantation a routine and frequent procedure [10]. Until recently, using bladder drainage was associated with a significantly lower technical failure rate according to the international pancreas transplant registry data. The drainage of the exocrine secretion into the bladder allows the possibility of monitoring the graft function by measuring the amount (not concentration) of amylase secretion in the urine in 24 hours. This advantage seems to be useful in PTA and PAK. However, owing to new immunosuppressive protocols and a reduction in rejection episodes, even for these procedures enteric drainage is favoured today.

Preparation for surgery

Preparation of the pancreas graft

The back-table preparation should start immediately after arrival of the procured organs. This procedure usually takes at least 1 hour. First, the organ is inspected for suitability for transplantation. Severe injuries of the parenchyma, damaged or missing blood vessels or a mesenteric root that is dissected too close to the pancreas can be excluded by inspection. A missing duodenal patch is observed very rarely but would be a contraindication to transplantation.

The duodenum is shortened to 6–8 cm using linear staplers. The staple line may be reinforced using absorbable interrupted sutures. In our own experience we mark the papilla with a suture to the duodenal wall after putting a probe into the common bile duct and Vater's papilla. An extension of the portal vein is rarely necessary. The splenic artery and superior mesenteric artery are linked with an iliac Y-graft from the donor.

Before implantation the vascular anastomoses are checked for leakage.

Preparation of the recipient

After arriving at the transplant centre the recipient has to be evaluated for three key issues.

- Is he/she in a transplantable condition or are there acute contraindications to transplantation (acute infection, diabetic foot syndrome with open wounds)?
- Is there a need for immediate pre-operative dialysis (high serum potassium, fluid overload)?
- Are the organs immunologically compatible (negative crossmatch)?

In the case of a non-immunised patient receiving their first transplant without a recent history of blood transfusion, a crossmatch can be performed with stored serum. In all other cases (sensitised recipient (known preformed HLA antibodies), recent blood transfusion, re-transplantation) the crossmatch has to be performed using fresh serum. A positive crossmatch is a contraindication to transplantation.

Specific operative concerns

Surgical access

The routine surgical access for pancreas transplantation is a midline incision. The distal margin of the incision is the symphysis. The supraumbilical extension depends on the patient's condition. For obese patients an incision to the xiphoid can be necessary. On the right side the common iliac artery and the common iliac vein and vena cava are dissected. A mobilisation of the right hemicolon is not mandatory.

For retroperitoneal placement of the pancreas according to Boggi the right colon has to be mobilised from the retroperitoneal space [8].

For a portal-venous drainage the superior mesenteric vein is dissected cranially to the origin of the ileocolic vein.

Surgical technique

An atraumatic, careful preparation is mandatory for a technically successful pancreas transplantation. This is not only important for the gentle handling of the graft during transplantation but for the preparation of the arteries. Owing to long-lasting diabetes mellitus with resulting weakness of the vessels' media or heavy calcification this can be demanding.

The portal vein should remain short to avoid postoperative kinking and lower the risk for venous thrombosis. After completion of the venous anastomosis, the arterial anastomosis is performed. Here again the vessels should not be too long to avoid kinking. The reperfusion always starts with the release of the venous clamp first before opening the arterial clamp. With this approach surgical problems with the vein can be solved more easily than starting with arterial reperfusion. Before starting the exocrine anastomosis, careful haemostasis is performed. Most bleeding following reperfusion is located periportal, at the mesenteric root and at the tail of the pancreas.

The anastomosis of the donor duodenum and the bladder or intestine is usually carried out as double layer using a monofilament, absorbable suture. Some authors prefer to use a Roux-en-Y loop. After performing the exocrine anastomosis, irrigation of the abdominal cavity is performed to avoid bacterial contamination. At the end of the operation two drains are placed around the pancreas graft after ensuring haemostasis.

Intraoperative medication

For kidney transplantation a central venous pressure of 8–10 cm H_2O and a mean arterial pressure above 80 mmHg is desirable. For further anaesthesia management see Chapter 13.

Immunosuppression

A detailed account of immunosuppressive therapy is found in Chapter 16. Immunosuppressive therapy for kidney/pancreas transplantation is based on four classes of drug:
- antibody induction
  - polyclonal anti-T-lymphocyte globulin (rabbit, ATG-Fresenius®) or antithymocyte globulin (rabbit, Thymoglobulin®) or
  - chimaeric monoclonal interleukin-2 receptor antibody (basiliximab, Simulect®)
  - alemtuzumab (anti-CD 52, Campath-1H®)
- calcineurin inhibitors
  - tacrolimus
  - ciclosporin
- antiproliferative drugs
  - mycophenolate mofetil (MMF) or enteric-coated mycophenolate sodium (MPA)
  - sirolimus
- steroids.

The long-term results of a European multicentre study (Euro SPK 001) comparing tacrolimus with ciclosporin both in combination with anti-T-cell induction, MMF and short-term steroids show a rejection rate of 27.2% (tacrolimus) and 38.2% (ciclosporin) after 1 year [11]. Pancreas graft survival at 1 year (91.3% versus 74.5%, p = 0.001) and 3 years (89.2% versus 72.4%, p = 0.002) was significantly higher with tacrolimus [11]. Thus although ciclosporin may have been chosen over tacrolimus owing to a lesser impact on glucose metabolism, these superior outcomes have led to tacrolimus being the calcineurin inhibitor of choice for pancreatic transplantation.

A study using a combination of tacrolimus with either MMF or sirolimus (Euro SPK 002) found more frequent study withdrawal in the sirolimus group as a result of toxicity [11]. With triple immunosuppression using tacrolimus, MMF and steroids in combination with antithymocyte globulin induction the rejection rate is as low as about 20%. Graft loss due to rejection has become very rare using this combination. Some centres now advocate the use of alemtuzumab, which results in extremely low rates of early rejection.

Antibiotic prophylaxis

There are some specific postoperative infections that affect pancreas recipients, as well as the general risk of opportunistic infection following organ transplantation (see Chapter 21). In pancreas transplantation, intra-abdominal infections are very dangerous, as they are associated with a high risk of graft loss [12].

The spectrum of postoperative infections is comparable to kidney transplantation. In the early postoperative course, urinary tract infections and cytomegalovirus (CMV) infection are most frequent followed by pneumonia and wound infections.

Intra-abdominal infections mostly occur in combination with graft pancreatitis. Risk factors for the occurrence of graft pancreatitis are long ischaemia time and old or obese organ donors. In our own practice, we give antibiotic prophylaxis with imipenem for 5 days.

Otherwise, postoperative anti-infective prophylaxis is the same as used in transplant recipients in general:
- *Pneumocystis jiroveci* (PJ)
- herpes simplex virus (HSV)
- CMV
- candidiasis.

To prevent infection with the above organisms, the following prophylaxis is recommended:
- trimethoprim (TMP) and sulfamethoxazole (SMX; TMP 80 mg/SMX 400 mg) three times a week for 6 months for PC pneumonia prophylaxis
- nystatin mouth washing for 6 weeks for prophylaxis of oropharyngeal candidiasis
- valganciclovir and IV or oral ganciclovir according to the kidney function for CMV prophylaxis.

Both prophylaxis and pre-emptive therapy are viable approaches for prevention of CMV disease [13,14]. For a detailed discussion of CMV prophylaxis, see Chapter 21).

The aggressive and early diagnosis and treatment of infections seems to be as important as prophylaxis. In the case of intra-abdominal infections, a CT- or ultrasound-guided drainage of localised fluid collections or relaparotomy in case of general abdominal infections is indicated.

Anticoagulation

Venous thrombosis of the pancreas graft is the most frequent cause of early graft loss. There is no evidence for any specific anticoagulation strategy to prevent this complication, with the exception of patients with known prothrombotic disorders [5].

Screening of pancreas transplant recipients revealed prothrombotic disorders in 34–53% of the patients, requiring anticoagulation [15].

For prevention of graft thrombosis, most centres use empirical peri-operative graft thrombosis prophylaxis protocols. Any anticoagulation protocol for pancreas recipients, however, is yet to be proven well tolerated and effective in a randomised study. Low-intensity perioperative anticoagulation using heparin, as practised by many centres, seems wise with discontinuation on postoperative day 7.

Postoperative treatment

Usually the pancreas graft starts functioning intraoperatively, shortly after reperfusion, leading to normoglycemia without need for exogenous insulin. In case of delayed graft function, the measurement of c-peptide can help to assess pancreas graft function.

After 2 or 3 days when peristalsis starts, oral food intake can be started.

Every SPK recipient should be seen by a transplant physician/surgeon twice a day during the initial hospital stay. The clinical examination is at least as important as the daily laboratory results.

Special postoperative complications

Graft pancreatitis
There is no uniformly accepted definition for graft pancreatitis and no limit values for amylase or lipase. Risk factors for the development of graft pancreatitis are donor derived [16] or caused by the procedure itself (cold ischaemia time, perfusion, intraoperative handling).

Like native pancreatitis, graft pancreatitis can be mild, or severe with necrosis. As the pancreas graft is usually placed intraperitoneally, retroperitoneal necroses are rare. Peritonitis can be the result of severe graft pancreatitis. Peripancreatic fluid collections can be infected and develop into an abscess or a pseudocyst. The decision for relaparotomy depends on the clinical appearance (signs of peritonitis) and laboratory results (C-reactive protein, leucocytes, amylase, lipase).

In the case of peritonitis, the indication for relaparotomy is mandatory even to rule out anastomotic leakage. The clinical signs of peritonitis can be uncertain owing to the immunosuppressive medication. Deterioration in renal function or confusion and sickness can be the first signs of developing peritonitis. Depending on the intraoperative finding, a lavage or resection of necrosis or resection of pancreas parenchyma or even graft pancreatectomy can be necessary during relaparotomy [17]. The most severe and frightening complication of a graft pancreatitis can be bleeding from the graft vessels because of erosion. These life-threatening complications are rare but can occur even after more than 4 weeks after transplantation. An immediate emergency operation is mandatory and removal of the pancreas graft is always indicated.

Graft pancreatitis is a consequence of ischaemia reperfusion leading to impaired microcirculation and organ damage [18]. Multiple drugs have been proven to reduce the ischaemia reperfusion pancreatitis in animal models [19]. There will be a European multicentre randomised study evaluating the influence of N-acetylcysteine and antithrombin III in clinical SPK (Euro SPK 003).

Graft thrombosis

Graft thrombosis of the portal vein or splenic vein are still the most frequent serious surgical complications, with an incidence of up to 10% [3,17]. With rare exceptions it results in the need for relaparotomy and transplant pancreatectomy [17]. Thus graft thrombosis is the most frequent cause of early graft loss following pancreas transplantation.

The aetiology of pancreas graft thrombosis is multifactorial. Donor risk factors include increased donor age, cardiocerebrovascular cause of death, significant haemodynamic instability and massive volume resuscitation [20]. Suboptimal surgical pancreas recovery, preservation and back-table preparation techniques have also been identified as risk factors [20].

Postreperfusion graft pancreatitis increases capillary flow resistance and creates a procoagulant, thrombogenic local milieu within the low-flow pancreas graft. Hypercoagulable recipients are also at higher risk for losing their pancreas graft [5]. Thus, pre-transplant screening for these prothrombotic disorders can lower the risk for thrombosis. A large European randomised prospective multicentre trial found an increased pancreas graft thrombosis rate in the study arm using ciclosporin (compared with tacrolimus) [11].

Clinical symptoms of pancreas graft thrombosis include sudden onset of otherwise unexplained hyperglycaemia. A decrease of c-peptide can be measured. Diagnosis of pancreas graft thrombosis can be established by imaging studies such as Doppler ultrasound, CT angiography, conventional angiography or magnetic resonance imaging. However, all of these tests may delay the relaparotomy where the graft could be salvaged. Once graft thrombosis is diagnosed the relaparotomy should be done promptly. Thrombectomy or resection of the pancreatic tail in the case of distal thrombosis can be performed and restore sufficient graft function [17]. However, for the vast majority of early post-transplant pancreas graft thromboses, treatment consists of transplant pancreatectomy. For highly selected thrombosed pancreas grafts, interventional approaches can yield successful long-term outcome [5]. For selected cases, an early pancreas re-transplantation at the time of pancreatectomy can be considered without increased morbidity and mortality.

Prevention of graft thrombosis includes besides postoperative anticoagulation, careful donor selection and atraumatic procurement techniques [20]. Furthermore, a back table preparation using arterial

Y-graft reconstruction and avoidance of portal vein extensions can prevent vascular problems.

Anastomotic leakage

Anastomotic leaks occur rarely but remain a clinically significant entity, as they are a risk factor for intra-abdominal infection. The impact on graft and patient survival is minimal if leaks are recognised early and managed properly.

As clinical appearance and therapeutic options are different, it is important to distinguish leaks in enteric- and bladder-drained grafts. Recipients of enteric-drained grafts develop early peritonitis and sepsis due to spillage of enteric contents. Further diagnostics may include abdominal CT scan with oral contrast to confirm the diagnosis. Treatment consists of relaparotomy with anastomotic revision or even transplant pancreatectomy. In the case of a localised abscess due to late leakage, percutaneous drainage may be sufficient. Bladder-drained graft leaks usually occur at the duodenocystostomy and are associated with a lower rate of serious infectious complications. Diagnosis can be made by cystogram or CT scan with retrograde bladder contrast. Treatment consists of prolonged bladder decompression with Foley catheterisation. In the case of peritonitis relaparotomy is indicated as well.

Complications of bladder drainage

The drainage of exocrine pancreas secretion through the bladder may cause several urologic complications of the urinary tract, such as haemorrhagic cystitis or recurrent urinary tract infections. Metabolic complications including hypovolaemia and metabolic acidosis occur as a result of loss of bicarbonate.

These complications lead to the need for conversion to enteric drainage in 18–30% of recipients. With the shift to primarily enteric-drained pancreas transplants the need for conversion operations has decreased [17].

References

1. Smets YF, Westendorp RG, van der Pijl JW, *et al.* (1999) Effect of simultaneous pancreas-kidney transplantation on mortality of patients with type-1 diabetes mellitus and end-stage renal failure. *Lancet* **353**, 1915–1919.
2. Tyden G, Tollemar J, Bolinder J. (2000) Combined pancreas and kidney transplantation improves survival in patients with end-stage diabetic nephropathy. *Clin Transplant* **5**, 505–508.
3. Gruessner AC, Sutherland DE, Gruessner RW. (2010) Pancreas transplantation in the United States: A review. *Curr Opin Organ Transplant* **15**, 93–101.
4. Sutherland DE, Gruessner RW, Gruessner AC. (2001) Pancreas transplantation for treatment of diabetes mellitus. *World J Surg* **25**, 487–496.
5. Wullstein C, Woeste G, Zapletal C, *et al.* (2003) Simultaneous pancreas-kidney transplantation in patients with antiphospholipid syndrome. *Transplantation* **75**, 562–563.

6. Bechstein WO. (2001) Long-term outcome of pancreas transplantation. *Transplant Proc* **33**, 1652–1654.

7. Stock PG, Roland ME, Carlson L, *et al.* (2003) Kidney and liver transplantation in human immunodeficiency virus-infected patients: A pilot safety and efficacy study. *Transplantation* **76**, 370–375.

8. Boggi U, Amorese G, Marchetti P. (2010) Surgical techniques for pancreas transplantation. *Curr Opin Organ Transplant* **15**, 102–111.

9. Gaber AO, Shokouh-Amiri H, Grewal HP, *et al.* (1993) A technique for portal pancreatic transplantation with enteric drainage. *Surg Gynecol Obstet* **177**, 417–419.

10. Sollinger HW, Odorico JS, Knechtle SJ, *et al.* (1998) Experience with 500 simultaneous pancreas-kidney transplants. *Ann Surg* **228**, 284–296.

11. Bechstein WO, Malaise J, Saudek F, *et al.* (2004) Efficacy and safety of tacrolimus compared with cyclosporine microemulsion in primary simultaneous pancreas-kidney transplantation: 1-year results of a large multicenter trial. *Transplantation* **77**, 1221–1228.

12. Troppmann C, Gruessner AC, Dunn DL, *et al.* (1998) Surgical complications requiring early relaparotomy after pancreas transplantation: A multivariate risk factor and economic impact analysis of the cyclosporine era. *Ann Surg* **227**, 255–268.

13. Kotton CN, Kumar D, Caliendo AM, *et al.* (2010) International consensus guidelines on the management of cytomegalovirus in solid organ transplantation. *Transplantation* **89**, 779–795.

14. Humar A, Lebranchu Y, Vincenti F, *et al.* (2010) The efficacy and safety of 200 days valganciclovir cytomegalovirus prophylaxis in high-risk kidney transplant recipients. *Am J Transplant* **10**, 1228–1237.

15. Wullstein C, Woeste G, Zapletal C, *et al.* (2003) Prothrombotic disorders in uremic type-1 diabetics undergoing simultaneous pancreas and kidney transplantation. *Transplantation* **76**, 1691–1695.

16. Humar A, Ramcharan T, Kandaswamy R, *et al.* (2004) The impact of donor obesity on outcomes after cadaver pancreas transplants. *Am J Transplant* **4**, 605–610.

17. Troppmann C. (2010) Complications after pancreas transplantation. *Curr Opin Organ Transplant* **15**, 112–118.

18. Benz S, Pfeffer F, Adam U, *et al.* (1998) Impairment of pancreatic microcirculation in the early reperfusion period during simultaneous pancreas-kidney transplantation. *Transpl Int* **11** (Suppl 1), 433–435.

19. Woeste G, Wullstein C, Meyer S, *et al.* (2008) Octreotide attenuates impaired microcirculation in postischemic pancreatitis when administered before induction of ischemia. *Transplantation* **86**, 961–967.

20. Troppmann C, Gruessner AC, Benedetti E, *et al.* (1996) Vascular graft thrombosis after pancreatic transplantation: Univariate and multivariate operative and nonoperative risk factor analysis. *J Am Coll Surg* **182**, 285–316.

12 Pancreatic islet transplantation

František Saudek

Introduction

Pancreatic islets of Langerhans are the site where the life essential hormone insulin, which controls glucose, protein and fat metabolism, is secreted. Human pancreatic islets are 0.1–0.4 mm large micro-organs scattered throughout the exocrine part of the pancreas. Their total number is estimated to be approximately 1 million, with the total mass of approximately 1–1.5 g. An average islet is composed of about 2000 endocrine cells, of which 65–80% represent insulin-producing β-cells, 15–20% glucagon-secreting alpha cells and the rest mainly delta, PP and gamma cells, which produce somatostatin, pancreatic polypeptide and ghrelin, respectively. Individual cells form irregular trabeculae and communicate with each other by paracrine and autocrine mechanisms. Pancreatic islets have a rich vascular and neural network, and the exocrine acinar tissue and pancreatic dusts are separated by a fine reticular capsule. Islet hormones are secreted into the portal venous system and achieve particularly high concentrations in the liver. Individual islets represent organised functional units, and impairment of their integrity may be reflected in their function.

Failure of islet β-cells to produce adequate amounts of insulin results in diabetes mellitus. Two main forms of diabetes are characterised by either absolute (type 1) or relative (type 2) lack of insulin. While type-1 diabetes is usually caused by a progressive autoimmune T-cell-mediated β-cell destruction, the underlying mechanism in type-2 diabetes consists of a combination of escalating peripheral insulin resistance and inability of β-cells to compensate for increasing metabolic demands. In type-1 diabetes, accounting for 5–10% of all diabetes cases, pharmacological insulin replacement represents the standard therapy, with the aim of mimicking physiological glucose control as closely as possible using subcutaneous insulin administration adjusted according to the results of frequent blood glucose self-monitoring. The main effort in type-2

Handbook of Renal and Pancreatic Transplantation, First Edition. Edited by Iain A. M. MacPhee and Jiří Froněk.
© 2012 John Wiley & Sons, Ltd. Published 2012 by John Wiley & Sons, Ltd.

diabetes is to improve insulin sensitivity and stimulate endogenous insulin secretion. However, insulin substitution is often needed in order to achieve good metabolic control.

The worldwide prevalence of diabetes is increasing, and it is estimated that from 2000 to 2030 it will double from 171 million to 366 million cases (see www.who.int). Despite evident improvement in diabetes care with the introduction of new pharmacological approaches and technical equipment, metabolic control remains far from perfect, and late microvascular and macrovascular complications, such as retinopathy, nephropathy, neuropathy and diabetic foot syndrome and accelerated atherosclerosis develop in most affected subjects. Consequently, although it is much more evident in type 1, biological replacement of the β-cell mass might represent the optimal way of treatment in both diabetes types, restoring the failing insulin secretion according to minute-to-minute metabolic needs and without the risk of iatrogenic hypoglycaemia. Currently, there are two methods for clinical β-cell replacement available, both being dependent on the supply of suitable deceased donors: whole-organ pancreas transplantation and transplantation of isolated islets of Langerhans. It is thus obvious that should β-cell-based therapy be adopted as a routine diabetes treatment on a larger scale, alternative sources of insulin-producing cells need to be found first.

The ability of transplanted tissue to normalise or near-normalise blood glucose concentrations and other metabolic parameters in diabetic recipients has been consistently demonstrated by whole-organ pancreas transplantation. This procedure, however, requires general anaesthesia and major surgery (discussed in detail in Chapter 11). Serious complications, including graft thrombosis, bleeding, infection, pancreatic leak and pancreatitis, are still frequent and may result in relaparotomy in as many as 35% cases in well-established centres [1]. Therefore, the idea to transplant only the missing endocrine part of the organ, representing no more than 1–2% of its volume, using a minimally invasive method, seems logical. Principal differences between islet and pancreas transplantation are summarised in Table 12.1.

History

Relevant experiments with islet transplantation date from the 1960s, when Lacy and Kostianovski succeeded in the separation of individual islets from the exocrine tissue using the enzyme collagenase. After the first series of seven human islet recipients in 1977 from Minneapolis had been published, many researchers thought that this method would soon replace the intricate organ pancreas transplantation – at that time the search of safer techniques for the management of the exocrine secretion was an ongoing challenge [2]. Potential advantages of islet transplantation seemed to be unequivocal: no need for major surgical

Table 12.1 Comparison of organ pancreas transplantation and islet transplantation.

		Pancreas transplantation	Islet transplantation
Current short-term success		>90%	50–80%
Current long-term success		>70%	<30%
Revascularisation		Perfect	Partial
Metabolic control		Normal or near-normal	Usually impaired glucose tolerance
Impact on diabetic microagiopathy		Stabilisation or improvement	Stabilisation
Donor criteria	Age	5–45 (50) years	18–65 years
	Obesity	Not acceptable	Acceptable
Islet count from one pancreas		Sufficient	Usually not sufficient
Procedure availability		In many transplant centres	Only in research centres
Long-term conservation		Impossible	Possible
Severe complications		Frequent	Rare
Costs		Similar	
Immunosuppression		Necessary	Necessary
Immuno-isolation		Impossible	Possible
Imuno-alteration		Impossible	Possible
Main perspectives		Less complication, safer immunosuppression	Immune tolerance Alternative tissue sources

procedure, the possibility of keeping the islets in culture or to store them for unlimited periods of time in a freezer, the chance to modify their immunologic properties in vitro and no complications resulting from the exocrine nature of the pancreas.

However, islet isolation in large animals or in humans led to a significant loss of endocrine tissue and to functional impairment. It soon turned out that isolated islets were at least as prone to immunological rejection as the whole organ and might be even more sensitive to the autoimmune milieu typical for type-1 diabetes [3]. In addition, the oxygenation and nutrition via diffusion from the blood before revascularisation with new vessels originating from the donor was shown to be insufficient owing to a completely disrupted vascular network. Subsequently, early graft loss due to ischaemia, coagulation and non-specific inflammation followed. Activation of the coagulation and inflammatory pathways following intravascular infusion of isolated islets has been called instant blood-mediated inflammatory reaction (IBMIR). IBMIR is initiated mainly by tissue factor, which is expressed on the surface of the islets and initiates the extrinsic coagulation cascade leading to islet injury, and which may account for considerable β-cell loss within minutes to hours following transplantation [4].

As late as 1979, Largiader in Switzerland reported the first successful islet transplantation in a C-peptide negative recipient, who remained insulin-independent for 1 year, but the number of such cases had been increasing only slowly. In 1988 Ricordi *et al.* [5] described a semi-automatic method for islet isolation, which lead to a substantially higher islet yield and enabled the first successful clinical transplants [6,7]. This technique, though subjected to many modifications and refinements, has still been in use up to the present. Nevertheless, unique islet transplants had been performed in several centres in the 1990s. However, the results were still beyond comparison with that in whole-organ transplantation and one-year independence from exogenous insulin was achieved only in isolated cases.

A landmark in the evolution of islet transplantation and encouragement for many laboratories worldwide was represented in the success of the Edmonton group at the University of Alberta, who achieved independence from insulin therapy with normal blood glucose concentrations in seven consecutive cases of brittle type-1 diabetes [8]. The Edmonton protocol introduced several modifications of the transplantation process, including the use of a potent immunosuppressive combination based on sirolimus, tacrolimus and an anti-CD25-receptor antibody, without steroids. The main reason for this success was considered to be the administration of a large number of islets (11,000 islet equivalents per kilogram), which was obtained by a refined isolation process beginning with careful organ selection and conservation through controlled collagenase digestion based on the Ricordi principle and high quality separation. In all recipients, two to four islet implantations were performed within several weeks until insulin independence was reached.

Over the following 7 years, many transplant centres increased their activity and initiated islet programmes, but not all procedures were properly documented on an international level. The Collaborative Islet Transplant Registry (CITR), established in the USA and working so far together with five European sites, evaluated in this period 325 recipients who received altogether 649 islet preparations (see www.citregistry.org). Unfortunately, data even from the most prominent centres showed that the results were inferior to those achieved by whole-organ pancreas transplantation and that islet transplantation still faced major challenges. At present, islet transplants are performed still only in the context of clinical experiments, and additional modifications seem to be necessary in the field of islet isolation, immunosuppression, implantation and post-transplant management, before this treatment might be considered not only as safer, but at least an equally effective substitute for whole-organ pancreas transplantation.

Recipient selection

With regard to lack of organ donors, risk of surgical complications and the necessity for life-long immunosuppressive therapy, transplant therapy of diabetes has been mostly limited for type-1 diabetic subjects suffering from end-stage diabetic nephropathy undergoing simultaneous kidney transplantation or who had already received a kidney graft. Of all pancreas transplants performed in the USA in 2008, only 7% were performed in subjects without end-stage kidney disease and without previous kidney transplant, and this percentage was even lower in Europe. For the vast majority of subjects with type-1 diabetes, intensive insulin therapy using several daily insulin doses or an insulin pump, systematic education and customised daily regimens represents the treatment of choice. This strategy helps to achieve acceptable metabolic control and to delay the development of late diabetic complications, but it is associated with an increased incidence of severe hypoglycaemic episodes [9], and in a substantial group of patients is difficult to apply successfully. Metabolic control is unstable, especially in subjects with prolonged diabetes duration who develop autonomic neuropathy with impaired hypoglycaemia counter-regulation, leading sometimes to the syndrome of hypoglycaemic unawareness. Typical for this situation are missing or delayed vegetative symptoms of hypoglycaemia due to blunted release of epinephrine. In addition to sometimes life-threatening hypoglycaemia, fear of hypoglycaemia often results in high mean blood glucose concentrations, with acceleration of the progression of other diabetic complications. In this 'nonuraemic' patient group, transplant therapy should be considered, despite the risks of long-term immunosuppression.

Islet transplantation now represents a realistic alternative to pancreas transplantation, and the selection criteria differ little between the two methods in most centres. When making a decision between them, three factors should be considered. Firstly, islet transplantation is much safer for the patient, and major surgical complications are exceptional. Secondly, while pancreas transplantation almost immediately establishes robust long-term normoglycaemia in most recipients, supplemental insulin doses are needed in many islet recipients after 1 year, and more than 90% require insulin at 5 years to maintain good metabolic control [10,11]. Thirdly, even partial restoration of endogenous insulin production is of great importance for type-1 diabetic subjects and in combination with intensive insulin therapy leads to near-perfect metabolic control, the reduction of the rate and severity of hypoglycaemic episodes and successful treatment of the hypoglycaemic unawareness syndrome in most islet recipients [10].

Typical current indications for islet allotransplantation are:
1. simultaneous allogeneic kidney transplantation in a type-1 diabetic recipient suffering from end-stage kidney disease
2. islet transplantation in a type-1 diabetic recipient with a functioning kidney graft from a deceased or living donor

3. hypoglycaemic unawareness syndrome with frequent severe hypoglycaemic episodes (coma or need for help from other person usually more than four times in the last year) in a type-1 diabetic subject in whom conservative measures, including qualified patient education and glucose monitoring, have failed
4. less frequently, poor metabolic control in type-1 diabetic patients (such as haemoglobin A1c >8%, frequent hypoglycaemic episodes interfering with daily life) with early development of diabetic complications, such as retinopathy and neuropathy, in whom qualified intensive insulin therapy has been failing.

Apart from general contraindications for transplant therapy, exclusion criteria for islet transplantation usually comprise conditions with impaired insulin sensitivity such as type-2 diabetes, obesity (BMI >28 kg/m^2) and high insulin need (usually >0.7 insulin units per kilogram), as a higher risk of graft exhaustion and treatment failure is expected. 'Islet transplant only' is usually not performed in subjects with incipient chronic renal insufficiency (creatinine clearance <60 mL/min) in whom the therapy with caclineurin or mammalian target of rapamycin (mTOR) inhibitors can accelerate progression to end-stage kidney failure [12,13]. In earlier stages of nephropathy, it is assumed that deterioration of kidney function may be prevented by careful follow-up and post-transplant management [14]. Attention must be also paid to individual psychological and social conditions that may lie behind the poor diabetes control but may also complicate treatment compliance following transplantation.

Pancreas allocation and procurement

Islet transplantation is still not a routine method, and allocation criteria differ among countries and centres. Priority is given to combined pancreas and kidney transplantation, which represents the treatment of choice for most type-1 diabetic subjects with end-stage kidney disease, who account for approximately 7–10% percent of all subjects listed for kidney transplant. Isolated pancreas transplantation is usually considered as the next step if a kidney is not available. Most of the pancreases selected for islet isolation thus recruit from those that do not match the rather strict criteria for organ transplantation. This concerns mainly donors older than 45–50 years, with body mass index (BMI) >30 kg/m^2 or with vascular abnormalities. Pancreata from high BMI donors have been successfully used for islet transplantation, with islet yield frequently better than from lean doors. Higher donor age (50–65 years) is not an obstacle to successful islet isolation, although the expected functional outcome is poorer. By contrast, islet isolation from very young donors (<18 years) is rarely successful, owing to the difficulty of separating the endocrine and exocrine tissue.

Pancreas procurement for islet isolation is by no means less demanding than in the case of whole-organ transplantation. Better results are usually achieved if the retrieval is done by the local surgical team. The pancreas can be excised en bloc with a segment of duodenum and spleen before or after the liver, but until removal it should be cooled with saline slush. Minimising warm ischaemia time and keeping the integrity of the pancreas capsule and of the ducts in order to prevent leak during the isolation process is of particular importance. Under specific conditions pancreata from non-heartbeating donors (donors after circulatory death) have been used, but in general, the detrimental effect of even short periods of warm ischaemia has been documented.

Most frequently, pancreata have been stored in University of Wisconsin (UW) solution, but histidine-tryptophan-ketoglutarate (HTK) solution may represent an alternative, provided the cold ischaemia time does not exceed 8–10 hours. A number of reports have shown that better islet viability and higher yield is achieved with the use of the two-layer method, which employs oxygenated perfluorocarbon overlaid with UW solution. Perfluorocarbon is a highly lipophilic compound that dissolves oxygen with a 25 times higher capacity than water and might help to maintain better oxygenation and higher ATP tissue concentrations during cold storage. Some recent clinical studies showed no beneficial effect of this technique compared with the simple UW storage, but the two-layer method is still used in many centres, especially if a longer cold ischaemia time is expected.

Islet isolation

Current isolation techniques are based on the principle that pancreatic islets do not directly communicate with the pancreatic duct system. One or two cannulae are inserted into the main pancreatic duct and the organ is distended with 250–350 mL of solution containing a highly purified, low-endotoxin, proteolytic enzyme blend containing class I and class II collagenase and neutral protease thermolysin. After distension the pancreas is trimmed from fat and vessels, cut into several pieces and processed for 10–30 min, until intact free islets are detected by microscopic monitoring. This phase is of critical importance, as the islets released earlier are subjected to prolonged proteolytic activity and mechanical stress while the others remain embedded within the exocrine tissue. Although the outcome depends upon the quality of the organ as well, the composition and activity of the enzyme blend plays an important role that can vary considerably, not only between producers but also lot-to-lot from the same producer. Selection of a suitable collagenase lot represents a problem, especially in smaller laboratories because it is still based mainly on individual experience, sometimes at the expense of time and wasted organs. Standardisation of the collagenase products and modification of the isolation process according to its activity assessed before isolation is of great importance [15].

At the end of the digestion process the collagenase is inhibited and washed out and the islets, dispersed in a tissue volume of 30–50 mL, are

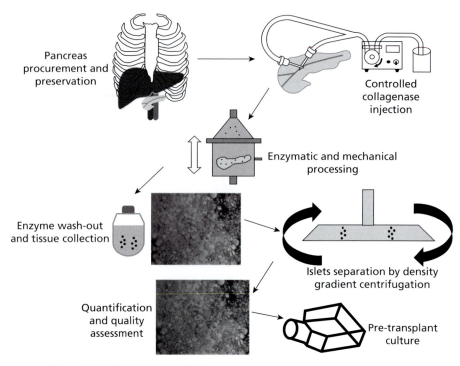

Figure 12.1 Scheme of islet isolation.

purified using a cell processor. Nearly all laboratories now use the semi-automated computerised cell processor COBE-2991, which allows purification in a closed system within a reasonable period of time. Exocrine tissue and islets with different grade of purity separate by centrifugation in different layers of a ficoll (or similar) continuous gradient, which makes it possible to prepare several islet fractions of different purity. Final packed islet volume then usually comprises 2–6 mL tissue volume with estimated purity of 30–70%. The isolation process is shown in Fig. 12.1.

Islet culture and quality assessment

Although only freshly isolated islets were used in the original Edmonton study [8], most transplant centres now culture the islets for at least 1 day before transplantation [16]. This option represents a major advantage that is not possible in the case of organ transplantation. First of all, it creates an opportunity for careful recipient selection, examination and pre-transplant conditioning and for exclusion of microbiological islet contamination. Islet viability may be assessed by intravital staining or by more complex methods, which include measurement of the mitochondrial membrane potential, ATP-to-ADP ratio and parameters of glucose-stimulated insulin secretion [17]. The islet mass is expressed in term of islet equivalents, corresponding to a number of islets with a diameter of 150 μm using digital image analysis [18]. In contrast to the previous report, it is now supposed that smaller islets survive better in culture and following transplantation than the large ones, which are vulnerable to central hypoxia and apoptosis.

Islet culture under specific conditions, such as under high partial pressure of oxygen, in low temperature (22 °C) or with a variety of growth factors and supplements, may improve islet purity, prevent apoptosis, improve resistance to oxidative stress, reduce the expression of tissue factor or modify the immunological properties. Cryopreservation and storage in liquid nitrogen is possible, but because of considerable tissue loss (~30%), mainly during the thawing procedure, it is now rarely used. What is becoming more frequent, however, is the cooperation of an experienced regional islet cell processing facility with several distant clinical islet transplant centres. After procurement, the pancreas is sent to the central isolation laboratory, and after processing the islet graft is either shipped back or is allocated according to a common waiting list. This cooperation improves the utilisation of available organs, allows tissue processing by an appropriately equipped and trained team and makes it easier to comply with complex cell-processing regulations. This concept has been recently used by the GRAGIL group (Group Rhin-Rhone-Alpes-Geneve pour la Transplantation d'Ilots de Langerhans) and the Nordic Network for Islet Transplantation, for example. Between these centres, islet preparations have been successfully transported in special media within hours, using gas-permeable bags, without compromising their mass and potency.

Transplant procedure

Although other alternative sites for islet transplantation are being tested, all successful islet transplants so far have been accomplished by islet implantation into the hepatic portal system. Most frequently, the access to the portal vein is obtained percutaneously through the liver under ultrasonographic and radiological control. Under local anaesthesia, a J-wire is introduced through a 21–22 gauge needle after radiological confirmation of its optimal position. The needle is then exchanged with a 4 Fr catheter. After measuring the portal pressure, the islets are gravity infused in one or two bags containing 150–250 mL of transplant medium supplemented with 2.5% human albumin and 35–70 units of heparin per kilogram in each bag over a period of 30–60 min. Islet infusion is interrupted or slowed down if portal blood pressure exceeds 20 mmHg, although this rarely happens. Bleeding from the liver parenchyma or from the portal vein, portal hypertension and portal vein thrombosis are potentially serious complications. Bleeding may be prevented by effective mechanical sealing of the puncture tract with thrombostatic coils and tissue fibrin glue or gelatin-sponge [19].

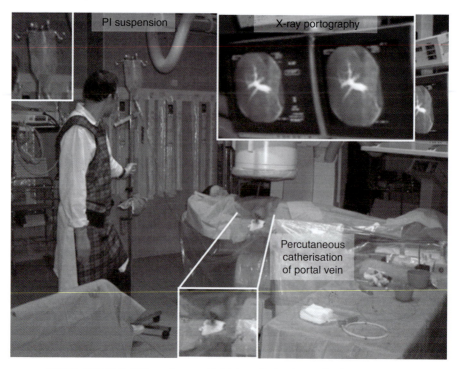

Figure 12.2 Implantation of pancreatic islets under local anaesthesia.

   Mini-laparotomy with introduction of the infusion catheter through a mesenteric vein is an alternative approach. This may be helpful, especially in simultaneous kidney and islet transplantation, as it brings only minimal additional risk. The islets are infused after completion of the kidney anastomoses and the site of venous puncture is safely sutured.

   Usually, insulin independence is not reached if fewer than 10,000 islet equivalents per kilogram of body weight are administered. Under current isolation protocols, such a yield is difficult to achieve from a single pancreas and as such usually one or two additional transplants within a reasonable period of time (usually up to 6 months) are necessary. A simplified scheme of islet implantation is shown in Fig. 12.2.

Post-transplant management and immunosuppression

Heparin or its low-molecular-weight analogues have been administered not only during the implantation procedure but also for several days following implantation in order to ameliorate the IBMIR and prevent portal thrombosis. This may be a problem in the case of suspicion of local bleeding, however. In addition, attention must be paid to tight glucose control in order to prevent exhaustion of the implanted β-cells and to improve their engraftment.

Immunosuppressive therapy in the original Edmonton protocol was based on a combination of sirolimus and low-dose tacrolimus [8]. Subsequent studies found tolerability problems with adverse effects of sirolimus such as oral ulcerations, diarrhoea, anaemia, proteinuria and hypercholesterolemia. Other researchers have also questioned its suitability for islet transplantation at all because of its potential negative effects on islet revascularisation due to inhibition of vascular endothelial growth factor (VEGF), β-cell regeneration and insulin action, which have been demonstrated in experimental studies. Nevertheless, mTOR and calcineurin inhibitors were the cornerstones in most islet programmes running in 2010, with mycophenolate as an alternative to mTOR inhibition. Typically, target trough tacrolimus and sirolimus blood concentrations are in the range 3–7 μg/L and 4–10 μg/L, respectively. In all cases a potent antibody induction, mostly with rabbit ATG or new monoclonal antibodies such as alemtuzumab (Campath-1H), humanised anti-CD3 (hOKT3γ 1 Ala-Ala), anti-C25-receptor and others) have been used. In order to prevent the detrimental effect of the cytokines released early following antibody administration and inthahepatic islet administration, anti-TNF γ (or its receptor) antibodies have been used frequently prior to islet infusion.

In general, islet implantation requires only a short hospital stay in order to exclude procedure-related complications, keep tight metabolic control and administer anticoagulation prophylaxis. Laboratory investigation usually shows transient elevation of liver enzymes (2–5-fold) with normalisation typically by 2 weeks.

Islet function is periodically assessed according to the fasting and stimulated (food, glucose challenge, glucagon IV) C-peptide concentrations, insulin requirement and haemoglobin A1c concentration. A more complex investigation may include intravenous arginine stimulation or a hyperglycaemic insulin clamp study.

Diagnosis of rejection is difficult to perform, as histological correlation is not possible with current methods of islet implantation into the portal system. Differential diagnosis includes IBMIR (early after implantation), recurrent autoimmunity and metabolic exhaustion with subsequent apoptosis, but mostly the reason remains unclear and is sometimes uncertainly called 'islet burn-out', which may include a combination of specific and non-specific factors in the absence of natural regeneration. Of help may be the follow-up of diabetes-related autoantibody tests or more complex autoreactive T-cell assays. Non-invasive in-vivo imaging of the islet graft is so far possible only if the islets are labelled in culture by contrast agent that incorporates into the islet cells before implantation. For short follow-up in terms of hours, positron emission tomography in combination with computed tomography has been used after in-vitro islet labelling with ^{18}F-2-fluoro-2-deoxy-D-glucose. It is now also possible to follow the presence of pancreatic islets labelled with superparamagnetic iron nanoparticles on serial magnetic resonance scans

[20] over a period of months. However, the significance of this investigation for diagnosis of islet rejection remains to be determined.

Clinical outcomes

Following the success of the Edmonton group published in 2000 [8], the number of active centres and islet recipients increased noticeably. In a multicentre trial testing the reproducibility of this protocol, insulin independence, at least for a short period of time, was attained in 21 of 36 recipients (58%) at 1 year and 16 (44%) were insulin-free [13]. The number of islet transplants performed since 2000 can only roughly be estimated according to individual reports in Europe and from CITR, which collected data from most North American programmes and from five European and three Australian centres (see www.citregistry.org). Between 1999 and 2008, CITR evaluated data from 412 islet recipients, of whom 84% received islet-alone infusions, whereas 16% had previously received a kidney transplant. Roughly half of them were treated by two islet transplants, a quarter by one transplant and another quarter by three consecutive transplants. Overall, 70% of all recipients achieved at least transient insulin independence (at least for 2 weeks), but only 70% and 55% of them remained insulin-free for 1 and 2 years, respectively. Measured from the recipient's last infusion, 35% of them had a total loss of C-peptide production by 3 years. Data from Edmonton evaluating 65 type-1 diabetic islet recipients shows that approximately 80% retained significant C-peptide production (>0.5 ng/mL) over 5 years, while the insulin independence rate decreased from 94% early post last infusion to 7.7% at 5 years. It is thus apparent that the success rate measured in terms of insulin independence still remains inferior to that achieved by whole-organ pancreas transplantation.

What is probably most important, for most recipients on insulin, is that excellent or good metabolic control and the almost complete elimination of severe hypoglycaemic episodes was achieved in all subjects with continuing C-peptide production [10]. In a similar way, islet transplantation simultaneously with the kidney does not always eliminate insulin injections but improves diabetes control significantly and reduces insulin requirements.

Nevertheless, the methods of islet isolation and peri-transplant management are steadily improving and 1-year insulin independence approaching 80% has been reported from most experienced centres using specific transplant regimens in selected patient groups [16,21]. Although robust long-term normoglycaemia without any exogenous insulin substitution still remains elusive on a larger scale, there is sufficient evidence to show that even incomplete islet graft function is of great importance for subjects with unstable type-1 diabetes. As long as significant endogenous C-peptide production is preserved, the recipients usually maintain much better metabolic control compared with before transplantation, do not suffer from severe hypoglycaemic events and enjoy a better quality of life. In addition, several studies demonstrated that the long-term improvement of metabolic control may improve the course of diabetic retinopathy and neuropathy as well as macroangiopathy in solitary islet or islet after kidney recipients [22]. This experience has led to the reconciliation of the realistic aims of islet transplantation, which are different from that in whole-organ pancreas transplantation and do not necessarily include insulin independence. The principal goals currently are to near-normalise glucose metabolism, get rid of severe hypoglycaemic episodes, ameliorate progression of chronic diabetic complication and improve quality of life.

Complications

Compared with whole-pancreas transplantation, islet implantation is a much safer procedure, and most complications are related to chronic immunosuppressive therapy. Liver puncture may be complicated by bleeding, which occasionally requires surgical intervention. Partial portal thrombosis is a rare complication under anticoagulant prophylaxis with heparin or its analogues. According to CITR, procedure-related serious adverse events occurred in less than 6% transplants and only two of 111 cases did not fully resolve. Immunosuppression-related complications (see Chapter 16) are similar to those for organ pancreas transplantation and include mainly specific drug-related toxicity, opportunistic infections and the risk of neoplasia. CITR recently reported only four cases of neoplasia possibly related to the immunosuppressive therapy; however, the experience is still limited, and it is necessary take into account that in principle, the treatment should be lifelong and should not only to suppress the allograft response but also the autoimmune process characteristic for type-1 diabetes. The potential benefit of islet transplantation must be carefully weighed in each recipient and the reasons for islet transplantation, such as hypoglycaemic unawareness syndrome, poor metabolic control under conventional treatment and progressive diabetic complications, need to be carefully documented and the patient informed. Also for consideration is the risk of accelerated progression of nephropathy under caclineurin or mTOR inhibitor treatment and the risk of allosensitisation after repeated islet implantations, which might represent a problem should the patient subsequently require kidney transplantation.

Autotransplantation

Following total pancreatectomy, insulin-dependent diabetes inevitably results. Metabolic control is frequently poor and hypoglycaemia counter-regulation is usually compromised because of complete absence of pancreatic glucagon secretion. Islet isolation and implantation into the liver may prevent overt diabetes in about a third of treated subjects and significantly stabilise glucose control in another third. The pancreas or its part is enzymatically processed in the same way as in allotransplantation; however, purification using the cell processor is usually not performed in order to get as many islets as possible. Although the final tissue volume is much higher, the procedure is usually well tolerated and therefore should be considered in any case of pancreatectomy for non-malignant reasons. The most typical situation in which this can be applied is a painful form of chronic pancreatitis or otherwise untreatable pancreatic leak after surgical interventions [23]. Sustained islet function following autotransplantation illustrates the so-far unmet challenges in the fight with allorecognition and autoimmunity, which despite elaborate immunosuppressive protocols still hampers the success in type-1 diabetic subjects treated by allogeneic islet infusion.

Future directions and perspectives in islet transplantation

At present, islet transplantation may represent an effective treatment option for a highly selected group of patients in whom conventional insulin therapy has been obviously failing. For type-1 diabetic subjects who already are, or are starting to be, on immunosuppressive therapy because of kidney transplantation, islet transplantation represents an alternative to whole-pancreas transplantation, especially for those with a higher surgical risk. However, before this method might be used on a larger scale for diabetes treatment, a series of hurdles needs to be overcome.

Isolation and purification techniques leading to higher islet yield are being developed so that a single pancreas might suffice to achieve insulin independence. Novel immunosuppressive protocols that are more efficient, less diabetogenic and potentially might induce long-term islet tolerance are being explored. Substances preventing β-cell apoptosis, supporting islet revascularisation, preventing the IBMIR reaction and potentially leading to β-cell regeneration are being studied. Under investigation are also new implantation sites, such as muscle, bone marrow, vascularised omental pouch, gastric mucosa or potentially even the pancreas. Several living donor islet transplants have been reported after partial pancreatectomy in a family member, mainly in Japan. This approach has not been ethically accepted in Europe so far. Sufficient β-cell mass for transplantation might be available from xenogeneic donors, but the risk of as-yet not fully defined infectious risk and the interspecies immunological barrier require development of novel safety strategies and potent immunosuppressive/modulatory protocols. Recent investigations also show that insulin-producing cells can be derived not only from the endocrine part of the pancreas but also from mesenchymal and haematopoietic stem cells, embryonic stem cells, induced pluripotent stem cells or transdifferentiated engineered cells. Although these approaches represent major hope for the not-too-distant future, no clinical study using in-vitro-developed β-cell lines has been initiated so far.

Acknowledgement

This work was supported by grant No. MZO 00023001 of the Czech Ministry of Health.

References

1. Troppmann C, Gruessner AC, Dunn DL, *et al.* (1998) Surgical complications requiring early relaparotomy after pancreas transplantation: A multivariate risk factor and economic impact analysis of the cyclosporine era. *Ann Surg* **227**, 255–268.
2. Largiader F. (1977) Farewell to pancreatic organ transplantation? *Eur Surg Res* **9**, 399–402.
3. Harlan DM, Kenyon NS, Korsgren O, *et al.* (2009) Current advances and travails in islet transplantation. *Diabetes* **58**, 2175–2184.
4. Johansson H, Lukinius A, Moberg L, *et al.* (2005) Tissue factor produced by the endocrine cells of the islets of Langerhans is associated with a negative outcome of clinical islet transplantation. *Diabetes* **54**, 1755–1762.
5. Ricordi C, Lacy PE, Finke EH, *et al.* (1988) Automated method for isolation of human pancreatic islets. *Diabetes* **37**, 413–420.
6. Ricordi C, Tzakis AG, Carroll PB, *et al.* (1992) Human islet isolation and allotransplantation in 22 consecutive cases. *Transplantation* **53**, 407–414.
7. Scharp DW, Lacy PE, Santiago JV, *et al.* (1990) Insulin independence after islet transplantation into type I diabetic patient. *Diabetes* **39**, 515–518.
8. Shapiro AM, Lakey JR, Ryan EA, *et al.* (2000) Islet transplantation in seven patients with type 1 diabetes mellitus using a glucocorticoid-free immunosuppressive regimen. *N Engl J Med* **343**, 230–238.
9. The Diabetes Control and Complications Trial Research Group. (1993) The effect of intensive treatment of diabetes on the development and progression of long-term complications in insulin-dependent diabetes mellitus. *N Engl J Med* **329**, 977–986.
10. Ryan EA, Paty BW, Senior PA, *et al.* (2005) Five-year follow-up after clinical islet transplantation. *Diabetes* **54**, 2060–2069.
11. Vantyghem MC, Kerr-Conte J, Arnalsteen L, *et al.* (2009) Primary graft function, metabolic control, and graft survival after islet transplantation. *Diabetes Care* **32**, 1473–1478.
12. Maffi P, Bertuzzi F, De Taddeo F, *et al.* (2007) Kidney function after islet transplant alone in type 1 diabetes: Impact of immunosuppressive therapy on progression of diabetic nephropathy. *Diabetes Care* **30**, 1150–1155.
13. Shapiro AM, Ricordi C, Hering BJ, *et al.* (2006) International trial of the Edmonton protocol for islet transplantation. *N Engl J Med* **355**, 1318–1330.
14. Leitao CB, Cure P, Messinger S, *et al.* (2009) Stable renal function after islet transplantation: Importance of patient selection and aggressive clinical management. *Transplantation* **87**, 681–688.
15. Balamurugan AN, Breite AG, Anazawa T, *et al.* (2010) Successful human islet isolation and transplantation indicating the importance of class 1 collagenase and collagen degradation activity assay. *Transplantation* **89**, 954–961.
16. Hering BJ, Kandaswamy R, Harmon JV, *et al.* (2004) Transplantation of cultured islets from two-layer preserved pancreases in type 1 diabetes with anti-CD3 antibody. *Am J Transplant* **4**, 390–401.
17. Hanson MS, Park EE, Sears ML, *et al.* (2010) A simplified approach to human islet quality assessment. *Transplantation* **89**, 1178–1188.

18. Girman P, Berkova Z, Dobolilova E, *et al.* (2008) How to use image analysis for islet counting. *Rev Diabet Stud* **5**, 38–46.
19. Villiger P, Ryan EA, Owen R, *et al.* (2005) Prevention of bleeding after islet transplantation: Lessons learned from a multivariate analysis of 132 cases at a single institution. *Am J Transplant* **5**, 2992–2998.
20. Toso C, Vallee JP, Morel P, *et al.* (2008) Clinical magnetic resonance imaging of pancreatic islet grafts after iron nanoparticle labeling. *Am J Transplant* **8**, 701–706.
21. Froud T, Ricordi C, Baidal DA, *et al.* (2005) Islet transplantation in type 1 diabetes mellitus using cultured islets and steroid-free immunosuppression: Miami experience. *Am J Transplant* **5**, 2037–2046.
22. Fiorina P, Shapiro AM, Ricordi C, *et al.* (2008) The clinical impact of islet transplantation. *Am J Transplant* **8**, 1990–1997.
23. Blondet JJ, Carlson AM, Kobayashi T, *et al.* (2007) The role of total pancreatectomy and islet autotransplantation for chronic pancreatitis. *Surg Clin North Am* **87**, 1477–1501.

13 Anaesthesia for renal transplantation

Nicoletta Fossati

Pre-operative assessment

Kidney transplantation (KT) recipients are assessed comprehensively before being listed. The attending anaesthetist should check their condition has not significantly changed since then. Also, some derangements may be recognised and treated prior to theatre.

End-stage renal disease (ESRD) patients with ischaemic heart disease (IHD), diabetes mellitus or who are over 50 years old will usually have had some form of stress test to define their cardiovascular reserve and risk (see Chapter 2). In the transplant setting, it is essential to confirm that the latest investigations are reasonably recent and match the current clinical status. A new 12-lead electrocardiogram (ECG) is imperative for all patients.

Chronic respiratory problems are an infrequent reason for turning down a potential KT recipient on the day of surgery. Moreover, as KT is an extraperitoneal procedure, the impact on post-operative breathing is likely to be limited. However, acute chest infections have to be excluded: if uncertainty persists after physical examination, a chest X-ray may be appropriate.

Fluid status in dialysed patients can shift from hypo- to hypervolaemia and KT recipients need to withstand a prolonged fluid challenge in the peri-operative period. Dialysis prior to transplant helps to minimise the chances of intra-operative fluid overload and attain acceptable plasma potassium concentrations, usually below 5.5 mmol/L: recent evidence points towards better outcomes with pre-operative dialysis [1]. However, this can worsen post-induction hypotension and cardiovascular instability. Antihypertensive drugs should not be discontinued peri-operatively, with the possible exception of angiotensin-converting enzyme (ACE) inhibitors and angiotensin-II receptor blockers. Discussion of this aspect with the renal medical team is recommended.

Handbook of Renal and Pancreatic Transplantation, First Edition. Edited by Iain A. M. MacPhee and Jiří Froněk.
© 2012 John Wiley & Sons, Ltd. Published 2012 by John Wiley & Sons, Ltd.

Some degree of chronic anaemia is not uncommon and is often well tolerated. Haemoglobin (Hb) levels lower than 6 g/dL should be treated with packed red cell transfusions: higher Hb levels may be needed in light of other co-morbidities, such as IHD. Further intra-operative transfusions are often unnecessary, but crossmatching should be arranged routinely, not least because of potential previous sensitisation to histocompatibility antigens: this can prolong crossmatch time significantly. Cytomegalovirus (CMV)-negative patients must receive CMV-negative blood units.

General considerations

General anaesthesia is the anaesthetic technique of choice for KT. Epidural analgesia can be considered, bearing in mind the possibility of platelet dysfunction, use of antiplatelet agents or anticoagulants, residual post-dialysis heparinisation or anticipated peri-operative administration of heparin and loss of sympathetic tone with potential difficulty in maintaining satisfactory blood pressure (BP) levels.

Because of the incidence of gastroparesis in diabetic ESRD patients and the erratic timing of KTs from deceased donors, the risk of aspiration of residual stomach contents at induction has to be assessed: a modified rapid sequence induction (RSI) technique may be appropriate in some cases. Suxamethonium is traditionally avoided in ESRD patients, given the potential risk of acute hyperkalaemia; rocuronium should be considered for RSI if a difficult airway is not anticipated [2].

Careful positioning is essential to avoid damage to peripheral nerves, especially in patients with poor nutritional status, or to an existing arteriovenous fistula (AVF): this should be protected with soft wrapping and the arm on that side not used for cannulation or BP measurements. Intramuscular anaesthetic premedication is generally avoided and tends to be given intravenously in the anaesthetic room.

Lines and monitoring

Peripheral intravenous cannulation may be difficult: AVFs also limit the options available. Starting with a small-bore peripheral cannula and postponing further cannulation until after induction is an acceptable strategy. If necessary, existing dialysis lines can be used, making sure to aspirate the indwelling heparin first and taking care to minimise line-related infection risks.

Non-invasive BP monitoring is acceptable in the majority of cases. Arterial cannulation may be difficult because of atherosclerosis or previous AVF attempts: it should be performed if high cardiovascular risk and/or frequent intra-operative blood sampling is anticipated.

The use of ultrasound is recommended to site and cannulate central veins, especially in patients with a previous history of dialysis lines. The use of less invasive haemodynamic monitoring tools, such as the oesophageal Doppler, is justified given the limitations of central venous pressure (CVP) as a guide to cardiovascular filling, potential cannulation difficulties and increased infection risk in immunosuppressed patients.

A urinary catheter is placed after induction. Routine monitoring should also include a temperature probe, as maintaining normothermia is crucial (see Maintenance section, below), and the use of a peripheral nerve stimulator for train-of-four monitoring of intra-operative paralysis: a steady level of muscle relaxation is needed, particularly during vascular anastomosis creation and upon kidney reperfusion, while avoiding drug overdosage.

Induction

Thiopentone is considered the induction agent of choice for KT; however, propofol is also used in clinical practice. Both should be carefully titrated to effect, to limit post-induction hypotension. Fentanyl is used to attenuate cardiovascular responses to laryngoscopy and tracheal intubation. Midazolam, a short-acting benzodiazepine with a relatively favourable cardiovascular profile, may add sedation and amnesia. As post-induction hypotension remains a common issue in ESRD patients, a co-induction strategy may be considered.

Maintenance

One of the main aims of anaesthesia for KT is to maintain cardiovascular stability and satisfactory BP levels. Volatile anaesthesia with isoflurane in a 50% O_2/N_2O or O_2/air mixture is an adequate option. Sevoflurane has been under scrutiny because of the nephrotoxic potential of Compound A, a significant by-product at low fresh gas flows, in some animals [3]. More recently, a potential role of sevoflurane in renal preconditioning and resistance to ischaemia has been suggested [4]. While further substantiation of sevoflurane-related effects on human kidneys is warranted, fresh gas flow rates of at least 2 L/min for exposures greater than 1 hour are considered a cautious approach.

Fentanyl can be used for analgesia during KT. Some of morphine's active metabolites are renally excreted, but this does not absolutely contraindicate its use in this setting.

Atracurium is the muscle relaxant of choice, as its metabolism does not depend directly on liver or renal function: Hofmann elimination, which is pH and temperature dependent, and ester hydrolysis both play a role. Where atracurium-mediated histamine release may be of concern, cisatracurium, an atracurium isomer, can be used where available; both drugs can be administered as boluses or continuous infusions. One of their metabolites is laudanosine, which has epileptogenic potential: this is usually not an issue in anaesthetic practice.

Normal (0.9%) saline (NS) has been challenged as an adequate replacement fluid, as it may induce metabolic, hyperchloraemic acidosis in normal patients and lead to hyperkalaemia. A recent study in live donor KT recipients has shown that intra-operative Ringer's solution administration was associated with less hyperkalaemia and acidosis than NS [5]. As the debate around peri-operative fluid management continues, it is still common practice to give KT patients potassium-free solutions intra-operatively. If monitored, a CVP between 12 and 15 mmHg (from the mid-axillary line) is an acceptable haemodynamic target, although trends may be more reliable. Colloids are not routinely used, except for the occasional fluid challenge in the post-operative period. The use of vasopressors should be kept to a minimum. There is lack of consistent evidence to support intra-operative use of diuretics to improve graft function, particularly for long-term results.

Maintaining normothermia prevents shivering and unwanted vasoconstriction upon emergence from anaesthesia; atracurium and cisatracurium elimination is also negatively affected by hypothermia. All the habitual temperature-preserving strategies should be deployed.

Anaesthetists are usually required to administer antibiotics and immunosuppressants during KT. It is important that immunosuppressants be administered ahead of kidney reperfusion. Muscle-relaxant reversal agents can be used: their elimination half-time may be prolonged.

For drug dosages, see Table 13.1.

Table 13.1 Drug dosages.

Drug	Timing	Dosage
Thiopentone	Induction	3–5 mg/kg*
Propofol	Induction	1.5–2.0 mg/kg*
Midazolam	Co-induction	0.04 mg/kg
Fentanyl	Induction	1 μg/kg
Fentanyl	intra-operative analgesia (every 30–60 min)	0.5–1 μg/kg
Fentanyl	PCA	up to 120–180 μg/h
Atracurium	Induction	0.3–0.6 mg/kg
Atracurium	Continuous infusion	5–8 μg/kg^{-1} min^{-1}
Cisatracurium	Induction	0.15–0.2 mg/kg
Cisatracurium	Continuous infusion	1–2 μg/kg^{-1} min^{-1}
Bupivacaine	End of surgery (local infiltration)	up to 2 mg/kg**
0.1% bupivacaine	Continuous infusion	4–15 mL/h**

*Titrated to effect.
**Maximum over 4 hours and total of 400 mg in 24 hours.

Post-anaesthesia care

Post-operative fluid therapy should aim to match urine output and replace insensible losses. Polyuria can occur, resembling acute tubular necrosis: if hourly urine output exceeds 500 mL, only 75% of the amount should be replaced. Local protocols may vary in the proportion and combination of different fluids electrolyte concentrations must be closely monitored. Oliguria should prompt investigations to exclude or treat hypovolaemia, vascular thrombosis or urinary catheter obstruction. BP levels should match at least those habitual for the patient: hypo- or hypertensive extremes must be avoided and treated aggressively.

Pain can be treated with opioid patient-controlled analgesia (PCA) and paracetamol. For fentanyl PCA, 15 microgram boluses with a delay of 5 minutes between doses is an acceptable regimen for most patients. Some potential for respiratory depression is inherent to opioid use: close patient observation and O_2 supplementation at least for the duration of PCA are advisable. Post-operative nausea and vomiting (PONV) can be prevented or treated with ondansetron, without dosage adaptation.

Local anaesthetic infusion may reduce opioid consumption: an epidural catheter can be positioned by the surgeon between muscle layers during wound closure. Bupivacaine is highly protein-bound and metabolised in the liver to inactive compounds, excreted by the kidney. An initial bolus of 0.25% or 0.5% bupivacaine, titrated to patient weight, is administered via the catheter at the end of surgery, followed by 0.1% bupivacaine via a syringe pump at a rate between 5 and 15 mL/hour. This infusion is maintained for the first 24 hours.

KT patients can usually be transferred back to the renal ward: admission to a high-dependency or intensive care unit is reserved to patients at higher risk of peri-operative complications or after an intra-operative adverse event. For an anaesthetic checklist, see Table 13.2.

Table 13.2 Kidney transplantation anaesthetic checklist.

Key area	Issues	Action(s)
Cardiovascular assessment	Too old? Reflecting current status?	Always new ECG Consider urgent echocardiogram
Fluid status (pre-operative)	Timing of last dialysis, hypo- or hypervolaemia	Early fluid infusion or dialysis session
Electrolyte status	Risk of hyperkalaemia	Consider dextrose and insulin, salbutamol, dialysis, alkalinisation

Continued

Table 13.2 *Continued*

Key area	Issues	Action(s)
Medications	β-blockers	Maintain*
	ACE-inhibitors	Withhold*
	Oral antidiabetics	Withhold
	Insulin	Sliding scale
Hb and blood transfusions	Chronic anaemia	Blood transfusion (threshold)
	IHD, peripheral vascular disease	Lower transfusion threshold
	HLA sensitisation	Discuss with haematologist/ arrange early crossmatch
	CMV status	CMV-negative blood for CMV-negative recipients
Platelets and clotting	Antiplatelet agents	Discuss with surgeon/ consider fresh platelets
	Warfarin	Vitamin K, consider fresh frozen plasma
	Residual heparin from dialysis	Consider protamine
Fasting status	Timing of last food, diabetic gastroparesis, acid reflux	Starve for 6 hours/ consider modified RSI
Monitoring	Presence of AVF	Avoid AVF side for cannulations/BP monitoring Warn recovery staff
	Significant IHD/poorly controlled BP levels	Consider invasive monitoring
	Filling status/cardiac output	Consider alternatives to CVP (e.g. oesophageal Doppler)
Induction	Post-induction hypotension	Titrate to effect Consider co-induction
Fluid status (intra-operative)	Adequate filling	CVP 12–15 mmHg Response to fluid challenge Consider trends Ask surgeon after reperfusion (Kidney 'floppy'? Anastomotic problems?)

Table 13.2 *Continued*

Key area	Issues	Action(s)
Maintenance	Varying stimulation levels	Avoid cardiovascular instability
Post-anaesthesia care	Pain control – PCA	O_2 while patient on PCA
	PONV prevention/ treatment	1st and 2nd line prescriptions

*Discuss with nephrologists.
ACE, angiotensin-converting enzyme; AVF, arterio-venous fistula; BP, blood pressure, CMV, cytomegalovirus; CVP, central venous pressure; ECG, electrocardiogram; HLA, human leucocyte antigen; IHD, ischaemic heart disease; PCA, patient-controlled analgesia; PONV, post-operative nausea and vomiting; RSI, rapid sequence induction.

References

1. Van Biesen W, Veys N, Vanholder R, *et al.* (2006) The impact of the pre-transplant replacement modality on outcome after cadaveric kidney transplantation: The Ghent experience. *Contrib Nephrol* **150**, 254–258.
2. Robertson EN, Driessen JJ, Vogt M, *et al.* (2005) Pharmacodynamics of rocuronium 0.3 mg kg^{-1} in adult patients with and without renal failure. *Eur J Anaesthesiol* **22**, 929–932.
3. Keller KA, Callan C, Prokocimer P, *et al.* (1995) Inhalation toxicity study of a haloalkene degradant of sevoflurane, Compound A (PIFE), in Sprague-Dawley rats. *Anesthesiology* **83**, 1220–1232.
4. Julier K, da Silva R, Garcia C, *et al.* (2003) Preconditioning by sevoflurane decreases biochemical markers for myocardial and renal dysfunction in coronary artery bypass graft surgery: A double-blinded, placebo-controlled, multicenter study. *Anesthesiology* **98**, 1315–1327.
5. O'Malley CM, Frumento RJ, Hardy MA, *et al.* (2005) A randomized, double-blind comparison of lactated Ringer's solution and 0.9% NaCl during renal transplantation. *Anesth Analg* **100**, 1518–1524.

14 Anaesthesia for pancreatic transplantation

Kai Zacharowski and Hans-Joachim Wilke

Pre-medication

The great majority of patients who present for pancreas transplantation suffer from advanced type-1 (juvenile) insulin-dependent diabetes mellitus (IDDM). Owing to significant diabetic nephropathy or end-stage renal failure requiring dialysis, they will generally also need simultaneous kidney transplantation. Although pancreas after kidney (PAK) transplantation or pancreas alone transplantation (PAT) are sometimes performed on these patients and do have their place, worldwide more than 80% of operative procedures are simultaneous pancreas and kidney transplants (SPK).

Any successful pancreas transplant leads to independence from exogenous insulin administration and, ideally, regression of diabetic neuropathy, retinopathy and nephropathy. Indeed, patients who have had SPK do not develop nephropathy in the graft kidney. Despite the burden of lifelong immunosuppression, outcome in patients after successful transplantation is far better in terms of overall morbidity and mortality than in patients who are managed only medically.

Despite these uncontroverted benefits, even in the hands of an expert, pancreas transplantation remains a high-risk surgical procedure, which often taxes the patient's physiological reserves to the utmost. Coronary artery disease causes most of the peri-operative morbidity and mortality in patients with IDDM and end-stage or near-end-stage renal disease. Consequently, it is crucial that the anaesthetist caring for these patients assesses the their cardiovascular status. Even patients who seem comparatively fit often suffer from asymptomatic but significant coronary and peripheral vascular disease. If the history, physical examination and/or routine tests such as electrocardiogram and chest X-ray of the patient suggest a cardiovascular problem, it is essential that it be investigated diligently with the help of the appropriate expert and, if possible, be corrected before transplantation.

Handbook of Renal and Pancreatic Transplantation, First Edition. Edited by Iain A. M. MacPhee and Jiří Froněk.
© 2012 John Wiley & Sons, Ltd. Published 2012 by John Wiley & Sons, Ltd.

Of course, equal attention must be paid to the patient's electrolyte, glucose, haemoglobin and acid-base status as well as time and type of last dialysis, if any.

In addition to the above, the anaesthetist must rule out the presence of diabetes-induced autonomic neuropathy and gastro-oesophageal reflux or gastroparesis. The autonomic neuropathy may manifest itself peri-operatively in exaggerated and sometimes refractory swings in heart rate or blood pressure in response to surgical stimulation and/or pharmacological interventions. Gastro-oesophageal reflux or gastroparesis predisposes the patient to pulmonary aspiration.

Finally, there is evidence that the incidence of difficult intubation is increased in patients presenting for pancreas transplantation. Hence, patients must be carefully checked for predictors of difficult intubation, such as stiffness of the temporomandibular and atlanto-occipital joints, retrognathia, prominent incisors, etc. If indicated, an alternative approach to airway management must be considered, such as video-assisted or awake fibre-optic intubation.

Planning of peri-operative anaesthesia

Regional anaesthesia

Although spinal anaesthesia, epidural anaesthesia or combined spinal–epidural anaesthesia (CSE) alone are theoretically possible, they are impractical in light of the long duration (5 hours or more) of the procedures, the frequent necessity for aggressive therapeutic interventions and the general need to properly secure the patient's airway. In addition, neuro-axial blocks with their attending sympathetic blockade may make fluid management more challenging. Similarly, patients suffering from diabetic polyneuropathy may wrongly attribute a peri-operative worsening of the condition to the block. Finally, nephropathy-induced coagulopathy may increase the risk of spinal cord injury.

These valid concerns must be balanced on a case-by-case basis against the well-documented benefits of (thoracic) epidural anaesthesia in major abdominal surgery (i.e. better autonomic stability and protection of the heart, superior peri-operative pain control, reduction of peri-operative intestinal paresis or paralysis and a shorter stay on the intensive-care/intermediate-care unit.

Combined epidural–general anaesthesia

At our clinic, a preferred method is a combined epidural-general anaesthetic that, in our opinion, is beneficial for the majority of patients. An epidural catheter is placed at the level of thoracic vertebrae 6 to 9 with the patient awake and either sitting or lying on their side. Meticulous attention is paid to proper technique and asepsis. Intraoperatively, the catheter is only used if the patient is haemodynamically stable. A mixture of ropivacaine plus sufentanil,

1.6 mg/mL and 0.5 μg/mL, respectively, is used; the rate of infusion is 4 to 8 mL/hour.

Induction of anaesthesia is done with propofol (1–2 mg/kg) and fentanyl (2–5 μg/kg). Prior to placement of the endotracheal tube, muscle relaxation is achieved by the administration of cis-atracurium (0.15 mg/kg), which offers the advantage of organ-independent Hoffmann degradation. If a patient is deemed at risk for pulmonary aspiration because of a full stomach (e.g. their last meal was less than 6 hours ago), or has a history of heartburn, early satiety and/or bloating, rapid sequence induction is performed, using rocuronium (0.6 mg/kg). The use of succinylcholine and pancuronium should be avoided. The former may lead to an unpredictable and potentially life-threatening rise in serum potassium concentration. The latter's duration of action is greatly prolonged in renal insufficiency.

Although anaesthesia could be maintained by a total intravenous technique such as continuous infusion of propofol plus repeat boluses of opioid and muscle relaxant, we maintain anaesthesia by the administration of desflurane. Desflurane's pharmacokinetic profile allows for rapid titration of anaesthetic depth and, as an added benefit, its hepatic metabolism is negligible. Sevoflurane's pharmacokinetic profile is similar and could also be used; however, up to 5% is metabolised, yielding inter alia inorganic fluoride, which is potentially nephrotoxic. Although there is no evidence in the literature that sevoflurane is detrimental in patients with compromised kidney function, we nonetheless believe it is prudent to avoid its use in cases of end-stage renal disease or a newly grafted kidney.

Appropriate antibiotic cover and immunosuppressant drugs are administered as per protocol. Placement of a nasogastric tube is routine. Throughout the procedure the patient is kept at normal body temperature by using a warming mattress, a forced air blower and warmed intravenous fluids. Finally, the site of a patient's arteriovenous fistula for dialysis is carefully protected by adequate positioning and cushioning.

Monitoring

In addition to standard monitoring consisting of pulse oximetry, electrocardiography with S-T segment analysis, non-invasive arterial blood pressure, temperature and urine output, we believe that it is mandatory to place both an arterial and a central venous line for continuous, beat-to-beat monitoring of arterial and central venous pressure (CVP). In the case of patients with limited cardiac reserve or extensive peripheral vascular disease, we place the arterial line prior to induction of anaesthesia, because prolonged hypotensive episodes right after induction are common in these patients and demand timely and decisive therapy.

The arterial line also permits frequent assessment of the adequacy of oxygenation and ventilation and allows tight control of blood glucose and haemoglobin concentrations as well as acid-base and electrolyte status. In turn, central venous access makes possible the rapid delivery of vasoactive and inotropic drugs in addition to determination of central venous oxygen saturation, which can be used as a surrogate measurement of cardiac output. These measures are necessary, as hypotension, hypoglycaemia, acidosis, anaemia and hyperkalaemia are common, in particular after unclamping and reperfusion of the allografts. These events must be treated timely and aggressively to ensure both the well-being of the patient and graft survival.

In patients with only marginal cardiac reserves, a transoesphageal echocardiography probe (TEE) or a Swan–Ganz catheter probe can be used in addition to the above monitoring devices. As a result, it is possible to achieve a more detailed analysis of cardiac function and performance and a more informed administration of fluid and inotropic and vasoactive drugs is possible.

Fluid management

To prevent the most common surgical complications, namely thrombosis of the pancreas graft and acute tubular necrosis of the kidney graft, there must be adequate graft blood flow, graft oxygen delivery and graft perfusion pressure. There is a consensus in the literature that to achieve these goals, CVP should be maintained at a high normal level of about 10–15 mmHg, haemoglobin concentration should be carefully monitored according to cardiovascular status and ischaemic tolerance, cardiac output be at least normal and systolic blood pressure between 120 to 140 mmHg. In practice, in an adult of average weight and height, this often means the administration of about 5 L of crystalloids, 1–2 L of colloids (albumin or hydroxyethyl starch) and 2–4 units of blood. If liberal fluid administration is not possible, or by itself insufficient to attain the aforementioned end points, the judicious use of inotropic and vasoactive drugs is recommended. Furthermore, to ensure kidney graft perfusion and reduce graft oedema, 20% mannitol is used by some centres during reperfusion of the kidney graft.

Needless to say, such aggressive volume loading in combination with the use of vasoactive drugs is not without risk to the patient. One does well not to follow 'numbers' blindly, but to use one's clinical judgment and experience. It is imperative to look at the 'whole picture' by communicating with the surgeon, by closely observing the surgical field and the appearance of the grafts, by noting the shape and the changes of the arterial and CVP curves and by meticulously monitoring urine output and changes in oxygenation and ventilation.

Pain management

Patients with diabetes mellitus often suffer from neuropathy. Pain is the most disturbing symptom of diabetic peripheral neuropathy. As many as

45% of patients with diabetes mellitus develop peripheral neuropathies. In addition to affected distal portions of neurones, axonal degeneration preferentially involves unmyelinated nerve fibres. This results in Schwann cell abnormalities, which translates into disturbances of nerve conduction of autonomic, motor and sensory fibres. Often a manifestation of bilateral peripheral neuropathy (motor and sensory) and various forms of dysautonomia can be observed, such as gastropathy, orthostatic blood pressure dysregulation, cardiac autonomic dysfunction, neurogenic bladder and sexual dysfunction. Several studies have analysed the beneficial effect of kidney–pancreas transplantation on diabetic neuropathy. It is undisputed that restoration of normoglycaemia is of benefit for the progression of neuropathy.

In great detail it was studied whether pancreas-transplanted patients have less diabetic autonomic and sensory motor neuropathy progression compared with a group receiving intensive insulin treatment. Following transplantation, the two groups were compared at 12, 24 and 42 months. In insulin-treated patients progression in diabetic autonomic and sensory motor neuropathy was seen, which was ameliorated in transplanted patients. Confirmation was delivered by more recent studies, also underlying an increase in nerve conduction velocity in combined pancreas–kidney transplanted patients with functioning pancreas grafts compared with those with a failed pancreas graft. Gastric neuropathy, which is estimated to occur in 20% of individuals with type-1 diabetes mellitus, causes gastroparesis accompanied by reduced motility and delayed emptying. This explains why blood glucose concentrations can be very difficult to control. Dehydration from persistent vomiting may lead to diabetic ketoacidosis, and diarrhoea is also often related to neuropathy. Symptoms of gastroparesis include abdominal bloating, nausea, vomiting and heartburn as a result of oesophageal regurgitation. Some patients suffer from severe, refractory pain requiring a special pain service. Usually, a single therapeutic agent is not sufficient, and simple analgesics are usually inadequate to control the pain. It is widely accepted that patients should be offered the available therapies in a stepwise fashion. However, following pancreatic transplantation pain control and therapy are often dominated by acute symptoms of surgical pain. After surgery, previously prescribed medication needs to be reviewed in terms of indication.

Thoracic epidural analgesia (TEA) has been demonstrated in our institution to be superior in comparison to intravenous opioids to achieve effective postoperative analgesia. Furthermore, TEA has been associated with a reduced rate of venous thromboembolic and respiratory failure events. We routinely use epidural analgesia as part of a combined general and regional anaesthetic technique. According to our standard procedure, we administer 10 mL of ropivacain 7.5% via the TEA prior to surgery. Thereafter, a mixture of ropivacain 0.16% and sulfentanil 0.5 μg/mL is given via a pump. Patients are followed up by our pain service twice a day.

Intensive-care/intermediate-care unit management

Following pancreas transplantation, patients should be cared for in a critical care unit. For the success of transplantation, excellent communication between the anaesthetic/critical care and surgical team is mandatory, as the most common cause of early graft lost in the first 6 months is technical failure (>50%), with thrombosis as the primary cause. Awareness and excellent training may help to diagnose early other causes of technical failure, such as infections, pancreatitis, bleeding and anastomotic leak. Technical reasons of graft failure are rare after 6 months.

Patients with diabetes undergoing pancreas transplantation usually suffer from additional conditions such as neuropathy, and microvascular and macrovascular changes that result in significant morbidity and mortality from complications of the kidneys, blood vessels, nerves and eyes. This translates into a 17 times higher incidence of kidney disease, a five times higher incidence of gangrene, and an incidence of heart disease that is doubled compared with non-diabetic patients. Approximately 34% of individuals with type-1 diabetes develop end-stage renal disease as a secondary complication within 15 years of disease onset. Diabetes accelerates atherosclerosis, resulting in cardiovascular disease, which is the leading cause of death in diabetic patients. Therefore, postoperative management needs to address these potential causes of complications early and sufficiently.

Treatment and monitoring includes acid–base management, analgesia, fluid balance, haemodynamics, oxygen and respiratory status. Peri-operative fluid management is guided by clinical judgement supported by urine output, various haemodynamic parameters and surgical circumstances (blood loss, larger wounds, long operation time, evaporative and nasogastric losses, and third space among others). Routine care includes blood glucose control, immunosuppression and steroid therapy, as well as guideline conformant and hospital-specific antibiotic therapy. Continuous monitoring of various parameters such as arterial gases, haemoglobin, serum electrolytes, amylase and clotting is important. Furthermore, a chest X-ray needs to be done to control/inspect CVP and nasogastric line position as well as lung fields. Anticoagulation with heparin (thromboprophylaxis) and total parenteral nutrition is usually started on the first day after surgery. Intensivists should be aware of the various potential complications following pancreas transplantation such as local and systemic infection, leaks from duodenum and/or ileum infection, side effects from immunosuppressive therapy, systemic inflammatory response syndrome and pancreatitis among others.

Pancreatic graft function is monitored by blood glucose, amylase, haemoglobin A1c, and C-peptide levels. If the systemic-bladder technique is used, the urinary amylase concentrations are monitored. Likewise, if the patient has a pancreatic drain, amylase concentrations in the drainage are monitored. Fluid-volume depletion can occur rapidly owing to fluid shifts, brisk diuresis, gastroparesis and, in patients with the bladder-diversion technique, loss of pancreatic fluid into the bladder. Laboratory findings include increased and serum urea and creatinine, decreased serum bicarbonate, and increased haematocrit due to haemoconcentration. Administration of albumin and intravenous fluids with or without bicarbonate prevents dehydration and corrects the metabolic acidosis associated with bladder drainage of pancreatic exocrine secretions. In patients with a duodenocystotomy, urinary catheter drainage is maintained for 5–10 days postoperatively. A cystogram or postvoid ultrasound is performed following removal of the catheter.

Key references

1. Pichel AC, Macnab WR. (2005) Anaesthesia for pancreas transplantation. Continuing Education in Anaesthesia. *Contin Educ Anaesth Crit Care Pain* **5**, 149–152.
2. Lima-Rodriguez JR, Garcia-Gil FA, Garcia-Garcia JJ, *et al.* (2008) Effects of premedication with tiletamine/zolazepam/medetomidine during general anesthesia using sevoflurane/fentanyl in swine undergoing pancreas transplantation. *Transplant Proc* **40**, 3001–3006.
3. Koehntop DE, Beebe DS, Belani KG. (2000) Perioperative anesthetic management of the kidney-pancreas transplant recipient. *Curr Opin Anaesthesiol* **13**, 341–347.
4. Halpern, H, Miyoshi E, Kataoka LM, *et al.* (2004) Anesthesia for pancreas transplantation alone or simultaneous with kidney. *Transplant Proc* **36**, 3105–3106.
5. Sealey MM. (1988) Anaesthesia for combined pancreatic and renal transplantation and potassium homeostasis. *Eur J Anaesthesiol* **5**, 193–206.
6. Backonja M, Beydoun A, Edwards KR, *et al.* (1998) Gabapentin for the symptomatic treatment of painful neuropathy in patients with diabetes mellitus. a randomized controlled trial. *JAMA* **280**, 1831–1836.
7. Kanji JN, Anglin RE, Hunt DL, *et al.* (2010) Does this patient with diabetes have large-fiber peripheral neuropathy? *JAMA* **303**, 1526–1532.
8. Martinenghi S, Comi G, Galardi G, *et al.* (1997) Amelioration of nerve conduction velocity following simultaneous kidney/pancreas transplantation is due to the glycaemic control provided by the pancreas. *Diabetologia* **40**, 1110–1112.
9. Ziegler D, Hidvegi T, Gurieva I, *et al.* (2010) Efficacy and safety of lacosamide in painful diabetic neuropathy. *Diabetes Care* **33**, 839–841.
10. Gruessner AC, Sutherland DE. (2005) Pancreas transplant outcomes for United States (US) and non-US cases as reported to the United Network for Organ Sharing (UNOS) and the International Pancreas Transplant Registry (IPTR) as of June 2004. *Clin Transplant* **19**, 433–455.

15 Anaesthesia for live donor nephrectomy

Rehana Iqbal and Karthik Somasundaram

Introduction

Renal transplantation was first attempted over 100 years ago and has been performed successfully for over 70 years. In the mid 1950s, the first successful kidney transplant from a live donor to his sibling was performed [1]. Since then, driven partly by increased transplant waiting times, as well as by demonstration of favourable outcomes compared with cadaveric donors, live donation has become a valuable treatment option for end-stage renal failure.

Anaesthetising a patient who is donating a kidney to another individual requires an understanding of the donor selection process, the surgical techniques used for nephrectomy, the specific anaesthetic issues related to the procedure and an appreciation that this major surgery is not of direct physical benefit to the patient. This enables the attending anaesthetist to address specific concerns of the patient with regard to anaesthesia that may not arise during discussions with patients preparing for other types of elective surgery.

Selection

British Transplantation Society guidelines recommend medical assessment of a live donor by a renal physician. This rigorous assessment takes into account all aspects of the patient's medical and social history, with emphasis on cardiovascular, renal, endocrine and psychiatric disease, as well as smoking and drug abuse.

Physical examination records body mass index (BMI) and identifies concomitant disease. Investigations include haematological and biochemistry profiles as well as screening for infectious diseases. ABO compatibility and HLA matching is mandatory, as are electrocardiography and chest X-ray. Renal anatomy including vasculature is assessed by ultrasound and computerised tomography scans prior to surgery.

Handbook of Renal and Pancreatic Transplantation, First Edition. Edited by Iain A. M. MacPhee and Jiří Froněk.
© 2012 John Wiley & Sons, Ltd. Published 2012 by John Wiley & Sons, Ltd.

Contraindications to donation include donor diabetes mellitus, evidence of end-organ hypertensive damage, glomerulonephritis, certain forms of nephrolithiasis, active malignancy, renovascular disease, BMI >35 and HIV infection. Patients should be warned in advance that screening may identify diseases that they were not previously aware of and this may have implications (for example, obtaining health insurance).

The purpose of the selection process is to ensure risks are minimal and inherent to general anaesthesia and the surgery.

Surgical technique

The technique used to anaesthetise for live donor nephrectomy is influenced by the planned method of surgery. It is common for the donor and recipient to be anaesthetised in parallel operating theatres for minimal ischaemic time.

Open nephrectomy involves a flank incision and occasionally rib resection for ease of access. It is associated with increased post-operative pain and potentially significant blood loss. Central access and intra-arterial access is obtained and the patient is usually positioned on their side. Large bore intravenous access is needed and a pre-operative blood sample for group and save is essential. An epidural catheter for postoperative pain relief is usual. Open nephrectomy has been largely superseded by laparoscopic techniques.

Laparoscopic donor nephrectomy has proven safe in experienced hands and associated with reduced blood loss and less postoperative pain [2]. Techniques vary and include both transperitoneal and retroperitoneal approaches with or without hand assistance [3,4].

Anaesthetic technique

The purpose of the anaesthetic technique is to provide anaesthesia with minimal risk to the donor, optimal conditions for surgical access and minimisation of physiological insult to the retrieved kidney. The procedure can be broadly classified into five stages.

Pre-operative assessment
It is increasingly common for live donors to meet their anaesthetist on the day of their operation at the pre-operative assessment. Patients presenting particular anaesthetic risks should be identified and discussed beforehand. Safety of the donor is paramount and anaesthesia and surgery should be postponed unless conditions are optimal to proceed on that particular day.

The pre-operative assessment provides an opportunity for the anaesthetist to assess the patient, plan the anaesthetic, develop a rapport with the patient, obtain consent for procedures and answer any specific questions or alleviate concerns.

Routine assessment includes an anaesthetic history, general medical questioning and relevant examination, medication history, allergies, functional history, starvation history and assessment of the airway. Patients should not ingest solids for 6 hours prior to surgery and clear fluids for two hours. All patients should have routine full blood count, biochemistry and a group and save sent.

Unidentified major disease is not usually discovered at the pre-operative visit but patients may still have conditions worth noting – for example, treated hypertension, osteoarthritis, obesity, active respiratory tract infection and potential difficult intubation may all be present in a live approved donor.

Patients have different concerns and questions about anaesthesia. It is important to note that the psychology of donation is complex. Patients are generally well and undertaking a procedure that carries a risk of mortality (1:3000) and potential major morbidity (1–2%) [5]. Although supported by transplant coordinators, the patients may remain apprehensive on the day and may not have discussed the risks of anaesthesia. Written information about anaesthesia may be provided prior to the surgery however meeting the anaesthetist may be their first opportunity to discuss anaesthetic plans and risks. Being aware of and addressing this with the patient should alleviate any concerns.

Other points to discuss with the patient will include the possibility of blood transfusion, central venous pressure (CVP)/arterial lines and postoperative high-dependency/intensive-care unit if complications arise.

Live organ donation is a topical issue with regard to consent. The concept of performing an unnecessary operation on a patient is potentially at odds with the *primum non nocere* doctrine of medical care. However, this may be overruled by both the patient's own autonomy and the fact that live organ donation may have psychological benefits for the donor as well as the recipient.

Nonetheless, it is crucial that patients are fully informed before consenting to live donor nephrectomy, and this includes the risks of anaesthesia. There is no evidence to suggest that anaesthesia for live donor nephrectomy carries any greater risk than anaesthesia for other elective surgery.

Induction of anaesthesia

The procedure is invariably undertaken with general anaesthesia. The choice of drugs used for induction and maintenance will depend on the experience and preference of the anaesthetist. Induction will tend to be with an intravenous induction agent such as propofol and anaesthesia maintained by continuing with an infusion of propofol or the use of an inhalational volatile agent. There is no evidence to suggest either technique is superior here. Following induction, an intubating dose of muscle relaxant is administered and the airway secured with a cuffed endotracheal tube (ET), allowing control of oxygenation and ventilation and protecting the airway from secretions and aspiration.

CVP/arterial lines are not routine but single large-bore peripheral intravenous access is established, as there is the potential for blood loss. Antibiotics are given depending on local protocols – infection rates for live donor nephrectomy are low. Given that there is potential for blood loss, patients should be group and saved.

Preparation of patient in theatre

A third of the time in theatre is spent positioning the patient. The importance of this cannot be underestimated. Care taken with positioning enables good surgical access and avoids complications related to surface or peripheral nerve injuries. The left kidney has a longer renal vein and is the preferred side to operate. For a left-sided nephrectomy patients are positioned in the right lateral position. Pressure areas are padded.

During positioning, patients are exposed and may drop their temperature significantly. It is not uncommon for core temperature to drop below 35 °C – which as well as being distressing for a patient once in recovery exposes them to increased risk of complications. For this reason it is advisable that warmed intravenous fluids are administered from the point of induction of anaesthesia and an underbody warming device used. Core temperature should be monitored for the duration of surgery and above and below warming blankets used.

Anaesthetic considerations during surgery

Fluid hydration
There is no set regimen for fluid hydration, either in terms of quantity of fluid and constituency of fluid. This may be an area for future research. These patients are often not starved for a prolonged period, have minimal insensible losses if the procedure is undertaken laparascopically and less than 100 mL of blood loss in uncomplicated surgery. Fluid administration is guided by the appearance of the kidney (an underfilled kidney is soft, vein is empty), surgical losses and physiological parameters (heart rate, blood pressure and urine output, which are influenced by the physiological consequences of laparoscopic surgery and the process of anaesthesia). The surgical time on average is 1.5–3 hours and patients typically receive between 2 and 3 litres of fluid.

Muscle relaxation
Adequate muscle relaxation is required for surgical access and the purposes of ventilation. The 'surgical space' is markedly reduced when relaxation is inadequate. Muscle relaxation should be monitored during the surgery with the use of a peripheral nerve stimulator.

Analgesia
Analgesia is provided with the use of intravenous opiates and paracetamol. Use of non-steroidal anti-inflammatory drugs is controversial and administration will depend on local policies.

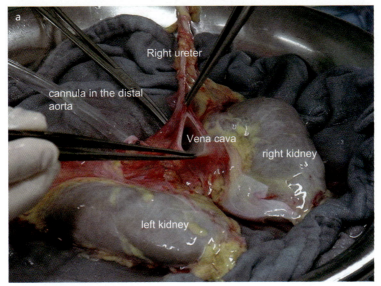

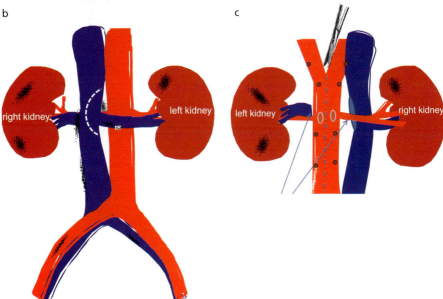

Figure 6.2 (a) Splitting of the en-bloc procured kidneys at the back table. Following en-bloc retrieval, the kidneys are first placed in a bowl in iced water in an anatomical position, and then both the ureters, the vena cava and the renal veins, as well as the aorta and the renal arteries, are identified. (b) After identification of all the renal vessels and structures, the left renal vein is first dissected free and divided (see dotted line) at the level of the vena cava, which remains with the right kidney (anterior view). (c) Following transection of the left renal vein from the vena cava (arrows), the kidney bloc is then turned upside down, so that the posterior surface of the aorta is laying anteriorly. The exact middle at the posterior surface of the aorta can be identified safely and easily by the presence of the lumbar arteries and is opened by cutting between the stumps of the lumbar vessels in a caudal to cranial direction. This allows a clear view of the exact vascular anatomy of the renal arteries and an easy and correct division of the aorta on the anterior surface can then be achieved (posterior view).

Handbook of Renal and Pancreatic Transplantation, First Edition. Edited by
Iain A. M. MacPhee and Jiří Froněk.
© 2012 John Wiley & Sons, Ltd. Published 2012 by John Wiley & Sons, Ltd.

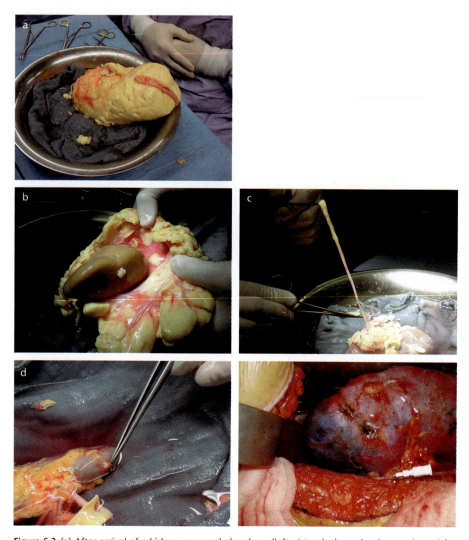

Figure 6.3 (a) After arrival of a kidney procured elsewhere (left picture), the redundant peri-renal fat is removed at the lower, middle and upper pole (but not around the pyelum, or pelvis) and between the lower pole and the upper ureter, revealing some unexpected and unreported lesions. Minimal defatting of the kidney immediately following the procurement will not only allow a better topical cooling but will also prevent unexpected findings to occur at the moment of unpacking the kidney at the recipient's centre; attention should be given not to devascularise the pyelum of the kidney. (b) During the removal of the fat, care must be taken not to cause any decapsulation that may render the renal graft no longer transplantable or compromise the transplantation. (c) One pitfall in the procurement of the ureter is to leave as much peri-ureteral tissue with the graft and not to dissect upon and to devascularise the ureter itself, resulting in the so-called 'spaghetti' ureter. (d) Image of a transected upper pole artery, which was responsible for a large zone of poorly vascularised renal parenchyma – this may be of particular importance for the lower pole, where the blood supply of the proximal ureter might be compromised. A vascular reconstruction was done using the inferior epigastric artery.

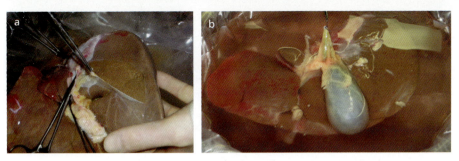

Figure 6.4 (a) An extensive capsular tear of the liver is shown. This may reflect the lack of gentle manipulation of the graft and its supplying blood vessels. (b) Example of an unflushed hepatic duct during procurement of the liver. Here, the common bile duct (CBD) was tied of instead of the cystic duct (CD). For more detailed examination of these issues, please see pp. 104–105.

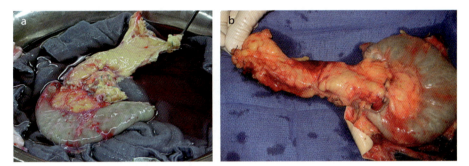

Figure 6.5 Representative image of a well-procured pancreas (a) and a pancreas that was discarded because of a large hematoma and capsular tear (b).

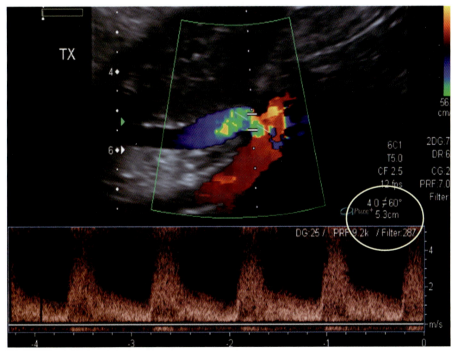

Figure 19.2 (a) Doppler ultrasound images showing a suspected stenosis just above the anastamosis, with an elevated velocity measured at around 4 m/s.

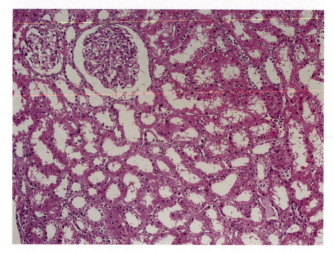

Figure 20.1 Ischaemic tubular injury with flattening of the epithelial cells and tubular dilatation (H&E).

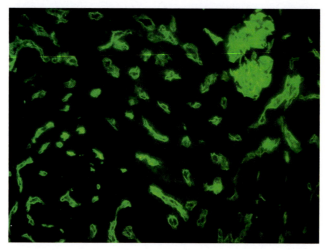

Figure 20.2 Diffuse positive staining of C4d along the peritubular capillaries (green) in immunofluorescence.

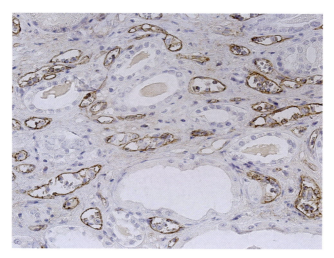

Figure 20.3 Deposition of C4d in peritubular capillaries detected by immunoperoxidase staining (brown) from paraffin-embedded tissue.

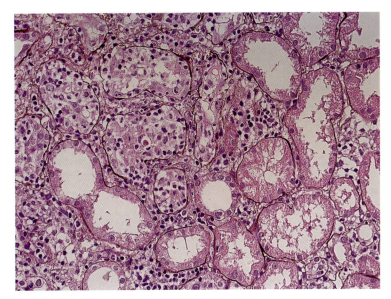

Figure 20.4 Interstitial inflammation with prominent tubulitis (mononuclear cells invade tubular epithelium, PASM).

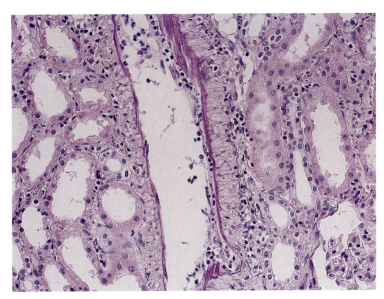

Figure 20.5 Intimal arteritis characterised by undermining of the endothelium by infiltrating lymphocytes (H&E with elastine).

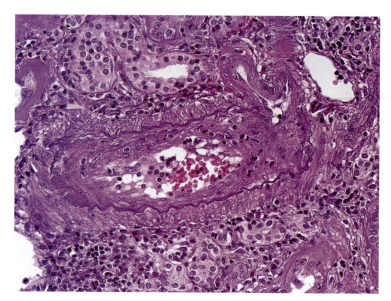

Figure 20.6 Advanced transplant arteritis with aggregates of mononuclear inflammatory cells and accumulation of fibrotic tissue in the intima (H&E with elastine).

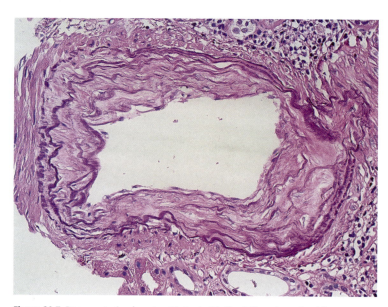

Figure 20.7 Donor arteriosclerosis with typical intimal fibroelastosis without inflammatory cells (H&E with elastine).

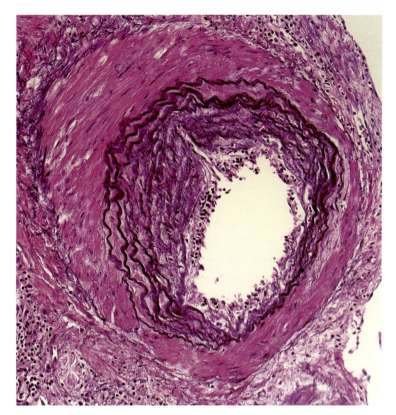

Figure 20.8 Transplant arteritis (early intimal arteritis) superimposed on pre-existing arteriosclerosis with intimal fibroelastosis (H&E with elastine).

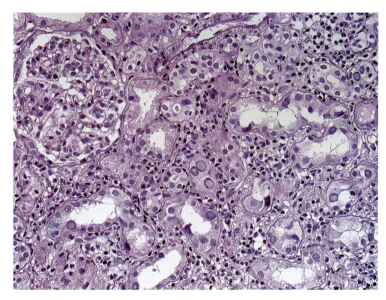

Figure 20.9 Polyomavirus nephropathy with nuclear inclusions in the epithelium and surrounding inflammation (H&E with elastine).

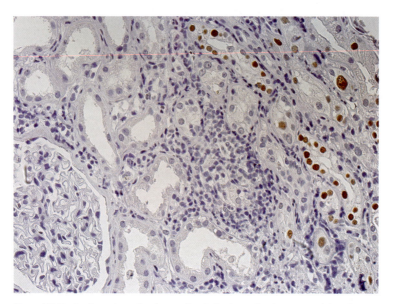

Figure 20.10 Confirmation of polyomavirus infection using immunostaining for SV40-T large antigen. Strong positive staining (brown) of the nuclei of infected tubular cells is demonstrated.

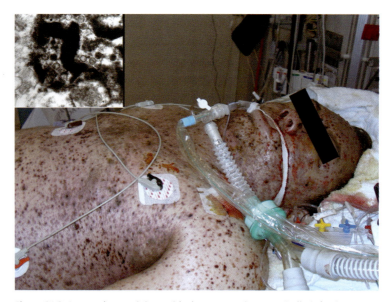

Figure 21.3 A transplant recipient with the severe primary varicella infection showing the characteristic skin eruption with associated respiratory failure, hepatic failure and disseminated intravascular coagulation. Insert: electron microscopy on liver tissue reveals viral nucleocapsids, typical of herpesviruses, associated with marginated chromatin.

Minimisation of insult to retrieved kidney

The anaesthetic technique should avoid hypotension and maintain oxygenation, normocarbia and hydration. This is for the purposes of minimising physiological insult to the patient but it also ensures that the retrieved kidney is in optimal condition for transplant.

Effects of laparoscopy

Physiological effects of laparoscopy can present certain issues to manage during the procedure [6]. These are broadly summarised below.

Cardiovascular

The effects of insufflating gas into the abdomen can cause a variety of haemodynamic effects.

Peritoneal stretch can be intensely stimulating, which can vary from vagally mediated bradycardia (and rarely ventricular standstill) to tachycardia and hypertension. Bradycardia can be treated with anticholinergics. It may be necessary to ask the surgeon to deflate the abdomen.

Pneumoperitoneum compresses the inferior vena cava and reduces venous return, which may cause hypotension. This may be partly offset by the fact that pneumoperitoneum will also increase systemic vascular resistance again by the effects of pressure. Consideration should be given to preloading the starved patient with fluid in the time between induction and insufflation.

Rarely, there is the potential for venous gas embolism or accidental insertion of the laparoscopic port directly into a major vessel. Both of these scenarios can lead to rapid cardiovascular collapse and require immediate resuscitation and treatment of the underlying cause.

Respiratory

Insufflation of the abdomen with CO_2 will splint the diaphragm and reduce functional residual capacity. Relatively high peak airway pressures may be needed to maintain minute ventilation and use of positve end-expiratory pressure is beneficial in maintaining small airway patency and reducing atelectasis.

Compression of the diaphragm by the insufflated abdomen can result in contents of the thorax being displaced cranially, occasionally causing an ET placed close to the carina to become an endobronchial one.

CO_2 used to insufflate the abdomen is gradually absorbed systemically, leading to a progressive rise in $PaCO_2$ and subsequently $ETCO_2$. This may be difficult to correct while the laparoscopy is ongoing because of balancing the needs of normocapnia against the risks of barotrauma. It is has been suggested that retroperitoneal CO_2 insufflation is associated with greater systemic CO_2 absorption than intraperitoneal procedures; however, the evidence for this is inconsistent [7,8]. It may be necessary to accept permissive hypercapnia for the duration of the procedure.

CO_2 may also pass through defects in connective tissue to cause carbothorax, which should be considered if the patient becomes suddenly difficult to ventilate, requiring higher pressures and desaturating.

Gastrointestinal

The pressure effects of CO_2 in the abdomen predispose to reflux of gastric contents. Laparoscopic surgery is associated with nausea and vomiting, and anti-emetics should be administered.

Renal

Pressure effects can reduce renal blood flow, which can be countered with fluid loading.

Emergence from anaesthesia and recovery

Patients can be recovered on the ward unless there is a specific indication for critical care. Early mobilisation, anti-emetics, analgesia, thromboprophylaxis and chest physiotherapy is undertaken routinely. Postoperative pain is usually managed with oral analgesics and opiates.

Although donors could be discharged at 24 hours, most donors live significant distances from the specialist centre in which the surgery is

Table 15.1 Summary of considerations for donor nephrectomy.

Stage of procedure	Approximate time (minutes)	Specific considerations
Pre-operative assessment	Extensive selection process	• Minimisation of risk to donor • Consent
Induction of anaesthesia	15	• Unanticipated airway problems or anaphylactic reactions • Warm intravenous fluids
Preparation of patient in theatre	30–45	• Positioning and padding • Urinary catheter • Antibiotic prophylaxis • Underbody warming mattress
Surgery	90–180	• Physiological effects of laparoscopic surgery • Adequate muscle relaxation for surgical access • Adequate fluid hydration • Avoidance of hypotension • Warming devices
Emergence and recovery	In-patient for approximately 24 hours to 3 days	• Anti-emetics • Analgesia • Early mobilisation • Chest physiotherapy

carried out. For this reason most donors would be discharged at 48 hours or later. For a summary of considerations for donor nephrectomy see Table 15.1.

In conclusion, anaesthesia for live donor nephrectomy is a relatively low-risk procedure; however, patients are having major surgery with the potential for significant complications. An awareness of the surgical options and potentially complex ethical and screening issues is vital to obtain informed consent. Specific consideration needs to be given to temperature control, physiological consequences of laparoscopic surgery, maintaining optimal condition of the retrieved organ, provision of optimal surgical conditions and – most importantly – minimisation of harm to the donor. The interests and safety of the donor have to be considered independently of the recipient.

References

1. Lawler RH, West JW, McNulty PH, *et al.* (1955) Successful homotransplantation of the kidney in an identical twin. *Trans Am Clin Climatol Assoc* **67**, 167–173.
2. Fabrizio MD, Ratner LE, Montgomery RA, *et al.* (1999) Laparoscopic live donor nephrectomy. *Urol Clin North Am* **26**, 247–256.
3. Challacombe B, Mamode N. (2004) Laparoscopic live donor nephrectomy. *Nephrology Dialysis Transplantation* **19**, 2961–2964.
4. Chandak P, Kessaris N, Challacombe B, *et al.* (2009) How safe is hand-assisted laparoscopic donor nephrectomy? Results of 200 live donor nephrectomies by two different techniques. *Nephrol Dial Transplant* **24**, 293–297.
5. British Transplantation Society. (2011) *UK Guidelines for Living Donor kidney Transplantation*. Available online from: http://www.bts.org.uk/transplantation/standards-and-guidelines/.
6. Perrin M, Fletcher A. (2004) Laparoscopic abdominal surgery. *Contin Educ Anaesth Crit Care Pain* **4**, 107–110.
7. Ng CS, Gill IS, Sung GT, *et al.* (1999) Retroperitoneoscopic surgery is not associated with increased carbon dioxide absorption. *J Urol* **162**, 1268–1272.
8. Streich B, Decailliot F, Perney C, *et al.* (2003) Increased carbon dioxide absorption during retroperitoneal laparoscopy. *Br J Anaesth* **91**, 793–796.

16 Immunosuppression

Iain A.M. MacPhee and Teun van Gelder

Overview

Immunosuppression for renal and pancreatic transplantation is based on multiple drug regimens [1] with wide variations between centres in the precise combinations used, reflecting the incomplete evidence base to guide practice. However, the majority of regimens are based on an induction antibody, calcineurin inhibitor (CNI), an antiproliferative agent and steroid. The point in the immune response targeted by each agent is summarised in Table 16.1. Use of synergistic combinations inhibiting different components of the anti-allograft response allows the minimisation of dose for each drug with the aim of reducing drug-specific side effects. Most episodes of acute rejection occur within the first month after transplantation and certainly within the first 3 months. A logical inference from this observation is that patients need more immunosuppression during the early period after the transplant and less after this point with the benefit of reduced long-term toxicity.

Complications of immunosuppression

The main consequence of suppression of the immune response to the graft is the concomitant inhibition of the response to intracellular pathogens resulting in opportunistic infection (covered in Chapter 21) and increased incidence of virus associated malignancy (covered in Chapter 23). The immunosuppressive drugs all have a narrow therapeutic index with a number of drug-specific side effects. As a general rule, more potent immunosuppressive combinations with low rates of acute rejection come at the expense of increased complications.

Monitoring of immunosuppression

Therapeutic drug monitoring
For the small-molecule drugs, total exposure over 24 hours measured as the area under the concentration-time curve (AUC) is the best predictor

Handbook of Renal and Pancreatic Transplantation, First Edition. Edited by Iain A. M. MacPhee and Jiří Froněk.

Table 16.1 Targets of the immunosuppressive drugs.

Site of action	Drugs
Inhibition of IL-2 production by T-lymphocytes	Ciclosporin Tacrolimus
Inhibition of T-lymphocyte response to IL-2	Basiliximab Sirolimus Everolimus
Inhibition of proliferation of T- and B-lymphocytes	Azathioprine Mycophenolate Leflunomide
Depletion of T- and B-lymphocytes	Polyclonal anti-lymphocyte antibodies (anti-thymocyte globulin, anti-lymphocyte globulin) Alemtuzumab
Depletion of T-lymphocytes	Muromonab CD3
Depletion of B-lymphocytes	Rituximab
Depletion of plasma cells	Bortezomib
Inhibition of complement-mediated cell lysis	Eculizumab
Inhibition of co-stimulatory signals	Azathioprine Belatacept Sotrastaurin

of efficacy. Measurement of full AUC is not practical for routine monitoring, and limited sampling strategies based on between one and three blood samples have been derived to estimate AUC. There is randomised controlled trial evidence to support therapeutic drug monitoring for mycophenolate, and measurement of blood concentrations of the CNI and mammalian target of rapamycin (mTOR) inhibitors has been widely adopted owing to the association between blood concentrations and efficacy or toxicity.

Prescribing clinicians should be aware of the type of assay being used. Immunoassays have the advantage of analysing samples as a batch, which facilitates same-day reporting of results. The disadvantage of the immunoassays is that the detection antibodies often cross-react with drug metabolites, which may be present at variable concentrations, resulting in assay variability. Some assays have substantial variability in the results obtained in different laboratories. Liquid chromatography-based assays offer greater accuracy and precision but with greater capital cost for equipment and a requirement for samples to be analysed in sequence, which may make same-day reporting more difficult. The results reported for chromatographic assays are usually lower than those for immunoassays owing to exclusion of cross-reacting metabolites. EDTA-anticoagulated blood is the standard blood sample used, allowing measurement of drug in whole blood or in plasma [2]. A recent development in blood sampling is the use of fingerprick sampling with measurement of the drug in dried blood spots. This approach allows the patient to collect multiple timed blood samples at home and has potential use in multicentre clinical trials, allowing the cards to be posted to a central laboratory [3].

Pharmacodynamic monitoring

With multiple drug therapy, measurement of blood concentrations of some, but usually not all, drugs in the regimen does not constitute a genuine assay of the overall degree of immunosuppression. A number of different approaches to pharmacodynamic monitoring are in development, but only the ImmuKnow assay (Cylex Inc.) based on inhibition of mitogen-driven T-lymphocyte proliferation has been licensed and adopted for routine clinical practice [4]. While the ranges of inhibition observed in patients with rejection indicating under-immunosuppression, stable patients and patients with infection indicating over-immunosuppression differ, there is wide variation between individuals in the assay. There may not be sufficient certainty in the target range to allow adjustments to therapy based on the assay, and a prospective trial of drug dosing based on the results is awaited. Several other approaches have been developed to the point of being ready for testing in prospective clinical trials. Use of intracellular cytokine expression in activated peripheral blood lymphocytes has been used as a read-out in assays validated for use in clinical trials [5]. Other approaches to pharmacodynamic monitoring include measurement of the degree of inhibition of inosine monophosphate dehydrogenase by mycophenolate and calcineurin by the CNIs. Residual expression of genes regulated by nuclear factor of activated T-cells may be a useful functional marker of the degree of calcineurin inhibition.

The drugs

Antibody induction

Antibodies can be used to intensify immunosuppression during the early period after transplantation, when there is the greatest risk of acute rejection. Therapeutic antibodies come in several forms. The first agents developed were polyclonal immunoglobulin preparations from the serum of animals immunised with human cells. Antithymocyte globulin (ATG) is the only polyclonal agent still in widespread use. The first monoclonal antibodies were raised in mice, yielding agents of defined specificity but retaining the immunogenicity of the mouse immunoglobulin, potentially leading to anaphylactic reactions and the generation of neutralising antibodies. Genetic engineering has allowed the antibody-binding domain (chimaeric) or the antibody-binding site (humanised) of the mouse molecule to be grafted onto the constant domains of a human IgG molecule, with minimisation but not elimination of immunogenicity.

Table 16.2 Therapeutic antibody nomenclature.

Type of antibody	Suffix	Examples
Polyclonal	. . . globulin	Thymoglobuline
Mouse monoclonal	. . . muromonab	Muromonab CD3
Chimaeric	. . . ximab	Basiliximab Rituximab
Humanised	. . . umab	Alemtuzumab Eculizumab

Terminology for describing these different types of antibody molecule is summarised in Table 16.2.

CD25 antibody

Basiliximab (Simulect) is a chimaeric monoclonal antibody that binds to the alpha chain of the interleukin 2 (IL-2) receptor, a molecule expressed on activated T-lymphocytes, and inhibits the response to IL-2. It is now the only available drug in this class following the withdrawal of daclizumab from the market. It is administered at a dose of 20 mg intravenously prior to revascularisation of the transplant with a second dose of 20 mg on day 4 after transplantation. The elimination half-life of basiliximab is around 7 days, with blood concentrations sufficient to saturate the IL2 receptors for 36 ± 14 days [6]. It has been shown to significantly reduce the rate of acute rejection in adult renal transplant recipients on CNI-based regimens. The increased efficacy brought by the addition of a CD25 antibody does not appear to come at the expense of increased risk of infection [7]. The incidence of a human anti-chimaeric antibody (HACA) response has been reported to be low (0.4%) and is not a major consideration in deciding whether to use basiliximab for a second or subsequent transplant when it was used previously.

Lytic induction

Antibodies that lyse lymphocytes and other bone-marrow-derived cells result in more profound immunosuppression but at the expense of increased rates of viral infection and malignancy. Cytokine-release syndrome with fever and hypotension is a feature seen after initial intravenous infusion with all of the lytic induction agents, in part because of cell activation prior to lysis. Infusion reactions can be minimised by the intravenous administration of chlorphenamine 10 mg and hydrocortisone 100 mg 1 hour prior to the infusion. First doses should be infused slowly, over 6–8 hours.

Antithymocyte globulin or anti-lymphocyte globulin

ATG and anti-lymphocyte globulin (ALG) preparations are derived by immunisation of rabbits or horses with human thymocytes or lymphocytes followed by preparation of the immunoglobulin fraction. An inevitable consequence of this process is some batch-to-batch variation. Administration of a foreign protein can result in serum sickness 5–15 days after starting treatment, presenting with fever, rash, arthralgia or myalgia. Symptoms tend to be self-limiting or respond to treatment with steroid. An immune response may generate neutralising antibodies, limiting subsequent use. They contain a broad range of antibody specificities including T- and B-lymphocytes and a number of adhesion molecules, including those expressed on vascular endothelium. This may explain the observed inhibition of ischaemia-reperfusion injury with a reduction in the incidence of delayed graft function if administered peri-operatively, although this has not been shown to translate into improved graft outcomes or function. There is sustained lymphopaenia that may take a year or longer to recover to normal levels.

The most widely used preparation is rabbit anti-human thymocyte immunoglobulin (Thymoglobuline). The standard recommended dosing regimen for induction therapy is 1–1.5 mg/kg/day for 3–9 days after transplantation and for treatment of steroid-resistant rejection 1.5 mg/kg/day for 7–14 days. For obese patients, ideal rather than actual weight should be used for the calculation. Ideally, ATG should be given via a central venous cannula, but it can be administered through a peripheral vein if required. The infusion time should be at least 6 hours. Infusion through a $0.22\,\mu m$ in-line filter to remove particulate material is recommended. Depletion of CD3-postive peripheral blood lymphocytes (T-lymphocytes) can be used for monitoring. The normal range is 1–30 cells/μL with a suggested algorithm for pre-dose count: <10 cells/μL, omit dose; 10–20 cells/μL, 50% usual dose; and >20 cells/μL, full dose. Dose omissions or adjustments are also required for severe haematological toxicity: platelet count $<50 \times 10^9$/L or white blood cell count $<2 \times 10^9$/L, omit; platelet count $50–75 \times 10^9$/L or white blood cell count $2–3 \times 10^9$/L, give 50% usual dose [8,9]. Consideration should be given to discontinuing mycophenolate or azathioprine for the duration of therapy to avoid profound haematological toxicity (neutropaenia or thrombocytopaenia).

Muromonab-CD3

Muromonab-CD3 (OKT3) is a murine monoclonal antibody to the CD3 component of the T-lymphocyte receptor complex that activates and then depletes T-lymphocytes. Muromonab-CD3 is a highly potent immunosuppressant with a high incidence of post-transplant lymphoproliferative disorder (PTLD) reported in some series. As a consequence, muromonab-CD3 has largely fallen from use. A standard regimen is daily doses of 5 mg given for 7–14 days, monitored as described above for ATG. Cytokine-release syndrome can be particularly severe, resulting in a capillary-leak syndrome with pulmonary oedema [10].

Alemtuzumab

This humanised monoclonal antibody, previously known as Campath-1H, binds to CD52, a molecule expressed on a wide range of peripheral blood mononuclear cells, including T- and B-lymphocytes and natural killer (NK) cells. Peripheral blood lymphocyte counts take between 3 months and 1 year after transplantation to return to normal. In tacrolimus- and mycophenolate-treated patients with early steroid withdrawal, alemtuzumab given as a single intravenous dose of 30 mg delivered lower rates of acute rejection than basiliximab in low-immunological-risk patients (5% versus 17%, $p < 0.001$ at 1 year) but at the expense of an increased infection rate. In high-risk patients, efficacy and safety were equivalent to those with ATG [11]. The cytokine-release syndrome that often follows initial intravenous administration can be avoided by subcutaneous administration with published data for 30 mg doses administered on day 0 and 1 following simultaneous pancreas kidney transplantation [12]. An increased incidence of relatively late episodes of acute rejection beyond the initial 3-month period has been reported for alemtuzumab-based regimens, which has implications for planning transplant follow-up schedules. Autoimmunity, including haemolytic anaemia, thrombocytopaenia and hyperthyroidism, is a rare complication of alemtuzumab therapy.

Rituximab

Rituximab binds to CD20, which is expressed on B-lymphocytes but not plasma cells. It has been used most widely in antibody incompatible transplantation to deplete B-lymphocytes. A typical dosing regimen would be a single dose of 375 mg/m^2 administered 2–4 weeks prior to transplantation. Circulating B-lymphocytes are depleted for 6–9 months, but treatment does not result in significant hypogammaglobulinaemia [13]. In studies of ABO-incompatible transplantation using rituximab there was a surprisingly low incidence of acute T-lymphocyte-mediated rejection, leading to the hypothesis that B-lymphocyte depletion interferes with antigen presentation to the T-lymphocyte. However, studies of rituximab administration at the time of transplantation have shown no clear benefit, possibly owing to delayed effect [14]. It is now being tested as an induction agent given several weeks prior to live donor renal transplantation. A high incidence of infectious complications has been reported for rituximab used in heavily immunosuppressed patients [15], including the rare but serious complication of progressive multifocal leucoencephalopathy. Rituximab bound to B-lymphocytes may lead to a false positive B-cell lymphocyotoxic or flow-cytometry crossmatch. Removal of the CD20 antibody using pronase has been employed as a strategy to allow meaningful crossmatch testing.

Small-molecule drugs

A summary of the pharmacological properties of the small-molecule drugs used for transplant immunosuppression is provided in Table 16.3. A summary of key drug interactions is provided in Table 16.4.

Calcineurin inhibitors

There are two drugs in the CNI class – ciclosporin and tacrolimus – with a third, voclosporin, currently undergoing clinical trials. The CNIs bind

Table 16.3 Pharmacokinetic properties of the small-molecule drugs.

	Tmax (hours)	Elimination half-life (hours)	Initial total daily oral dose	Dosing frequency	Oral bioavailability (%)	Proportion of oral dose for intravenous equivalence (%)
Ciclosporin microemulsion	2	6–20	5–10 mg/kg	Twice daily	25–30	30
Tacrolimus (immediate release)	1–2	3.5–40	0.1–0.2 mg/kg	Twice daily	20–30	20
Tacrolimus (sustained release)	2	3.5–40	0.1–0.2 mg/kg	Once daily	20–30	20
Azathioprine	1–2	0.5–2	1–3 mg/kg	Once daily	90	100
Mycophenolate mofetil	2	9–17	2000 mg (consider 3000 mg in ciclosporin-treated patients)	Twice daily	80–95	100
Enteric-coated mycophenolate sodium	1.5–5.0	9–17	1440 mg (consider 2160 mg in ciclosporin-treated patients)	Twice daily	80–95	n/a
Sirolimus	2–6	46.1–78.5	2–4 mg od	Once daily	10–14	n/a
Everolimus	1.5–2	18–35	1.5 mg	Twice daily	16	n/a
Prednisolone	1–2	2.5–4.5	20 mg	Once daily	100	See text

Tmax, time after dosing of maximum concentration in blood.

Table 16.4 Key drug interactions.

Interacting drug	Drug	Influence on drug	Mechanism of interaction
Ciclosporin	Everolimus Sirolimus	Increased exposure	Possibly due to inhibition of P-gp
Ciclosporin	Mycophenolate	Reduced MPA exposure	Inhibition of biliary excretion of MPAG resulting in loss of enterohepatic recirculation
Sirolimus	Tacrolimus	Reduced tacrolimus exposure	Unclear
Sirolimus	Ciclosporin	Enhanced nephrotoxicity	Inhibition of P-gp leading to increased concentrations of ciclosporin in tubular epithelial cells
Allopurinol	Azathioprine	Inhibition of metabolism with drug accumulation and severe myelotoxicity	Inhibition of xanthine oxidase
Steroid	Tacrolimus	Reduced exposure	Induction of metabolism by cytochrome P450
Calcium channel blockers Verapamil Diltiazem Macrolide antibiotics Clarithromycin Erythromycin Imidazole antifungals Fluconazole Ketoconazole Ritonavir Grapefruit juice	Ciclosporin Tacrolimus Sirolimus	Increased exposure	Inhibition of cytochrome P450 and P-gp
Rifampicin Anti-convulsants Carbamazepine Phenytoin St John's wart	Ciclosporin Tacrolimus Sirolimus	Reduced exposure	Induction of cytochrome P450 and P-gp

to cytoplasmic proteins: cyclophilin for ciclosporin and FK-binding protein 12 (FKBP-12) for tacrolimus. The resultant complexes inhibit the phosphatase calcineurin, which is required for activation of the transcription factor nuclear factor of activated T-cells, which activates the *IL-2* gene. These cyclophilins are peptidyl prolyl cis-trans isomerases, which have a key role in the folding of proteins. Some replicating viruses depend on cyclophilin for effective protein synthesis, and there is evidence for reduced rates of recurrent hepatitis C virus infection in ciclosporin-treated liver transplant recipients [16]. Toxicity, in particular nephrotoxicity, has led to a widespread aspiration to avoid CNIs, but their effective control of early acute rejection has maintained their place at the core of most current immunosuppressive regimens. Nephrotoxicity is manifest both as a reversible vasospastic response in the kidney that may be ameliorated by the co-prescription of calcium channel blockers and a more chronic arteriopathy with renal fibrosis. Acute tubular toxicity may be manifest as tubular vacuolation. There is probably no difference between the CNIs in degree of nephrotoxicity. Some would advocate delayed introduction of CNIs in patients either with, or at high risk of, delayed graft function, but clinical trials have shown no benefit from this approach [17]. The CNIs are diabetogenic – tacrolimus more so than ciclosporin, with approximately twofold higher incidence of new-onset diabetes after transplantation (NODAT) [18].

The CNIs are metabolised by the oxidative enzymes cytochrome P450 (CYP) 3A4 and 3A5 in the enterocyte and liver and are substrates for the drug transporter P-glycoprotein (P-gp) encoded by the *ABCB1* gene (formerly known as *MDR1*). Oral bioavailability is only 25–30%, in part due to the active barrier to drug absorption formed by CYP3A4 and CYP3A5 and P-gp [19]. Inhibitors of these proteins (e.g. macrolide antibiotics (erythromycin, clarithromycin) and imidazole antifungals (fluconazole, ketoconazole)) increase the oral bioavailability of the CNIs by around twofold. If these treatments are required, reducing the CNI dose to 50% with careful monitoring and return to the original dose on stopping therapy will generally maintain blood concentrations within the therapeutic range. Inducers of CYP and P-gp (e.g. rifampicin, carbamazepine, phenytoin) reduce CNI exposure, and doubling of the current dose with careful monitoring should avoid underexposure, again with return to the original dose on stopping treatment. Grapefruit juice significantly inhibits CYP3A with increased CNI exposure, although this is not a consistent phenomenon owing to batch-to-batch variability for grapefruit. Patients taking CNIs should be advised to avoid grapefruit [20]. The main route of elimination is the secretion of CYP3A metabolites into bile.

Ciclosporin

Ciclosporin is a fungally produced cyclical undecapeptide. It was initially available formulated in corn oil as Sandimmun, but variable absorption was a problem that was improved by the introduction of microemulsion preparations such as Neoral. Ciclosporin microemulsion is administered twice daily. Peak blood concentration is at around 2 hours with an elimination half-life of 6–20 hours. The majority of ciclosporin in blood is present in erythrocytes (60–70%), with only 4% in the plasma, of which 60–70% is bound to protein.

Ciclosporin is measured in whole blood, usually on an EDTA-anticoagulated blood sample. Initially, measurement of blood concentrations immediately before the morning dose (12 hour post-dose, trough or C0) was adopted routinely. A limitation of this approach is the relatively poor correlation with AUC with R^2 values from most studies being 0.5 or less. Most of the interpatient variability in drug exposure is accounted for by differences in drug absorption rather than the rate of elimination. Ciclosporin blood concentrations collected during the absorption phase, 2 hours after drug dosing (C2), provide a significantly better estimate of AUC. Monitoring C2 poses some logistic problems, as samples must be collected within the time interval of 15 minutes before or after the 2-hour post-dose time to remain within a 10% margin for error [21]. Ciclosporin concentrations in samples collected 2 hours post-dose are usually outside the range of detection of standard assays and require dilution. The laboratory needs to be informed that a C2 sample has been sent and requires a validated dilution method. If C2 samples are run on the standard assay calibrated for C0 samples, they will generate results above the range of measurement of the assay.

The conventional therapeutic range for ciclosporin C0 concentrations is 150–300 µg/L during the first 3 months after transplantation and 100–200 µg/L thereafter. A lower target of 50–150 µg/L has provided comparable results in regimens using mycophenolate and anti-CD25 induction therapy [22]. A target of 75–125 µg/L rather than 150–250 µg/L from month 12 in renal transplant recipients significantly reduced the incidence of malignancy with no loss of efficacy [23]. Several studies have attempted to define a therapeutic range for C2. A randomised controlled trial of two different ranges for C2 concentrations delivered good results with: 1600–2000 µg/L during month 1; 1400–1600 µg/L during month 2; 1200–1400 µg/L during month 3; 800–1000 µg/L in months 4–6; and 600–800 µg/L thereafter. [24]. A conventional initial daily dose for ciclosporin is 5–10 mg/kg.

Several toxicities are more common with ciclosporin than tacrolimus. Hypertension is more prevalent, being almost ubiquitous in ciclosporin-treated patients. Cosmetic impact tends to be greater with hypertrichosis and gum hypertrophy and a tendency to coarsen features. Gum hypertrophy is particularly common if the patient is co-prescribed a dihydropyridine calcium channel blocker (e.g. nifedipine, amlodipine). Although improved dental hygiene and antibiotic therapy have been advocated as management strategies, switching to an alternative agent such as tacrolimus is the most effective approach. Plasma uric acid concentrations are often elevated, with increased incidence of gout.

Tacrolimus

Tacrolimus is a macrolide, and there is occasional cross-reaction with allergy to the macrolide antibiotics (e.g. erythromycin, clarithromycin). Tacrolimus is available as twice daily (Prograf and a number of generic preparations) and a once-daily sustained release preparation (Advagraf). Oral bioavailability is 20–30%. Peak blood concentration occurs at 1–2 hours, with an elimination half-life of 3.5–40 hours (usually towards the upper end of this range). Most of the tacrolimus in blood (95%) is present in erythrocytes, and of the 5% in plasma 99% is bound to protein. Given the high proportion of the drug in erythrocytes, blood concentration measurements in the presence of anaemia should be interpreted with caution [2]. Taking tacrolimus along with food markedly reduces absorption, reducing peak concentrations and AUC but with relatively little impact on the trough concentration. It is important that patients adhere to the guidance to take tacrolimus either 1 hour before or 2 hours after eating [25]. With twice-daily Prograf there is always less absorption following the evening dose, possibly owing to food intake during the day. Exposure is always greater in fasted patients, which is of particular relevance in the immediate post-transplant period, when the first sample after transplantation in a fasted patient should be interpreted with caution, as it is likely to overestimate exposure when the patient starts eating again. Diarrhoea generally results in increased tacrolimus absorption, possibly through loss of the active barrier to drug absorption formed by CYP3A4/3A5 and P-gp. Hepatic CYP3A metabolites are eliminated via biliary excretion in stool.

There are several toxicities that are more common with tacrolimus than ciclosporin. Rates of NODAT in tacrolimus-based regimens are twofold higher than with ciclosporin-based regimens. Steroid avoidance (see below) reduces this risk to some degree but does not eliminate it. Hypertension is common but not universal. Hyperkalaemia and hypophosphataemia are commoner than with ciclosporin. Serum phosphate concentrations below 0.32 mmol/L may result in skeletal muscle weakness and cardiac dysfunction. Advice should be given on a high-phosphate diet, the reverse of that probably taking when on dialysis, and oral phosphate supplements should be administered (40–100 mmol phosphate daily in divided doses). Cosmetic effects are uncommon but there is occasional hair loss. Neurotoxicity is common, most frequently manifest by paraesthesia or tremor, which resolves on dose reduction. Acute confusion is occasionally observed, perhaps owing to synergy with high-dose steroid and appears to be more of a problem for elderly patients.

There is a paucity of data to define the therapeutic range for tacrolimus precisely. The target range in *de novo* patients in the Symphony study, where excellent results for tacrolimus treatment were reported, was 3–7 ng/mL, but the range actually achieved in the study was closer to 5–10 ng/mL [22]. There are data indicating increased toxicity, in particular NODAT at concentrations above 15 ng/mL. A reasonable estimate for the therapeutic range is 5–15 ng/mL for *de novo* patients over the first 3 months after transplantation and 3–10 ng/mL subsequently.

An initial dose of 0.1–0.2 mg/kg daily is followed by dose adjustments based on blood concentrations. The AUC over 24 hours correlates with efficacy. Trough concentrations measured either 12 hours (±2 hours) after dosing with twice daily preparations or 24 hours (±2 hours) for once daily correlate well with the AUC, although the strength of correlation varies in the published literature [2]. However, unlike ciclosporin, there is no practically applicable alternative sampling strategy that is more predictive. Tacrolimus is measured in whole blood by either immunoassay or liquid chromatography. The immunoassays perform poorly at the lower end of the therapeutic range. Based on elimination half-life and time to reach steady state, there is no value in taking measurements more frequently than on alternate days.

Individuals who are genetically sub-Saharan African in origin (Black) require, on average, twofold higher doses of tacrolimus to achieve target blood concentrations of tacrolimus than other ethnic groups. The ethnic difference is entirely due to oral bioavailability, with no difference in exposure after intravenous administration and no difference in the elimination half-life when compared with White patients [26]. In order to avoid delay in achieving target blood concentrations in Black patients, consideration should be given to using a higher initial dose than for other groups: 0.3 mg/kg. Individuals from other ethnic groups who possess at least one *CYP3A5*1* allele, predicting expression of the enzyme cytochrome P4503A5 also have a twofold higher dose requirement for tacrolimus. Initial dosing of CYP3A5 expressers with a total daily dose of 0.3 mg/kg and non-expressers (homozygous for the *CYP3A5*3* mutation) with 0.15 mg/kg has been shown to result in earlier attainment of target blood concentrations [27], although it remains to be shown that this improves outcomes.

Choice of calcineurin inhibitor

Tacrolimus has emerged as the most widely used CNI for *de novo* kidney and pancreas transplant recipients. The benefits of tacrolimus are lower rates of acute rejection and absence of some of the cosmetic side effects of ciclosporin. However, this comes at the expense of a twofold higher rate of NODAT when compared with ciclosporin-based regimens and more neurotoxicity. CNI side effects are compared in Table 16.5. If converting between CNIs, in general the dose of ciclosporin required to

Table 16.5 Calcineurin inhibitor side effects.

Side effect	Ciclosporin	Tacrolimus
Nephrotoxicity	++	++
Hypertension	+++	++
NODAT	+	++
Hyperkalaemia	+	++
Hypophosphataemia	−	+
Neurotoxicity	+	++
Gum hyperplasia	+	−
Hypertrichosis	+	−
Hair loss	−	+

achieve the therapeutic range is 30-fold higher than the dose of tacrolimus [28].

Antiproliferative agents

The antiproliferative agents are generally used as adjunctive therapy along with a CNI or mTOR inhibitor. Azathioprine has generally been superseded by mycophenolate for *de novo* transplants but remains a useful agent after the initial post-transplant period. Once daily dosing may be an advantage, but the financial benefit compared with mycophenolate is now much less than in the past owing to the availability of generic mycophenolate preparations.

Azathioprine

The purine analogue azathioprine inhibits the *de novo* and salvage pathways of purine synthesis, inhibiting the proliferation of T- and B-lymphocytes and also inhibits the co-stimulatory signal delivered by CD28 [29]. Azathioprine is well absorbed orally and is rapidly reduced by glutathione and other sulphydryl-containing compounds to 6-mercaptopurine, with subsequent metabolism along three competing pathways. The active agents, 6-thioguanine nucleotides, are generated initially by hypoxanthine phosphoribosyl transferase. Inactive metabolites are catalysed by xanthine oxidase and thiopurine-S-methyltransferase (TPMT). Co-administration of allopurinol, a xanthine oxidase inhibitor, prevents the generation of inactive metabolites and should be avoided. Likewise, co-prescription of other drugs that inhibit TPMT, including the 5-aminosalicylic acid derivatives, may cause problems. The half-life of 6-mercaptopurine (6-MP) is short (38–114 min), but the 6-thioguanine nucleotides persist in the tissues, allowing once daily dosing. A typical initial daily dose is 1–3 mg/kg body weight given either orally or intravenously (no adjustment required for parenteral administration) with dose adjusted according to toxicity. Dose-related myelosuppression is the commonest problem, and macrocytosis is an expected observation. Hepatotoxicity, including cholestasis and hepatic veno-occlusive disease, is uncommon. Measurement of plasma concentrations of azathioprine or 6-MP is of no value but it has been suggested that erythrocyte 6-thioguanine nucleotide concentrations may be helpful [30]. Monitoring of full blood count and liver blood tests are essential, weekly for at least the first 4 weeks after initiation followed by a reduced frequency but not less than every 3 months. Dose reduction should be considered with white blood cell counts below 4×10^9/L or platelets below 100×10^9/L or evidence of hepatic injury.

Variable TPMT activity is genetically determined [31]. Approximately 90% of the population are homozygous for normal alleles with normal enzyme activity; 10% are heterozygotes with reduced enzyme activity; and 0.3% are homozygotes for non-functional alleles with functional enzyme deficiency. TPMT deficiency predicts myelotoxicity but not hepatotoxicity. Patients with TPMT deficiency require 5–10% standard dose of azathioprine, and heterozygotes can be treated with standard doses but are more likely to require dose reduction. TPMT deficiency can be identified by measurement of enzyme activity in erythrocytes (avoiding assay within 30–60 days of blood transfusion) or by genotyping. Screening for TPMT deficiency before treatment may not be cost-effective in the presence of regular monitoring for myelosuppression.

Mycophenolate

The active agent mycophenolic acid (MPA) is currently available as mycophenolate mofetil (MMF), the morpholinoethyl ester of MPA) or enteric-coated mycophenolate sodium (MPS). The bioequivalent dose for 1 g MMF is 720 mg MPS. These preparations have been shown to have equivalent efficacy and safety [32]. MPA inhibits the enzyme inosine monophosphate dehydrogenase, in particular the IMPDH-II isoenzyme. IMPDH is involved in the salvage pathway of purine synthesis blocking the proliferation of both T- and B-lymphocytes and downregulates expression of some inflammatory adhesion molecules. Mycophenolate has been shown to have superior efficacy to azathioprine in preventing acute rejection in CNI-treated renal transplant recipients [33].

The pharmacokinetics of mycophenolate are complex (Fig. 16.1) and have resulted in common misconceptions on optimal drug dosing. Both

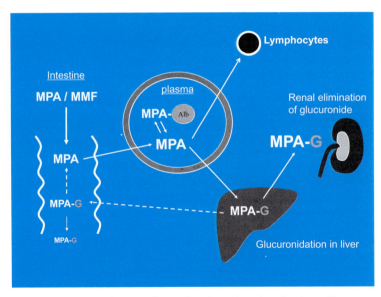

Figure 16.1 Pharmacokinetics of mycophenolate. Mycophenolate is readily absorbed from the gut and is highly protein-bound in plasma. The unbound (free) fraction is available to enter lymphocytes with inhibition of IMPDH or to enter hepatocytes, where it is conjugated to a glucuronide, which is then eliminated either in urine or by active transport by ABCC2 into bile. Intestinal bacteria then cleave some of the glucuronide groups, resulting in a second peak in MPA absorption 6–8 hours after drug dosing that is inhibited by ciclosporin. Adapted from a figure originally drawn by Dr Andrew Watts.

forms have excellent oral bioavailability of almost 100%. The mofetil group is cleaved in the gut and is not detectable in the blood. For MMF the peak MPA blood concentration is at around 2 hours, occurring later and with greater variation for MPS. Co-administration of antacids reduces MPA absorption. The plasma half-life is around 17 hours. MPA is glucuronide conjugated in the liver to generate the pharmacologically inactive phenolic glucuronide (MPAG) and small amounts of the active and probably pro-inflammatory acyl glucuronide. The glucuronide conjugates are then eliminated either in urine or through active transport by the drug transporter ABCC2, previously known as MRP2, into bile. Intestinal bacteria remove some of the glucuronide groups leading to a second peak of MPA absorption at around 6–8 hours. This second peak contributes 30–50% of the total AUC. Ciclosporin, but not tacrolimus or sirolimus, inhibits ABCC2, resulting in lower MPA exposure for a given dose than in patients not taking ciclosporin [34]. Likewise, other drugs inhibiting enterohepatic recirculation, such as colestyramine, may reduce MPA exposure. MPA is highly bound to protein, typically >98%. A number of factors increase the 'free' fraction that is not protein-bound, including high concentrations of MPAG retained due to renal impairment, acidaemia, uraemia and hypoalbuminaemia. Increase in the 'free' fraction results in increased glucuronide conjugation with increased secretion into bile. This is the underlying explanation for the observed gradual increase in total plasma MPA concentration with time after transplantation as renal function improves with increased protein binding and less glucuronide formation [35]. Counter-intuitively, efficacy is associated with total MPA rather than the 'free' fraction. Factors increasing free MPA result in a fall in total plasma MPA, with an increase in the gastrointestinal tract leading to gastrointestinal toxicity. This can result in the unusual situation of a patient with dose-limiting toxicity but insufficient systemic exposure for efficacy. It has been suggested that Black patients require higher doses of mycophenolate, but this has no pharmacokinetic basis, nor any well-founded pharmacodynamic basis [36].

Based on studies of therapeutic drug monitoring for mycophenolate mofetil, the optimal dose is 3 g/day for the first month followed by 2 g/day in ciclosporin-treated patients and 2 g/day for the first month followed by 1–1.5 g/day in patients on tacrolimus or mTOR inhibitor [37,38]. This suggested dosing strategy differs from the recommended licensed doses, which do not take recently published pharmacokinetic data into account. Slavishly aiming at a daily dose of 2 g/day in the long term in tacrolimus-treated patients, as is often advocated, has no rational basis and is likely to result in over-exposure in the majority of patients. There is some controversy as to whether therapeutic drug monitoring for MPA is of benefit, although there is one randomised controlled trial demonstrating benefit [38], which is one more than is available to support use with the other drugs. MPA is measured in plasma (EDTA blood). Twelve-hour post-dose trough concentrations do not correlate sufficiently well with AUC to be clinically useful. Limited sampling

> **Box 16.1 Algorithms for calculating AUC for MPA from blood samples collected 0, 0.5 and 2 hours after drug administration.**
>
> 1. For fasted adults on MMF+ Tacrolimus:
> $$AUC = 7.75 + 6.49 \times C0 + 0.76 \times C0.5 + 2.43 \times C2$$
> $$r^2 = 0.862$$
> 2. For fasted adults on MMF+ CsA:
> $$AUC = 11.34 + 3.1 \times C0 + 1.102 \times C0.5 + 1.909 \times C2$$
> $$r^2 = 0.752$$
> 3. For not fasted pediatric patients on MMF and Tacrolimus:
> $$AUC = 10.01391 + 3.94791 \times C0 + 3.24253 \times C0.5 + 1.0108 \times C2$$
> $$r^2 = 0.800$$
> 4. For fasted pediatric patients on MMF and CsA:
> $$AUC = 18.609 + 4.309 \times C0 + 0.536 \times C0.5 + 2.148 \times C2$$
> $$r^2 = 0.72$$
>
> Algorithms used in the FDCC study [37].

strategies have been developed to estimate the AUC, based for example on samples collected pre-dose, then 30 and 120 mins after dosing. A Bayesian estimator for use with samples collected at various time points after drug dosing is available online at: https://pharmaco.chu-limoges.fr. The equations used to estimate AUC in the fixed-dose versus concentration-controlled (FDCC) study are shown in Box 16.1 [37]. The therapeutic range in the early period after transplantation on CNI treatment is 30–60 mg.hr/L and possibly higher in patients on CNI minimisation regimens. If trough concentrations are used, the suggested lower end of the therapeutic range is 1.3 μg/mL for ciclosporin-treated patients and 1.9 μg/mL for tacrolimus-treated patients with an upper limit of 3.5–4.0 μg/mL [39]. These limited sampling strategies cannot be applied to enteric-coated MPA and a full 12-hour AUC is the only reliable way of measuring MPA exposure. Measurement of the degree of inhibition of IMPDH in peripheral blood is a potentially useful pharmacodynamic assay that has yet to be translated to clinical practice.

The main toxicities with MPA are myelosuppression and gastrointestinal toxicity, manifest most commonly by diarrhoea. Full blood count should be monitored weekly during the first month of treatment, twice monthly during the second and third months and then monthly throughout the first year. Dose reduction should be considered when the white blood cell count falls below 4×10^9/L or platelets below 100×10^9/L. An approach to managing gastrointestinal symptoms sometimes employed is split dosing with administration three or four times daily. However, there is no evidence that this preserves efficacy. A better approach is to reduce the dose until the symptoms resolve and then check exposure. If inadequate, then consideration should be given to an alternative agent. It has been suggested that enteric coating may reduce gastrointestinal side effects, although the evidence for this is weak and it is unlikely to influence the effects of increased secretion of MPAG in bile.

Other antiproliferative agents

Leflunomide is a long-acting orally absorbed dihydroorotate dehydrogenase inhibitor that inhibits pyrimidine synthesis. It is licensed for use in treating inflammatory rheumatological diseases. It has come to attention recently owing to activity against BK polyomavirus [40].

Mammalian target of rapamycin (mTOR) inhibitors

Mammalian target of rapamycin (mTOR) is an intracellular signalling molecule involved in a number of processes including the response of lymphocytes to cytokines and pro-fibrotic processes such as those involved in wound healing. The first drug in this class was sirolimus (known previously as rapamycin), a fungal product from *Streptomyces hygroscopicus*. The closely related drug, everolimus, was derived by conjugation of a 2-hydroxyethyl group to sirolimus. They bind to the same immunophilin, FKBP-12, as tacrolimus but with different molecular consequences. They are less efficacious than the CNIs but are more potent in preventing rejection than the other antiproliferative drugs. A key benefit of the mTOR inhibitors is the absence of nephrotoxicity, although they do enhance the nephrotoxic effect of the CNIs, probably through inhibition of P-gp, resulting in increased intracellular concentrations of the CNI [41]. Medium-term (3–5 years) graft function and histological changes on protocol biopsy were better in sirolimus- than in ciclosporin-treated patients [42]. Although they are not nephrotoxic, the mTOR inhibitors do delay recovery from acute tubular necrosis and are not an ideal agent in patients with delayed graft function.

Sirolimus has a very long half-life in adults, of around 60 hours, but a much shorter half-life in children, closer to 10 hours [43]. Thus, although once-daily dosing is standard for adults, twice-daily dosing may be required in children. Everolimus has a significantly shorter half-life of 16–19 hours and requires twice-daily dosing. When sirolimus was introduced it was hoped that it would offer a non-nephrotoxic alternative to the CNIs. Unfortunately a number of toxicities make this a difficult class of drugs to use. It has been suggested that everolimus has a better toxicity profile than sirolimus, but this remains to be demonstrated conclusively.

Use of mTOR inhibitors in the *de novo* setting immediately after transplantation without a CNI has fallen from favour owing to an increased rate of acute rejection compared with CNI-based regimens and impaired wound healing with increased incidence of lymphoceles [44,45]. The wound complications are a particular issue in obese patients. In patients chronically treated with an mTOR inhibitor, consideration should be given to discontinuation prior to any elective surgery and replacement with a CNI followed by reinstatement after 6 weeks to facilitate wound healing. Alternative strategies involve the use of low-dose mTOR inhibitor along with a CNI or initial use of a CNI with later switch to an mTOR inhibitor (discussed in more detail below).

Early studies suggested that sirolimus was less diabetogenic than tacrolimus, but recent studies have demonstrated that this is not the case. mTOR is involved in downstream signalling from the insulin receptor, resulting in insulin resistance [46]. Hyperlipidaemia is almost universal owing to changes in lipid distribution and may not result in increased atherosclerotic risk but is likely to trigger prescription of lipid-lowering therapy. Haematological toxicity, including thrombocytopaenia and anaemia, is common, in particular in combination with another antiproliferative agent. Inhibition of vascular endothelial growth factor (VEGF) may be responsible for the increased incidence of proteinuria that is often problematic when using mTOR inhibitors. They should be avoided in individuals with >800 g protein in urine/24 hours [47]. Other common toxicities are mouth ulcers, which may be more common in patients not also treated with corticosteroid and skin rashes. Ankle oedema is common with severely disabling lymphoedema in a small number of cases that may not resolve on drug discontinuation. Sirolimus pneumonitis is a rare but serious complication that can mimic a number of other opportunistic infections or malignancy, presenting with dyspnoea, dry cough, fever or generalised fatigue. mTOR inhibitors should be avoided in individuals with pre-existing pulmonary pathology, where the incidence is increased. The reported incidence is higher in individuals with late switch and significantly impaired renal function. Typically, investigations reveal bronchiolitis olibertans-organizing pneumonia and lymphocytic alveolitis. Diagnosis is based on a high index of suspicion with thoracic computerised tomography scanning and possibly bronchoscopy to confirm the diagnosis. The pneumonitis usually resolves on drug discontinuation, and it is best to discontinue mTOR inhibitors in patients with respiratory pathology of uncertain aetiology [48]. Reduced fertility in male patients has been reported [49].

A benefit of the mTOR inhibitors is a reduced incidence of malignancy; indeed, sirolimus derivatives have been licensed for the treatment of renal cell carcinoma. Kaposi's sarcoma is highly responsive to mTOR inhibition [50] and the rate of recurrence of non-melanoma skin cancer reduces following introduction of sirolimus [51]. This is probably the immunosuppressive class of choice in patients with previous malignancy. Both sirolimus and everolimus retard cyst growth in patients with autosomal dominant polycystic kidney disease, probably more so in the liver than in the kidney. Although this was not shown to result in preservation of glomerular filtration rate, this may be a benefit for patients suffering significant symptoms due to mass effect [52].

The therapeutic range for sirolimus measured in whole blood (EDTA-anticoagulated) is probably 5–15 ng/mL during the first 3 months after transplantation and then 5–10 ng/mL [45,53]. The poor results for the sirolimus-treated group in the Symphony study may be due to inadequate sirolimus exposure, with a target of 4–8 ng/mL in *de novo* patients [22]. The *CYP3A5* genotype has a similar influence on pharmacokinetics of sirolimus to that observed for tacrolimus, with reduced exposure in CYP3A5 expressers, but not everolimus [54]. This may explain the higher sirolimus dose requirement in Black patients. There are no clinical trials of pharmacogenetic dosing strategies. The recommended therapeutic range for everolimus measured in whole blood 12 hours after dosing (trough concentration) is 3–8 ng/mL.

Corticosteroids

Corticosteroids have a broad spectrum of immunosuppressive and anti-inflammatory activity that reduces the innate immune response to ischaemia-reperfusion injury in the peri-transplant period and possibly reduces chronic rejection, perhaps through limiting response to inflammatory stimuli such as infection. Steroids have a broad spectrum of toxicity, including impaired glucose tolerance, hypertension, adverse effect on lipid profile, osteoporosis, cosmetic effects due to redistribution of body fat, acne and increased appetite contributing to obesity. Sleep disturbance may be a problem that can be ameliorated by ensuring that the steroid is all taken in the morning rather than in the evening. Most immunosuppressive regimens include a bolus of high-dose intravenous steroid at the time of transplantation followed by oral prednisolone.

Prednisolone is well absorbed, with maximum blood concentrations at 1–2 hours after dosing and an elimination half-life of 2.5–4.5 hours. Prednisolone exposure in renal transplant recipients is up to 50% higher for a given dose than in normal control subjects [55]. Enteric coating results in reduced and unpredictable absorption of prednisolone and should be avoided. In considering alternative steroids (e.g. if intravenous administration is required), the following doses have equivalent glucocorticoid effect to 5 mg prednisolone: hydrocortisone 20 mg, methylprednisolone 4 mg, dexamethasone 0.75 mg.

The hypothalamic pituitary adrenal axis is suppressed in patients on long-term steroid therapy, and steroid dose should be increased at times of physiological stress, including surgery.

Co-stimulatory blockade

Belatacept, a fusion protein between a modified CTLA4/CD152 molecule and an immunoglobulin domain, has been licensed recently for use as an alternative to the CNIs. It has been engineered to have greater affinity for CD80 and CD86 than the natural ligands CD28 and CD152 and inhibits delivery of the second (co-stimulatory) signal required to activate T lymphocytes following cross-linking of the antigen receptor. In Phase III studies, there was more acute rejection and PTLD than in the ciclosporin group but better renal function and less interstitial fibrosis with tubular atrophy in protocol biopsies. The increased incidence of PTLD occurred mostly, although not exclusively, in Epstein–Barr virus naïve patients [56]. The requirement for monthly intravenous infusions will require appropriate facilities.

Kinase inhibitors

The orally active protein kinase C inhibitor Sotrastaurin and the JAK 3 inhibitor Tasocitinib (CP-690,550) are currently in development with the aim of replacing either the CNI or mycophenolate.

Choice of regimen

The range of available drugs offers a wide range of different potential combinations, and very few transplant centres employ exactly the same regimen. The current standard of care immunosuppressive regimen based on anti-CD25 antibody, tacrolimus, mycophenolate and steroid is based on the results of the Symphony study. The drug regimen with the lowest acute rejection rate and best 1-year renal function was based on a CD25 antibody, low-dose tacrolimus MMF and steroid. However, this did come at the expense of a higher rate of NODAT and diarrhoea than in ciclosporin-treated patients [22].

Steroid minimisation

In an attempt to avoid steroid side effects a number of approaches have been tried across the spectrum of complete steroid avoidance, short courses of steroids (typically 7 days) and later steroid withdrawal from 3 months post-transplantation onwards. Disappointing results with late steroid withdrawal leading to loss of transplant function have directed efforts towards steroid avoidance or early withdrawal. In a randomised controlled trial using a ciclosporin-based regimen, conventional long-term steroid treatment was compared with complete steroid avoidance (including omission of bolus steroids at the time of surgery) and a 7-day course of steroids followed by withdrawal. Somewhat disappointingly, the incidence of NODAT was only significantly lower in the group in which steroids were avoided completely, and this came at the expense of an increased rate of acute rejection [57]. In tacrolimus-treated patients with steroid withdrawal after 7 days, there was no difference in the overall rate of NODAT, but fewer patients required insulin therapy in the steroid-withdrawn group. Again, this came at the expense of an increased rate of acute rejection [58].

Should CNI and mTOR inhibitor be given together?

There is no consensus on whether CNIs and mTOR inhibitors should be given together, and everolimus is licensed to be used along with a CNI. Although there were initial concerns that sirolimus and tacrolimus would not synergise, owing to both agents binding to FKBP-12, these concerns have now been shown to be unfounded. The key argument against this combination is the enhancement of CNI nephrotoxicity by the mTOR inhibitors, mediated by inhibition of P-gp, leading to increased intracellular CNI concentrations. However, there are studies that have yielded excellent results with the drugs used in combination.

CNI-free regimens

Several CNI avoidance strategies have been tried, but none has yet achieved widespread adoption. CD25 induction followed by mycophenolate and steroids resulted in unacceptably high rates of acute rejection but good 1-year renal transplant outcomes [59]. Regimens based on sirolimus, mycophenolate and steroids suffer from higher acute rejection rates than seen typically with CNI-based regimens and an increased incidence of lymphoceles and wound-healing complications. Potent induction therapy, with alemtuzumab for example, has been used as an approach to reduce the incidence of acute rejection. The recently introduced Belatacept does allow a CNI-free regimen, but at the expense of an acute rejection rate of around 20% and increased incidence of PTLD. At present CNI-minimisation regimens are more feasible.

Calcineurin inhibitor minimisation

Initial calcineurin inhibitor therapy with subsequent withdrawal

A therapeutic strategy employing the efficacy of the CNIs to prevent rejection early after transplantation with subsequent replacement by a non-nephrotoxic agent has evolved. There is some debate as to the optimal time to convert when this strategy is employed. Late conversion, from 1 year after transplantation, does not appear to confer any benefit, possibly through irreversible established renal damage. By 3 months after transplantation, the risk of acute rejection is minimal except in regimens based on alemtuzumab. Protocol biopsies at this point usually demonstrate minimal chronic damage. The optimal time to make the switch from CNI probably lies somewhere between 6 weeks and 6 months after the transplant.

Early (3–6 months after transplantation) CNI withdrawal to a dual drug regimen comprising mycophenolate and steroids resulted in an unacceptable rate of acute rejection [60]. Later switch to azathioprine or prednisolone may be an option for low-risk patients and does come at some risk of acute rejection at the time of CNI withdrawal but yields excellent long-term outcomes [61].

Early CNI replacement by an mTOR inhibitor has proved to be a more successful strategy, with a very low incidence of acute rejection at the time of switch with improved renal function at 1 year compared with patients continuing on CNI, although this improvement was not maintained at 2 years in the recently published Spare the Nephron study [42,44,62–64]. Initial studies employing overlap of the CNI and mTOR inhibitor resulted in infectious complications related to over-immunosuppression, and an abrupt switch is the safest and most straightforward approach.

Pharmacokinetic interactions between the immunosuppressive drugs

Key drug interactions are summarised in Table 16.4. High-dose steroid therapy has been reported to reduce the oral bioavailability of tacrolimus, probably through the induction of CYP3A. There are experimental, but not clinical, data to suggest that this may be the case for ciclosporin, and it is not an issue for sirolimus. Patients treated for rejection may require an increased tacrolimus dose to maintain blood concentrations in the desired range. Conversely, there may be a need to reduce the dose following steroid withdrawal. Ciclosporin increases sirolimus exposure, whereas tacrolimus has no effect. Co-administration of sirolimus reduced tacrolimus exposure in paediatric and adult renal transplant recipients [43].

Generic preparations

Generic preparations are now available for most of the immunosuppressive drugs used for transplantation. New preparations do not require efficacy and safety data in transplant patients, requiring only pharmacokinetic bioequivalence to be demonstrated after a single dose in normal human volunteers. Although generic preparations may be therapeutically equivalent, this has not always transpired to be the case, and care should be applied in choosing immunosuppressive preparations. The CNIs are lipid-soluble drugs, and their pharmacokinetics are very dependent on formulation. A key example of this is the differing influence of taking the drug in the fed versus fasted state for different ciclosporin preparations. It is essential that patients are not switched from one preparation to another without careful monitoring. Branded prescribing for the CNIs, even when generic preparations are used, minimises the risk of inadvertent switching. Preparation is probably less of an issue for mycophenolate, with excellent oral bioavailability and large intrapatient variability in exposure, even with the original branded preparations based on patient rather than formulation factors. However, repetitive switching from one formulation to another should be avoided, as this may confuse patients and may lead to mistakes, potentially with serious consequences.

Treatment of acute rejection

Acute cellular (T-lymphocyte-mediated) rejection

T-lymphocyte-mediated acute cellular rejection (Banff grade 1) is usually treated with high-dose steroid. A conventional regimen would be three daily intravenous doses of 500–1000 mg methylprednisolone. High-dose oral steroid therapy is equally effective in reversing acute rejection but does increase the risk of dyspeptic problems. In the case of more severe rejection, opinion is split as to whether more potent agents such as ATG should be used as first-line therapy or reserved for steroid-resistant rejection. In the event of serum creatinine not falling within 5 days of initiating steroid therapy, re-biopsy to confirm ongoing rejection is indicated to confirm steroid-resistant rejection followed by more intensive therapy such as ATG.

Antibody-mediated rejection

A different approach is required for humoral or antibody-mediated rejection, with morphological changes, C4d deposition and the presence of donor-specific antibody (see Chapter 20). A number of approaches to remove and prevent re-synthesis of antibody have been employed. Plasma exchange along with administration of intravenous immunoglobulin is the basis for most regimens to remove antibody [65]. ATG and rituximab have activity against B lymphocytes and may prevent re-synthesis. Recent data using bortezomib to remove plasma cells are promising. Complement is a key effector mechanism in antibody-mediated rejection and the antibody to C5, eculizumab, which inhibits the formation of the membrane attack complex, has been effective in reversing humoral rejection.

Increase in maintenance immunosuppression and reinforcement of compliance

An episode of acute rejection is the most direct bioassay for under-immunosuppression. The intensity of maintenance immunosuppression should be increased after an episode of rejection. Several changes have been shown to reduce the incidence of recurrent rejection, including changing from ciclosporin to tacrolimus or replacing azathioprine with mycophenolate. If patients have rejected following withdrawal of steroids or CNIs the drug should probably be re-instituted. Poor compliance with immunosuppressive treatment is a significant problem, particularly in health-care economies that do not fund life-long immunosuppressive treatment. The possibility of poor compliance should be considered, in particular for late episodes of acute rejection. There are data from other therapy areas to suggest that once-daily dosing results in improved compliance but robust data supporting this concept for transplant immunosuppression are lacking.

HIV-infected patients: interaction with antiretrovirals

Ritonavir, given along with protease inhibitors to treat HIV infection, is an extremely potent inhibitor of cytochrome P4503A, resulting in a massive increase in the elimination half-life of the CNIs. Some patients need as little as 1 mg tacrolimus once per week to achieve blood concentrations within the desired range [66]. Ideally, HIV-infected patients should undergo a trial period of immunosuppression prior to either living donor transplantation or listing for deceased donor transplantation to optimise exposure to both antiviral and immunosuppressive drugs. Use of alternative antiretroviral regimens that do not include ritonavir (e.g. by using raltegravir) makes the pharmacology much less complex.

Immunosuppression and pregnancy

Although none of the immunosuppressive drugs are considered to be 'safe' in pregnancy, there has been no reported increased incidence of fetal malformations or teratogenicity with azathioprine, corticosteroids, ciclosporin or tacrolimus, and regimens based on these drugs would generally be regarded as acceptable. They are present in breast milk, and breastfeeding is best avoided. Although blood concentrations in the baby are small, there is a theoretical risk of drug accumulation due to the immature cytochrome P450 system. Mycophenolate and sirolimus are teratogenic and should be avoided.

References

1. Halloran PF. (2004) Immunosuppressive drugs for kidney transplantation. *N Engl J Med* **351**, 2715–2729.
2. Holt DW, Armstrong VW, Griesmacher A, *et al.* (2002) International Federation of Clinical Chemistry/International Association of Therapeutic Drug Monitoring and Clinical Toxicology working group on immunosuppressive drug monitoring. *Ther Drug Monit* **24**, 59–67.
3. Hoogtanders K, van der HJ, Christiaans M, *et al.* (2007) Dried blood spot measurement of tacrolimus is promising for patient monitoring. *Transplantation* **83**, 237–238.
4. Kowalski RJ, Post DR, Mannon RB, *et al.* (2006) Assessing relative risks of infection and rejection: A meta-analysis using an immune function assay. *Transplantation* **82**, 663–668.
5. Bohler T, Nolting J, Kamar N, *et al.* (2007) Validation of immunological biomarkers for the pharmacodynamic monitoring of immunosuppressive drugs in humans. *Ther Drug Monit* **29**, 77–86.
6. Kovarik JM, Kahan BD, Rajagopalan PR, *et al.* (1999) Population pharmacokinetics and exposure-response relationships for basiliximab in kidney transplantation. The U.S. Simulect Renal Transplant Study Group. *Transplantation* **68**, 1288–1294.
7. Adu D, Cockwell P, Ives NJ, *et al.* (2003) Interleukin-2 receptor monoclonal antibodies in renal transplantation: Meta-analysis of randomised trials. *Br Med J* **326**, 789.

8. Peddi VR, Bryant M, Roy-Chaudhury P, *et al.* (2002) Safety, efficacy, and cost analysis of thymoglobulin induction therapy with intermittent dosing based on CD3+ lymphocyte counts in kidney and kidney-pancreas transplant recipients. *Transplantation* **73**, 1514–1518.

9. Brennan DC, Flavin K, Lowell JA, *et al.* (1999) A randomized, double-blinded comparison of Thymoglobulin versus Atgam for induction immunosuppressive therapy in adult renal transplant recipients. *Transplantation* **67**, 1011–1018.

10. Norman DJ, Kahana L, Stuart FP Jr, *et al.* (1993) A randomized clinical trial of induction therapy with OKT3 in kidney transplantation. *Transplantation* **55**, 44–50.

11. Hanaway MJ, Woodle ES, Mulgaonkar S, *et al.* (2011) Alemtuzumab induction in renal transplantation. *N Engl J Med* **364**, 1909–1919.

12. Clatworthy MR, Sivaprakasam R, Butler AJ, *et al.* (2007) Subcutaneous administration of alemtuzumab in simultaneous pancreas-kidney transplantation. *Transplantation* **84**, 1563–1567.

13. Clatworthy MR. (2011) Targeting B cells and antibody in transplantation. *Am J Transplant* **11**, 1359–1367.

14. Tyden G, Genberg H, Tollemar J, *et al.* (2009) A randomized, doubleblind, placebo-controlled, study of single-dose rituximab as induction in renal transplantation. *Transplantation* **87**, 1325–1329.

15. Kamar N, Milioto O, Puissant-Lubrano B, *et al.* (2010) Incidence and predictive factors for infectious disease after rituximab therapy in kidney-transplant patients. *Am J Transplant* **10**, 89–98.

16. Liu Z, Yang F, Robotham JM, *et al.* (2009) Critical role of cyclophilin A and its prolyl-peptidyl isomerase activity in the structure and function of the hepatitis C virus replication complex. *J Virol* **83**, 6554–6565.

17. Kamar N, Garrigue V, Karras A, *et al.* (2006) Impact of early or delayed cyclosporine on delayed graft function in renal transplant recipients: A randomized, multicenter study. *Am J Transplant* **6**, 1042–1048.

18. Kasiske BL, Snyder JJ, Gilbertson D, *et al.* (2003) Diabetes mellitus after kidney transplantation in the United States. *Am J Transplant* **3**, 178–185.

19. Ware N, MacPhee IA. (2010) Current progress in pharmacogenetics and individualized immunosuppressive drug dosing in organ transplantation. *Curr Opin Mol Ther* **12**, 270–283.

20. Lown KS, Bailey DG, Fontana RJ, *et al.* (1997) Grapefruit juice increases felodipine oral availability in humans by decreasing intestinal CYP3A protein expression. *J Clin Invest* **99**, 2545–2553.

21. Levy G, Thervet E, Lake J, *et al.* (2002) Patient management by Neoral C(2) monitoring: An international consensus statement. *Transplantation* **73**, S12–S18.

22. Ekberg H, Tedesco-Silva H, Demirbas A, *et al.* (2007) Reduced exposure to calcineurin inhibitors in renal transplantation. *N Engl J Med* **357**, 2562–2575.

23. Dantal J, Hourmant M, Cantarovich D, *et al.* (1998) Effect of long-term immunosuppression in kidney-graft recipients on cancer incidence: Randomised comparison of two cyclosporin regimens. *Lancet* **351**, 623–628.

24. Stefoni S, Midtved K, Cole E, *et al.* (2005) Efficacy and safety outcomes among de novo renal transplant recipients managed by C2 monitoring of cyclosporine a microemulsion: Results of a 12-month, randomized, multicenter study. *Transplantation* **79**, 577–583.

25. Bekersky I, Dressler D, Mekki Q. (2001) Effect of time of meal consumption on bioavailability of a single oral 5 mg tacrolimus dose. *J Clin Pharmacol* **41**, 289–297.

26. Mancinelli LM, Frassetto L, Floren LC, *et al.* (2001) The pharmacokinetics and metabolic disposition of tacrolimus: A comparison across ethnic groups. *Clin Pharmacol Ther* **69**, 24–31.

27. Thervet E, Loriot MA, Barbier S, *et al.* (2010) Optimization of initial tacrolimus dose using pharmacogenetic testing. *Clin Pharmacol Ther* **87**, 721–726.

28. Higgins RM, Morlidge C, Magee P, *et al.* (1999) Conversion between cyclosporin and tacrolimus–30-fold dose prediction. *Nephrol Dial Transplant* **14**, 1609.

29. Tiede I, Fritz G, Strand S, *et al.* (2003) CD28-dependent Rac1 activation is the molecular target of azathioprine in primary human CD4+ T lymphocytes. *J Clin Invest* **111**, 1133–1145.

30. Gearry RB, Barclay ML. (2005) Azathioprine and 6-mercaptopurine pharmacogenetics and metabolite monitoring in inflammatory bowel disease. *J Gastroenterol Hepatol* **20**, 1149–1157.

31. Evans WE. (2004) Pharmacogenetics of thiopurine S-methyltransferase and thiopurine therapy. *Ther Drug Monit* **26**, 186–191.

32. Salvadori M, Holzer H, de Mattos A, *et al.* (2004) Enteric-coated mycophenolate sodium is therapeutically equivalent to mycophenolate mofetil in de novo renal transplant patients. *Am J Transplant* **4**, 231–236.

33. A blinded, randomized clinical trial of mycophenolate mofetil for the prevention of acute rejection in cadaveric renal transplantation. The Tricontinental Mycophenolate Mofetil Renal Transplantation Study Group. (1996) *Transplantation* **61**, 1029–1037.

34. Hesselink DA, van Hest RM, Mathot RA, *et al.* (2005) Cyclosporine interacts with mycophenolic acid by inhibiting the multidrug resistance-associated protein 2. *Am J Transplant* **5**, 987–994.

35. Kuypers DR, Vanrenterghem Y, Squifflet JP, *et al.* (2003) Twelve-month evaluation of the clinical pharmacokinetics of total and free mycophenolic acid and its glucuronide metabolites in renal allograft recipients on low dose tacrolimus in combination with mycophenolate mofetil. *Ther Drug Monit* **25**, 609–622.

36. Shaw LM, Korecka M, Aradhye S, *et al.* (2000) Mycophenolic acid area under the curve values in African American and Caucasian renal transplant patients are comparable. *J Clin Pharmacol* **40**, 624–633.

37. van Gelder T, Silva HT, de Fijter JW, *et al.* (2008) Comparing mycophenolate mofetil regimens for de novo renal transplant recipients: The fixed-dose concentration-controlled trial. *Transplantation* **86**, 1043–1051.

38. Le Meur Y, Buchler M, Thierry A, *et al.* (2007) Individualized mycophenolate mofetil dosing based on drug exposure significantly improves patient outcomes after renal transplantation. *Am J Transplant* **7**, 2496–2503.

39. Gaston RS, Kaplan B, Shah T, *et al.* (2009) Fixed- or controlled-dose mycophenolate mofetil with standard- or reduced-dose calcineurin inhibitors: The opticept trial. *Am J Transplant* **9**, 1607–1619.

40. Liacini A, Seamone ME, Muruve DA, *et al.* (2010) Anti-BK virus mechanisms of sirolimus and leflunomide alone and in combination: Toward a new therapy for BK virus infection. *Transplantation* **90**, 1450–1457.

41. Anglicheau D, Pallet N, Rabant M, *et al.* (2006) Role of P-glycoprotein in cyclosporine cytotoxicity in the cyclosporine-sirolimus interaction. *Kidney Int* **70**, 1019–1025.

42. Mota A, Arias M, Taskinen EI, *et al.* (2004) Sirolimus-based therapy following early cyclosporine withdrawal provides significantly improved renal histology and function at 3 years. *Am J Transplant* **4**, 953–961.

43. Schachter AD, Meyers KE, Spaneas LD, *et al.* (2004) Short sirolimus half-life in pediatric renal transplant recipients on a calcineurin inhibitor-free protocol. *Pediatr Transplant* **8**, 171–177.

44. Flechner SM, Glyda M, Cockfield S, *et al.* (2011) The ORION Study: Comparison of two sirolimus-based regimens versus tacrolimus and mycophenolate mofetil in renal allograft recipients. *Am J Transplant* **11**, 1633–1644.

45. Campistol JM, Cockwell P, Diekmann F, *et al.* (2009) Practical recommendations for the early use of m-TOR inhibitors (sirolimus) in renal transplantation. *Transpl Int* **22**, 681–687.

46. Di Paolo S, Teutonico A, Leogrande D, *et al.* (2006) Chronic inhibition of mammalian target of rapamycin signaling downregulates insulin receptor substrates 1 and 2 and AKT activation: A crossroad between cancer and diabetes? *J Am Soc Nephrol* **17**, 2236–2244.

47. Diekmann F, Budde K, Oppenheimer F, *et al.* (2004) Predictors of success in conversion from calcineurin inhibitor to sirolimus in chronic allograft dysfunction. *Am J Transplant* **4**, 1869–1875.

48. Weiner SM, Sellin L, Vonend O, *et al.* (2007) Pneumonitis associated with sirolimus: Clinical characteristics, risk factors and outcome–a single-centre experience and review of the literature. *Nephrol Dial Transplant* **22**, 3631–3637.

49. Zuber J, Anglicheau D, Elie C, *et al.* (2008) Sirolimus may reduce fertility in male renal transplant recipients. *Am J Transplant* **8**, 1471–1479.

50. Stallone G, Schena A, Infante B, *et al.* (2005) Sirolimus for Kaposi's sarcoma in renal-transplant recipients. *N Engl J Med* **352**, 1317–1323.

51. Salgo R, Gossmann J, Schofer H, *et al.* (2010) Switch to a sirolimus-based immunosuppression in long-term renal transplant recipients: Reduced rate of (pre-) malignancies and nonmelanoma skin cancer in a prospective, randomized, assessor-blinded, controlled clinical trial. *Am J Transplant* **10**, 1385–1393.

52. Qian Q, Du H, King BF, *et al.* (2008) Sirolimus reduces polycystic liver volume in ADPKD patients. *J Am Soc Nephrol* **19**, 631–638.

53. Kahan BD, Napoli KL, Kelly PA, *et al.* (2000) Therapeutic drug monitoring of sirolimus: Correlations with efficacy and toxicity. *Clin Transplant* **14**, 97–109.

54. Anglicheau D, Le Corre D, Lechaton S, *et al.* (2005) Consequences of genetic polymorphisms for sirolimus requirements after renal transplant in patients on primary sirolimus therapy. *Am J Transplant* **5**, 595–603.

55. Potter JM, McWhinney BC, Sampson L, *et al.* (2004) Area-under-the-curve monitoring of prednisolone for dose optimization in a stable renal transplant population. *Ther Drug Monit* **26**, 408–414.

56. Vincenti F, Charpentier B, Vanrenterghem Y, *et al.* (2010) A phase III study of belatacept-based immunosuppression regimens versus cyclosporine in renal transplant recipients (BENEFIT study). *Am J Transplant* **10**, 535–546.

57. Vincenti F, Schena FP, Paraskevas S, *et al.* (2008) A randomized, multicenter study of steroid avoidance, early steroid withdrawal or standard steroid therapy in kidney transplant recipients. *Am J Transplant* **8**, 307–316.

58. Woodle ES, First MR, Pirsch J, *et al.* (2008) A prospective, randomized, double-blind, placebo-controlled multicenter trial comparing early (7 day) corticosteroid cessation versus long-term, low-dose corticosteroid therapy. *Ann Surg* **248**, 564–577.

59. Vincenti F, Ramos E, Brattstrom C, *et al.* (2001) Multicenter trial exploring calcineurin inhibitors avoidance in renal transplantation. *Transplantation* **71**, 1282–1287.

60. Bemelman FJ, de Maar EF, Press RR, *et al.* (2009) Minimization of maintenance immunosuppression early after renal transplantation: An interim analysis. *Transplantation* **88**, 421–428.

61. Gallagher MP, Hall B, Craig J, *et al.* (2004) A randomized controlled trial of cyclosporine withdrawal in renal-transplant recipients: 15-year results. *Transplantation* **78**, 1653–1660.

62. Lebranchu Y, Thierry A, Toupance O, *et al.* (2009) Efficacy on renal function of early conversion from cyclosporine to sirolimus 3 months after renal transplantation: Concept study. *Am J Transplant* **9**, 1115–1123.

63. Weir MR, Mulgaonkar S, Chan L, *et al.* (2011) Mycophenolate mofetil-based immunosuppression with sirolimus in renal transplantation: A randomized, controlled Spare-the-Nephron trial. *Kidney Int* **79**, 897–907.

64. Budde K, Becker T, Arns W, *et al.* (2011) Everolimus-based, calcineurin-inhibitor-free regimen in recipients of de-novo kidney transplants: An open-label, randomised, controlled trial. *Lancet* **377**, 837–847.

65. Archdeacon P, Chan M, Neuland C, *et al.* (2011) Summary of FDA antibody-mediated rejection workshop. *Am J Transplant* **11**, 896–906.

66. Frassetto LA, Browne M, Cheng A, *et al.* (2007) Immunosuppressant pharmacokinetics and dosing modifications in HIV-1 infected liver and kidney transplant recipients. *Am J Transplant* **7**, 2816–2820.

17 Antibody-incompatible kidney transplantation

Nicos Kessaris and Nizam Mamode

ABO-Incompatible kidney transplantation

Introduction

Until recently, ABO-I transplantation was not carried out due to the high risk of hyperacute rejection due to preformed IgG and IgM antibodies against A or B blood group antigens found on the kidney allograft. As 30% of potential living donors are ABO-I to their recipient, this is a significant issue. Over the last few years, many transplant units have started using new techniques allowing ABO-incompatible renal transplantation with excellent results.

Experience and results

The largest experience in ABO-I transplantation comes from Japan, where organ transplantation from brain-dead donors was not common practice until the late 1990s. More than 1000 such cases have been performed in Japan since 1989, and they account for 18% of all living donor kidney transplants [1]. Initially, 1-year and 3-year graft survival rates were 84% and 80%, but since 2001 they have increased to 96% and 94%, respectively. These results are comparable to ABO-compatible transplant outcomes. Early approaches included splenectomy shortly before or at the time of transplantation to remove some of the plasma cells producing blood group antibody. More recently, this has been substituted by giving rituximab, a chimeric monoclonal antibody against the CD20 antigen on B cells. It prevents the formation of new antibody-producing plasma cells but does not remove existing plasma cells.

In addition to rituximab, ABO-incompatible transplantation includes pre-transplant plasmapheresis (PP) or immunoadsorption (IA) to remove IgG and IgM antibodies against the ABO group of the potential recipient to a concentration below a clinically significant titre (typically IgG titre ≤1 in 8). Immunoadsorption using GlycoSorb ABO columns (Glycorex Transplantation AB, Lund, Sweden) has the advantage over PP in that it specifically depletes anti-A or anti-B antibodies only (Fig. 17.1).

Handbook of Renal and Pancreatic Transplantation, First Edition. Edited by Iain A. M. MacPhee and Jiří Froněk.
© 2012 John Wiley & Sons, Ltd. Published 2012 by John Wiley & Sons, Ltd.

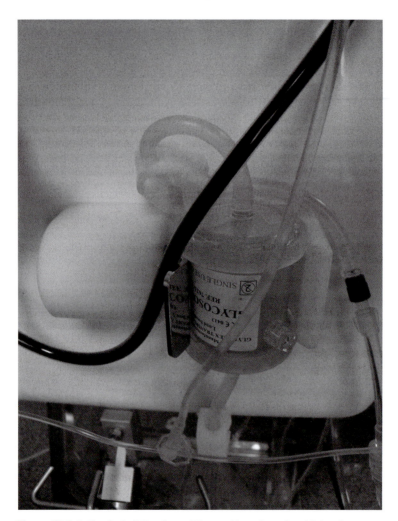

Figure 17.1 A GlycoSorb ABO column (Glycorex Transplantation AB, Lund, Sweden).

This reduces the potential for bleeding due to removal of clotting factors as well as infectious complications due to the removal of protective antibody.

The first ABO-I transplant using rituximab and IA was performed by Tyden *et al.* in Sweden in 2001 [2]. The original protocol evolved over time. The current one includes the administration of rituximab (375 mg/m²) 1 month before transplantation. Conventional immunosuppression using tacrolimus (0.2 mg/kg, target trough concentration 15 ng/mL), mycophenolate mofetil (2 g daily) and prednisolone (30 mg) is started 10 days before transplantation. Immunoadsorption using GlycoSorb ABO columns is then performed four times before surgery and three times after surgery. Intravenous immunoglobulin (IVIg) (0.5 g/kg) is given the evening before transplantation.

The largest study involving rituximab and immunoadsorption in ABO-I transplantation comes from Sweden and Germany [2]. This describes a three-centre experience of 60 ABO-incompatible transplants. Two of these grafts were lost after a mean follow-up of 17.5 months (non-compliance and death with a functioning graft). These cases were compared with 274 patients who underwent ABO-compatible kidney transplantation. Graft survival was 97% for the ABO-incompatible compared with 95% for the ABO-compatible. Patient survival was 98% in both groups. There was no late rebound of antibodies and there were no humoral rejections.

Three-year results of 20 ABO-I transplant patients from Sweden, with more than 1 year follow-up, were compared with 48 ABO-compatible ones [3]. Patient and graft survival were comparable, as well as the incidence of acute rejection. In a similar study from Germany, with an average follow-up of just over 3 years, 40 patients were compared with 43 ABO-compatible ones [4]. Again, patient and graft survival were comparable, as well as the incidence of acute rejection.

The Johns Hopkins team first used rituximab together with PP and low-dose cytomegalovirus (CMV) hyperimmunoglobulin (CMVIg) to accomplish ABO-I transplantation successfully. Subsequently, they eliminated the use of rituximab and continued with PP and CMVIg, even for the high-titre patients, successfully. The 1-, 3- and 5-year graft survival rate for 60 patients from this group were 98.3, 92.9 and 88.7%, respectively [5]. Less than 15% of patients experienced antibody-mediated rejection. This was not increased after the elimination of rituximab. CMVIg is not available in Europe at present.

At the West London Transplant Centre in the UK, alemtuzumab is currently used instead of rituximab for ABO-I transplantation, together with tacrolimus monotherapy. Antibody removal is accomplished with plasma exchange. Each session is followed up with IVIg. Graft function was 93.3% at 1-year follow-up out of 23 patients treated with this protocol compared with 91.3% in a similar number of ABO-I transplant patients who received rituximab in the same study at 1 year [6].

Method of ABO-I transplantation

In the UK, 44% of the population has blood group A, 8% has blood group B, 3% has blood group AB and 45% has blood group O [7]. Blood group A is subdivided into A1 and A2. There is less A2 antigen on the allograft and the affinity of antibodies is weaker than with the A1 subtype. Therefore, ABO-I transplantation across the A2 blood group barrier is easier than the A1 subtype.

The method of ABO-I transplantation described here is based on the Swedish protocol [2,3]. This is summarised in Table 17.1. Rituximab is preceded with the final crossmatch, as this can interfere with the result owing to rituximab in the recipient's serum binding to B lymphocytes, leading to a false positive crossmatch. This is given in a single dose as an

Table 17.1 ABO-I transplant protocol used at St George's Hospital based on the Swedish protocol.

Time	Steroids	Tacrolimus	MMF	Rituximab 375 mg/ m² IV	IA and IVIg 0.5 g/kg	Titres
Day −30				Rituximab		
Day −10	30 mg pred	0.2 mg/kg	1 g bd			
Day −6	30 mg pred	Aim level 10–15 ng/ mL until end of first month	1 g bd For 3 months		IA	Before and after IA
Day −5	30 mg pred	As above	As above		IA	Before and after IA
Day −4	30 mg pred	As above	As above			
Day −3	30 mg pred	As above	As above			
Day −2	30 mg pred	As above	As above		IA	Before and after IA
Day −1	30 mg pred	As above	As above		IA followed by IVIg if titres ≤1:8	Before and after IA*
Day −0 (before Tx)	1 g methyl pred	As above	As above			Check titres before Tx
Day 1	100 mg pred	As above	As above			Check titers
Day 2	90 mg pred	As above	As above		IA	Before and after IA
Day 3	80 mg pred	As above	As above			Check titres
Day 4	70 mg pred	As above	As above			Check titres
Day 5	60 mg pred	As above	As above		IA	Before and after IA
Day 6	50 mg pred	As above	As above			Check titres
Day 7	40 mg pred	As above	As above			Check titres
Day 8	30 mg pred	As above	As above		IA	Before and after IA
Day 9	20 mg Pred	As above	As above			Check titres
Day 14	15 mg pred	As above	As above			Check titres every OPD
Day 28	10 mg Pred, as per standard protocol	aim level 8–12 ng/mL	As above			Check titres once a week

Table 17.1 *Continued*

Time	Steroids	Tacrolimus	MMF	Rituximab 375 mg/m² IV	IA and IVIg 0.5 g/kg	Titres
Month 1	As per standard protocol	As above	Check conc. & adjust dose to achieve 45 mg/h/L (range 30–60)			Check titres once every 2 weeks

intravenous infusion at a dose of 375 mg/m² made up in 500 mL of 0.9% saline. Methylprednisolone (100 mg) is given intravenously, 30 minutes prior to rituximab with oral chlorphenamine (4 mg) and paracetamol (1 g).

An alternative approach, used at Guy's Hospital, involves double filtration plasma exchange (DFPE) in patients with antibody titres ≤1 in 64 to reduce financial cost. Although with double filtration part of the plasma is returned to the patient, attention should be paid to the plasma fibrinogen concentration to avoid the risk of bleeding. Guy's Hospital has eliminated the use of IVIg the day before transplantation without any obvious clinical consequences but introduced basiliximab at induction in order to reduce the risk of acute rejection. Graft survival rates of 97% were obtained at 2 years in 54 patients undergoing ABO-I using this tailored regimen, which was comparable to a control group of 139 blood group compatible patients [8].

HF440 (L.IN.C Medical Systems Ltd, Loddington, UK) is a multi-therapy extracorporeal filtration device (Fig. 17.2) that can be used to perform IA (Fig. 17.3) and DFPE. During IA, blood passes through a primary plasma filter before passing through the Glycorex column, where the unwanted anti-A/B antibody is removed. If the patient is on an angiotensin-converting enzyme (ACE) inhibitor, this should be stopped a week before as it may potentiate problems related to kinin production as a consequence of the extracorporeal blood circuit. Ten litres of plasma are processed each time. A citrate-heparin protocol is used for anticoagulation. Acid-citrate dextrose solution is given at 10% of plasma flow rate (270–297 mL/h). 5 mL of heparin is given for rinsing the circuit followed by 1 mL/h. Calcium is replaced with intravenous 10% calcium gluconate at a rate of 5–10 mL/h. Clotting and serum calcium is monitored before and after IA. If the patient is already on haemodialysis (HD), IA is performed before HD. DFPE involves separating plasma with the primary filter before passing it through a secondary filter with

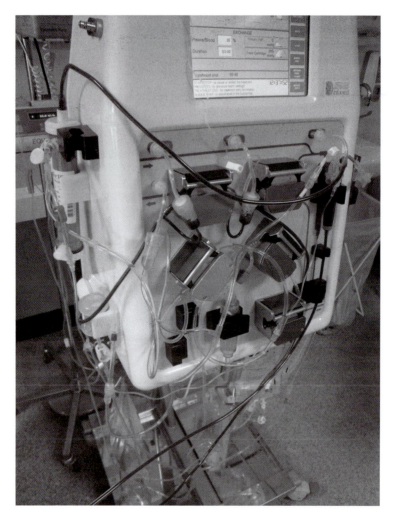

Figure 17.2 The HF440 multi-therapy extracorporeal filtration device (L.IN.C Medical Systems Ltd, Loddington, UK). On the left side, the plasma filter and the GlycoSorb ABO column can be seen.

smaller-sized pores called a fractionator. This allows complement components and some clotting factors to be retained. 250 mL/kg of plasma can be treated per day. Anticoagulation is not usually necessary, as the procedure lasts only 1.5 hours. 1–1.5 litres of 5% albumin is used as a replacement fluid, although coagulation factors are commonly replaced before surgery using fibrinogen or fresh frozen plasma (FFP). Another way of removing unwanted antibody is using the Life 18 Apheresis unit (Fig. 17.4) with TheraSorb adsorbers (Miltenyi Biotec GmbH, Germany). These reduce immunoglobulin concentrations in the patient's blood in a less specific way than Glycorex. Conventional plasma exchange (PE)

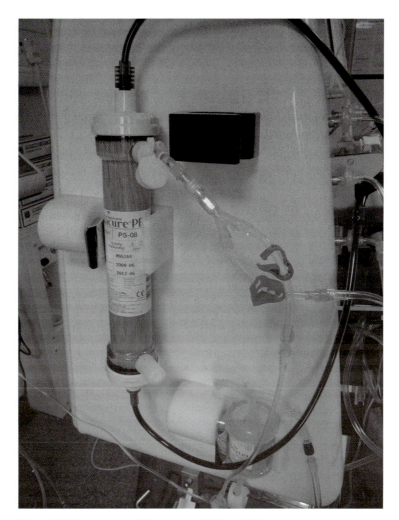

Figure 17.3 The process of IA using the HF440 multi-therapy extracorporeal filtration device. The plasma filter is seen on the left and the GlycoSorb ABO column on the right.

techniques can also be used but are even less specific and result in a higher incidence of coagulopathy, infection and hypocalcaemia.

Titres should be measured using the gel hemagglutination technique [9]. This has the least variability when compared among different units. Titres are monitored postoperatively as shown in Table 17.1. Even though both of our centres used to perform IA routinely post-transplantation, it is currently only performed in cases where there is a deterioration of renal function and a rise in anti-A/B IgG concentration by two dilutions or more. Rejection should always be proven by biopsy and treated according to standard methods depending on the histological findings.

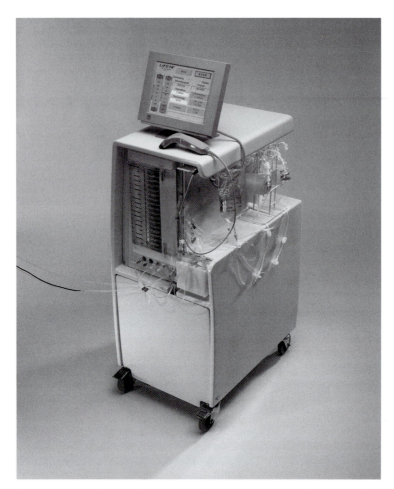

Figure 17.4 The Life 18 Apheresis unit (Miltenyi Biotec, Germany). Reproduced by permission of Miltenyi Biotec Ltd.

If blood transfusion is required after ABOI transplantation, the following policy can be followed:

- for emergency
  - red cells: high titre (HT)-negative red cell units, ABO/D compatible with renal transplant recipient
  - platelets: (HT)-negative platelet units, ABO compatible with renal transplant donor
  - plasma: FFP, type AB
- in all other cases
  - red cells: washed red cells, ABO/D compatible with renal transplant recipient
  - platelets: platelets in platelet suspension medium (PSM), ABO compatible with renal transplant recipient (at Guy's Hospital,

Table 17.2 Summary of ABOI transplant results from Guy's and St George's Hospitals.

Hospital	Patients	Death-censored graft Survival (%)	Patient survival (%)	Mean creatinine (μmol/L)	Mean follow-up (days)	Rejection episodes (patients)
Guy's	59	98	93	143	705	19*
St George's	6	100	100	126	227	3*

*None of these was related to blood group antibodies.

> platelets are ABO compatible with the renal transplant donor instead)
> plasma: FFP, type AB or donor group specific

Results from the authors' units using these protocols are summarised in Table 17.2.

HLA-I transplantation

Introduction

Results from HLA-I transplantation have been similar to deceased rather than live donor renal transplantation [10]. Such a transplant should be undertaken when the patient has not been successful in having a kidney through 'kidney paired donation' in countries where this is available [11]. Donor-specific HLA antibodies (DSA), arise through different sensitisation events such as pregnancy, blood transfusion and previous transplants. These increase the risk of a patient having a positive crossmatch. Therefore, such patients have to wait longer on the deceased donor transplant waiting list before receiving a transplant.

Experience and results

There have been two major desensitisation protocols produced over the last few years from the USA. The first one involves giving high-dose IVIg and the second one low-dose IVIg and PP [11].

The high-dose IVIg protocol entails giving monthly infusions (2 gm/kg) of IVIg. This continues until the crossmatch has become negative or a total of four doses has been given. This protocol has increased the transplantation rate from 17 to 35% in a multicentre, double-blinded, placebo-controlled study by Jordan *et al.* involving deceased donor transplantation in highly sensitised patients [12].

The low-dose IVIg protocol involves PP with low-dose IVIg (100 mg/kg) after each session. Rituximab is sometimes included in these protocols. At Johns Hopkins more than 200 such transplants have been performed. The original protocol has evolved. Only high-risk patients currently receive rituximab the night before transplantation. Induction includes CD25 antibody. Rescue splenectomy is required for resistant antibody-mediated rejection in 5% of cases [11].

The Mayo group has compared high-dose IVIg with low-dose IVIg and PP. The latter method was found to be superior, with 84% desensitisation success versus 36% in the former group [13]. Rituximab was given between 4 and 7 days before transplantation with the low-dose IVIg and PP treatment.

In Newcastle, UK, rituximab is given 1 month before transplantation followed by alemtuzumab on induction to accomplish HLA-I transplantation. Unwanted antibody is removed using the TheraSorb adsorbers. Out of six such transplants (two of which were both HLA-I and ABO-I) there have been no episodes of acute rejection at a mean follow-up of 5 months [14]. These results are very good, as the rate of antibody-mediated rejection in HLA-I transplantation has been reported at between 30 and 50% [11].

Interestingly, Bohmig's group from Austria has successfully applied peritransplant IA (protein A) to enable deceased donor kidney transplantation in patients with a positive complement-dependent cytotoxicity (CDC) crossmatch [15]. Some 68 deceased donors underwent IA between 1999 and 2008. The overall graft survival and death-censored graft survival was 63% and 76%, respectively, at 5 years. Legendre's group from France has successfully combined post-transplant prophylactic IVIg, rituximab and PP in kidney recipients with preformed donor-specific antibodies [16]. The rate of early antibody-mediated rejection was 16.6%, whereas the rate of chronic antibody-mediated rejection at 1 year was 13.3%. DSA-median fluorescence intensity (MFI) declined by 80% ($\pm$8%) over the first year. Finally, the glomerular filtration rate at 1 year was $54 \pm 16 \, \text{mL/min/1.73} \, \text{m}^2$.

Method

Assessment of immunological risk for transplantation is performed by evaluating the sensitisation history and by crossmatching. The sensitisation event is defined. As explained above this may be due to a previous transplant, blood transfusion or pregnancy. The risk is higher with the second or third transplant, if the new transplant shares mismatched HLA antigens with a previous one, if the previous graft was lost due to rejection, the presence of high DSA or of multiple DSA.

Crossmatching is performed using cell-based and solid-phase assays. CDC and flow cytometry (FC) crossmatch (XM) are cell-based assays. Results are differentiated according to T- and B-cell positivity. Immunological risk is higher when CDC-XM and FC-XM are positive versus negative CDC-XM and positive FC-XM. HLA antibody specificities are defined using solid-phase assay techniques such as Luminex technology. The strength of these antibodies is defined by dilution of the recipient serum. The highest dilution at which the crossmatch remains positive is measured. HLA antigen repeat mismatches are defined. The maximum DSA titre for eligibility for desensitisation is 1/32 for a non-HLA antigen repeat mismatch and 1/4 if there is a direct HLA antigen repeat mismatch, although this may vary among groups.

At Guy's Hospital the aim is to proceed with transplantation when a confirmatory negative FC-XM has been achieved. Occasionally the FC crossmatch may be positive due to non-HLA autoantibodies – then an auto crossmatch is performed. If this is positive, it indicates an autoantibody, and this result can be deducted from the positive donor cells versus recipient serum crossmatch result to give a clinically negative crossmatch.

A test PE or DFPE of 3 L, with crossmatch before and after, is initially performed to assess the feasibility of transplantation. The number of such plasma exchanges prior to transplantation depends on the baseline titre and specificities. Post transplantation DFPE is performed if the titres begin to rise.

In Newcastle, UK, the goal is to have a negative CDC, a significantly reduced T-cell FC-XM titre and DSA titre less than 3–4000 MFI by Luminex. The B-cell XM is difficult to interpret after rituximab, so for HLA class II DSA the decision to transplant is based solely on DSA titre.

The protocol used at Guy's Hospital is summarised in Table 17.3, with a summary of results in Table 17.4. Changes in HLA antibody measured by the Luminex assay for a typical transplant are shown in Fig. 17.5.

Table 17.3 Current HLA-I transplant protocol used at Guy's Hospital.

Time	Steroids	Tacrolimus	MMF	Alemtuzumab* 30 mg sc	DFPE and IVIg 0.5 g/kg	FC-XM and titres
Day −10						
Day −6	25 mg pred	aim level 10–12 ng/mL until end of first month	1 g bd For 3 months		DFPE	Before and after DFPE
Day −5	25 mg pred	As above	As above		DFPE	Before and after DFPE
Day −4	25 mg pred	As above	As above			
Day −3	25 mg pred	As above	As above			
Day −2	25 mg pred	As above	As above		DFPE	Before and after DFPE
Day −1	25 mg pred	As above	As above		DFPE followed by IVIg 0.5 g/kg	Before and after DFPE
Day 0 (before Tx)	1 g methyl pred	As above	As above	Alemtuzumab 30 mg sc		Check titres before Tx

Continued

Table 17.3 *Continued*

Time	Steroids	Tacrolimus	MMF	Alemtuzumab* 30 mg sc	DFPE and IVIg 0.5 g/kg	FC-XM and titres
Day 1	20 mg pred	As above	As above			
Day 2	20 mg pred	As above	As above			
Day 3	20 mg pred	As above	As above			Check titres
Day 4	20 mg pred	As above	As above			
Day 5	20 mg pred	As above	As above			
Day 6	20 mg pred	As above	As above			
Day 7	20 mg pred	As above	As above			Check titres
Day 8	20 mg pred	As above	As above			
Day 10	20 mg pred	As above	As above			Check titres
Day 14	10 mg pred	As above	As above			Check titres weekly
Day 28	15 mg Pred, as per standard protocol	aim conc. 8–12 ng/mL	As above			Check titres weekly
Month 1	As per standard protocol	As above	As above			Check titres weekly

*Alemtuzumab is also used for induction in patients having combined ABO-I and HLA-I transplantation at Guy's Hospital.

Table 17.4 Summary of HLA-I transplant results from Guy's Hospital.

Hospital	Patients	Death-censored graft survival (%)	Patient survival (%)	Mean creatinine (μmol/L)	Mean follow-up (days)	Rejection rate
Guy's*	26	77%	88%	196	713	50%

*The last six transplants from Guy's were performed using alemtuzumab for induction. The rest were performed using basiliximab. On two occasions rituximab was also given.

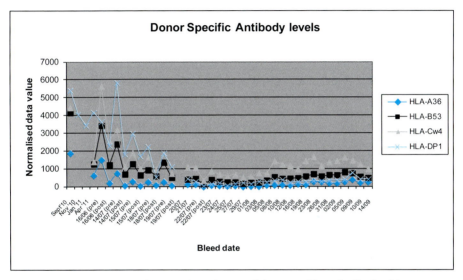

Figure 17.5 The graph shows the reduction of donor-specific antibodies (MFI) in a patient following treatment and transplant on the 20 July.

Conclusions

ABO-I and HLA-I transplantation is now possible through a variety of different protocols. The short-term results from the former are comparable to live-donor antibody-compatible transplantation. Short-term results from the latter are comparable to deceased-donor renal-transplantation outcomes and long-term allograft survival is affected by the process of antibody-mediated rejection. These new techniques, which are both cost-effective compared with long-term dialysis, have opened the pathway for more transplants to be achieved, but they also have their limitations. These always need to be explained to the patients. Other more compatible donors and options such as 'kidney paired donation' should be explored at all times.

Acknowledgements

Special thanks to Steven Wiltshire, Blood Bank Manager for formulating the St George's Hospital blood transfusion policy for ABO-I transplantation.

References

1. Takahashi K. (2007) Recent findings in ABO-incompatible kidney transplantation: Classification and therapeutic strategy for acute antibody-mediated rejection due to ABO-blood-group-related antigens during the critical period preceding the establishment of accommodation. *Clin Exp Nephrol* **11**, 128–141.
2. Tydén G, Donauer J, Wadström J, *et al.* (2007) Implementation of a Protocol for ABO-incompatible kidney transplantation–a three-center experience with 60 consecutive transplantations. *Transplantation* **83**, 1153–1155.
3. Genberg H, Kumlien G, Wennberg L, *et al.* (2008) ABO-incompatible kidney transplantation using antigen-specific immunoadsorption and rituximab: A 3-year follow-up. *Transplantation* **85**, 1745–1754.
4. Wilpert J, Fischer KG, Pisarski P, *et al.* (2010) Long-term outcome of ABO-incompatible living donor kidney transplantation based on antigen-specific desensitization. An observational comparative analysis. *Nephrol Dial Transplant* **25**, 3778–3786.
5. Montgomery RA, Locke JE, King KE, *et al.* (2009) ABO incompatible renal transplantation: A paradigm ready for broad implementation. *Transplantation* **87**, 1246–1255.
6. Galliford J, Chan E, Lawrence C, *et al.* (2010) Campath induction and Tacrolimus monotherapy: A novel and effective immunosuppressive regime for ABO incompatible live donor renal transplantation. Abstract O40, British Transplantation Society 13th Annual Congress.
7. British Transplantation Society. (2011) UK Guidelines for Living Donor kidney Transplantation. Available online from: http://www.bts.org.uk/transplantation/standards-and-guidelines/.
8. Mamode N, Hadjiansastassiou V, Dorling A, *et al.* (2011) Successful outcomes after minimising antibody modulation in blood group incompatible kidney transplantation. Abstract O-134, European Society for Organ Transplantation Congress 15th Congress.
9. Kumlien G, Wilpert J, Säfwenberg J, *et al.* (2007) Comparing the tube and gel techniques for ABO antibody titration, as performed in three European centers. *Transplantation* **84** (12 Suppl), S17–19.
10. Higgins R, Hudson A, Johnson R, *et al.* (2011) National Registry of ABO and HLA Antibody Incompatible Renal Transplantation. *Am J Transplant* **11** (s2), 109.
11. Montgomery RA. (2010) Renal transplantation across HLA and ABO antibody barriers: Integrating paired donation into desensitization protocols. *Am J Transplant* **10**, 449–457.
12. Jordan SC, Tyan D, Stablein D, *et al.* (2004) Evaluation of intravenous immunoglobulin as an agent to lower allosensitization and improve transplantation in highly sensitized adult patients with end-stage renal disease: Report of the NIH IG02 Trial. *J Am Soc Nephrol* **15**, 3256–3262.
13. Stegall MD, Gloor J, Winters JL, *et al.* (2006) A comparison of plasmapheresis versus high-dose IVIG desensitization in renal allograft

recipients with high levels of donor specific alloantibody. *Am J Transplant* **6**, 346–351.

14. Torpey N, Talbot. (2011) HLA antibody incompatible live donor renal transplantation with and without T-cell depleting induction immunosuppression. Abstract O57, British Transplantation Society, 13th Annual Congress.

15. Lorenz M, Regele H, Schillinger M, *et al.* (2005) Peritransplant immunoadsorption: A strategy enabling transplantation in highly sensitized crossmatch-positive cadaveric kidney allograft recipients. *Transplantation* **79**, 696–701.

16. Loupy A, Suberbielle-Boissel C, Zuber J, *et al.* Combined posttransplant prophylactic IVIg/anti-CD 20/plasmapheresis in kidney recipients with preformed donor-specific antibodies: A pilot study. *Transplantation* **89**, 1403–1410.

18 Renal transplantation in children

Luisa Berardinelli and Luciana Ghio

Introduction

In Europe, the incidence rate of end-stage renal disease (ESRD) in children up to 16 years of age is very low – approximately one to two children per million general population or four to six children per million childhood population per year [1]. Kidney transplantation in paediatric patients is the treatment of choice for children with ESRD, owing to better patient survival at 5 years (95% versus 80%) and psycho-physical rehabilitation compared with those remaining on dialysis [2].

Kidney transplantation in paediatric patients has become a routinely successful procedure [3], with overall patient survival at 5, 10 and 20 years being 97, 94 and 72%, respectively, transplant survival (first transplant) for deceased and living-related donors being 66% and 87% at 5 years ($p < 0.01$), 51% and 54% at 10 years, and 36% at 20 years (deceased-donor transplants only) [4].

The causes of ESRD are markedly different in children from those in adults: in contrast to adult patients, primary renal diseases responsible for ESRD in children are mostly (60%) congenital and hereditary disorders [1], and the precise cause of ESRD should be well defined preoperatively in order to assess the risk of recurrent disease [5].

All children with ESRD should be considered as candidates for transplantation. Very young children are generally treated by peritoneal dialysis, deferring transplantation until body weight has reached at least 8–10 kg in order to reduce the risk of vascular complications. Pre-transplant bilateral nephrectomy of the native kidney should be considered in the case of severe arterial hypertension, heavy proteinuria or renal cancer. The only circumstances in which a child would not be an appropriate candidate for kidney transplantation would be an overall poor prognosis, history of cancer, uncontrolled viral infection (human immunodeficiency, hepatitis B (HBV), Epstein–Barr (EBV)), very young age (<6 months), severe mental retardation and/or additional disabilities

Handbook of Renal and Pancreatic Transplantation, First Edition. Edited by
Iain A. M. MacPhee and Jiří Froněk.
© 2012 John Wiley & Sons, Ltd. Published 2012 by John Wiley & Sons, Ltd.

limiting potential quality of life, according to the European guidelines [1]. However, transplantation in very young children remains controversial, as recipients under 5 years of age are at higher risk of graft failure than older children [4,6]. A recipient age under 2 years is a significant negative prognostic factor, as well as that of a donor age below 6 years [7].

Routine childhood vaccination should be completed whenever possible prior to transplantation, in addition to vaccination against HBV, pneumococcus and varicella.

Growth is adversely affected by uraemia, and children younger than 6 years exhibit the best statural growth when they are transplanted early [6].

The mean waiting time for children is much lower than that of adults (300 days versus more than 900 days), as kidney allocation rules are specifically designed to favour children because of the necessity of enhancing their psycho-physical development with renal transplantation (see Chapter 8).

Recently an increasing number of children have undergone 'pre-emptive' transplantation – that is before being submitted to dialysis, mostly using a living donor [8].

Living donation delivers better results in the paediatric population than deceased donor transplantation. Pretransplant recipient preparation must include a thorough urologic evaluation, as many paediatric recipients have hidden lower urinary tract abnormalities [9]. The bladder must be distensible, the residual volume should be less than 30 mL and the end-filling pressure less than 30 cm H_2O. A poor flow rate may be due to urethral or bladder outlet obstruction. Detrusor malfunction, very low capacity or high pressure of the bladder may require augmentation cystoplasty, which must be performed at least 3 months before transplantation. Intermittent catheterisation through native urethra or using a Mitrofanoff procedure prevents urine stasis and infection after transplantation. Whenever the bladder is unusable for enterocystoplasty or the recipient is unwilling or unable to perform self-catheterisation, an ileal conduit may be useful in case of neurogenic bladder dysfunction.

The heightened immune response in young children that leads to increased graft loss after the initial rejection episode is partly due to differences in pharmacokinetics [10].

Induction therapy with anti-CD25 antibody is associated with significantly increased graft survival in children [11]. HLA mismatch for deceased donor transplants should be minimised in order to reduce the risk of sensitisation that would render re-transplantation later in life difficult.

Surgical technique of transplantation in children

It is mandatory to pay attention to every single minimal detail: the ambient temperature in the operating room must be set at approximately

a   b   c   d   e

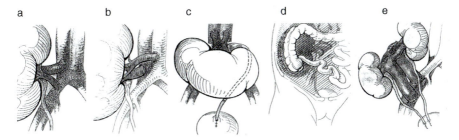

Figure 18.1 Surgical techniques of kidney transplantation in children. Reproduced from Vegeto A, Berardinelli L. (1999) *Il Trapianto di Rene*, with permission from UTET, Periodici Scientifici, Torino.

32 °C and all intravenous solutions/transfused blood products must be warmed to 35 °C to prevent arterial spasm, which is a relatively common finding in children and may lead to organ failure. Partial occluding clamps are preferred in children to avoid risks of intravascular coagulation and acidosis, and at least half of the arterial anastomosis should be performed using interrupted sutures to prevent the development of stenosis.

The surgical technique of transplantation in children varies according to the donor age, donor size and recipient size.

A small kidney or a kidney coming from a deceased donor of similar age allows use of the less invasive retroperitoneal approach in small recipients. In the case of a big kidney, the left side of a small recipient should be preferred, as the retroperitoneal space may provide more room without the right lobe of the liver. If the kidney has been recovered without an aortic patch, the internal iliac artery (which in small children is often larger than the external iliac artery) can be safely used for an end-to-end anastomosis with the renal artery. However, the use of more proximal arteries is recommended, as a vascular spasm of the small external iliac artery can compromise the outcome of the transplant. If an adult kidney must be implanted, an end-to-side anastomosis of the donor renal vein to distal vena cava and of renal artery to the recipient common iliac artery (Fig. 18.1a) may be performed. In very young recipients, the distal aorta and vena cava can be adopted for the anastomosis (Fig. 18.1b), using a transverse position in the case of a very big kidney (Fig. 18.1c), to limit the risks of vascular thrombosis and surgical complications [12]. Children whose lower limb vessels had been previously cannulated for hemodialysis must be submitted to a careful evaluation for patency of iliac vessels and vena cava.

Transperitoneal approach

A midline incision from xyphoid to the pubis is mandatory for children weighing less than 15 kg who receive the kidney from an adult donor. For living donation, the smallest compatible relative is first evaluated as the preferred candidate and the smaller of the two kidneys is chosen to reduce technical problems.

The posterior peritoneum is opened lateral to the right colon, which is reflected medially to expose the terminal aorta and vena cava. Native kidney removal may make room for a bigger kidney. A slow infusion of furosemide (1 mg/kg) and mannitol (12.5 g/kg) may be given to promote diuresis before the renal vein is anastomosed in an end-to-side fashion to the vena cava (or the common iliac vein). Then, an end-to-side anastomosis is made between the renal artery and the terminal aorta (or the common iliac vein) (Fig. 18.1d). The greater the size discrepancy between graft and recipient, the higher the target central venous pressure should be, aiming for values up to 17 cm of water before revascularisation. Maintenance of adequate intravascular volume with supplemental fluid boluses is mandatory to prevent hypotension and to avoid postoperative acute tubular necrosis, using an additional 300 mL of albumin solution or blood products, the amount that is sequestered by an adult donor kidney after revascularisation. The donor kidney is then replaced beyond the right and ascending colon (Fig. 18.1d) and the right parietocolic incision is sutured.

The ureter is re-implanted into the bladder according to an antireflux ureterocystoneostomy, after having brought it down retroperitoneally to favour the development of collateral circulation. As a last step, it may be useful to remove the appendix to avoid problems of diagnosis between appendicitis and rejection crisis presenting with right-sided abdominal pain.

En-bloc transplantation

The number of paediatric donors <6 years used as single transplant in children is nowadays declining because of higher rate of primary non-function and poor results. The use of a single kidney from very young donors is now controversial, although significant hypertrophy of infant kidneys is described after transplantation and good results are described from some transplant centres [13].

In the case of an infant donor younger than 2 years, weighing less than 15 kg [14] and with a polar length of the organ less than 6 cm [15], an 'en-bloc' transplant of both kidneys into bigger children or into adults is advisable, thus providing a sufficient nephron mass.

Organs are recovered maintaining liberal segments of aorta and vena cava, and careful preparation at the bench, specific to the transplant technique that will be employed, must precede implantation. All lumbar and gonadal vessels located on the anterior and posterior surface of the donor aorta and vena cava are ligated with 6/0 polypropylene stitches. The suprarenal aorta and vena cava are oversewn with two running 6/0 polypropylene sutures and the distal ends are anastomosed end-to side to the recipient iliac vessels (Fig. 18.1e), or, if the recipient is very small, to infrarenal aorta and vena cava. It is advisable to fix the kidneys to the psoas muscle to prevent kinking of the renal vessels.

One of the disadvantages of this en-bloc technique consists in the formation of thrombi in the cul-de-sacs of cranial ends of donor aorta and cava, due to turbulent blood flow inside. This complication may be avoided by interposing the en-bloc specimen into the transacted external iliac vessels with end-to-end anastomoses of the proximal and distal donor aorta and vena cava.

The two ureters should be anastomosed separately from the bladder, to limit damage to the other kidney in case of urological complications.

Immunosuppressive treatment

The transplant immunosuppression used in children is the same as that used in adults (see Chapter 16). It is noteworthy that children have an increased metabolic rate, and the standard doses used in adults are not always appropriate. The standard recommended mycophenolate mofetil dose for children is 600 mg/m^2 twice daily. Therapeutic drug monitoring is a particularly important tool in this so-called 'new era of immunosuppression minimisation' [16].

In fact, the young infant is the most favoured for best long-term graft survival, and now an inverse relationship has been noted between recipient age and graft acceptance rates across many types of solid organ transplants. Kidney allograft half-life for an adult sized kidney in a recipient <5 years old is 31 years, far better than the 23-year graft half-life reported for the 'gold-standard' adult HLA identical sibling transplant. The greatest benefit of immunosuppression minimisation for children may lie in reducing patient morbidity, by the elimination of the inherent side effects of steroid and calcineurin inhibitors (CNIs). However, this is in the population at greatest risk of acute rejection and requires a cautious approach.

Steroid minimisation strategies overall offer this young age group a substantive growth boost, with a possible positive impact on final adult height. Furthermore, the adolescents may have an incentive for improved compliance with immunosuppression minimisation trials, if these reduce the number of daily medications, and particularly if they reduce or eliminate cosmetic side effects.

An intermediate strategy has been to develop alternative-day steroid regimes. This approach improves growth without compromising graft function but may favour accidental non-compliance in adolescents.

It is possible also to perform steroid withdrawal after initial steroid-based immunosuppression [17]. A number of authors have attempted steroid withdrawal in paediatric recipients, with variable rates of early and late acute rejection episodes after non-randomised steroid discontinuation. In addition, a number of adverse effects develop very early after transplantation, and late withdrawal of steroids fails to prevent their occurrence.

The use of humanised or chimaeric anti-CD25 antibodies, lymphocyte depletion strategies and the increasing use of tacrolimus, mycophenolate and other antiproliferative agents, offer the transplant physician the possibility of immunosuppressive protocol, with steroid avoidance, but until now there are only preliminary findings and additional studies are required for paediatric patients.

CNIs have changed the short-term outcomes in transplantation, with their biggest impact being on the reduction in the incidence of acute rejection and short-term graft survival. However, the benefit of minimising early alloimmune response is offset by the burden of nephrotoxicity. Elimination of these aspects thus carries the potential of minimising nephrotoxicity and also hypertension, diabetes and hyperlipidemia, but there is a risk of acute rejection and consequently an increase immune chronic graft injury.

CNI minimisation has been tested extensively in adult transplantation, but in the paediatric population only some observational uncontrolled studies have been performed. Improvements in graft function were seen following these strategies in patients who tolerated the treatment – although in all studies, patients who had no benefit or did poorly with CNI minimisation were difficult to predict.

Safe CNI elimination in children remains an aspiration that has yet to be fully realised.

Morbidity

The first aspect that must be examined is growth. In fact, a major distinguishing feature of paediatric from adult recipients is the need for children to grow. The growth failure commonly observed in children at the time of transplantations is multifactorial. It is caused by nutritional deficiencies, metabolic disturbances and effects on the growth hormone axis. Dialysis does not improve growth velocity or pubertal development. Despite the pre-transplant use of growth hormone, the majority of young adults with end-stage renal failure have a height below -25 SD score.

Renal transplantation may increase growth velocity in children with ESRD with a natural increase in adult height. Factors that influence catch-up growth are age and height at the moment of renal failure, the moment of transplantation, level of transplant function and dose and frequency of corticosteroid treatment. Children younger than 4 years have the largest benefit from transplantation. Their growth time increases by more than 3 cm/year compared with that of children on dialysis. In children who receive a transplant post-puberty, acceleration of growth velocity and adult height are much lower than in children who are transplanted at a younger age. Despite the positive influence of renal transplantation on growing speed, the final adult height of children with ESRF remains lower than that of healthy subjects.

Corticosteroids given after transplantation have a negative influence on longitudinal growth, which can be diminished by steroid-free immunosuppression or by the reduction of the frequency of administration from once daily to once every other day. An alternative method of attaining catch-up growth after transplantation would be the use of growth hormone. At present, rhGH is not approved for use in children after transplantation; however, several uncontrolled studies have shown its ability to accelerate growth in this setting, but with potential for toxicity. The role of rhGH after transplantation has yet to be defined.

Post-transplant lymphoproliferative disease and malignancy

The incidence of post-transplant lymphoproliferative disease (PTLD) is increasing, and this may be the unfortunate consequence of 'improved', more potent, immunosuppressive regimens. The frequency is higher in children than in adults because children are frequently 'naïve' for EBV, with primary EBV infection as a key risk factor for PTLD.

Most of these are B lymphocyte in origin and are related to EBV infection.

The diagnosis of PTLD has generally been made on the basis of characteristic pathologic findings, and the diagnosis cannot be made without biopsy material. However, in cases of persistent EBV DNA polymerase chain reaction, it is advisable to taper the immunosuppression to allow the immune system to clear the viral load prior to the development of monoclonal B-lymphocyte proliferation. It is important to carefully monitor the incidence of PTLD (al least an abdominal ultrasound and chest X-ray once a year), particularly in patients with a raised EBV viral load or unexplained symptoms such as bloody diarrhoea or lymphadenopathy. For intestinal PTLD a contrast computerised tomography scan, and in other cases magnetic resonance imaging investigation, can be helpful for early diagnosis. The treatment consists of lowering the intensity of immunosuppression, rituximab, virus-specific cytotoxic T lymphocytes and chemotherapy.

The risk for development of other malignant disease after transplantation is higher than in the normal population. Therefore it is important to advise on factors that increase the risk – for example, skin cancer after excessive exposure to sunlight. In adults the overall risk is estimated to be 6%, and in childhood approximately 2–3%.

Other infections

The infections that arise in children are the same as for adults, but it is necessary to pay attention to the fact that infection is generally the major cause of death, particularly in the first year after transplantation.

Two particular infections may have to be faced in children with renal transplant: cytomegalovirus (CMV) infection and varicella. In children, CMV infection is frequently a primary infection. Therefore, a prophylactic therapy with valganciclovir in these children is important. Varicella is one of the constant worries of both the transplant physician and the patient's family, because exposure in the paediatric age range is extremely common. The rash in an immunocompromised patient may become confluent, bullous and haemorrhagic. If the disease becomes systemic, the fatality rate can be high. Treatment of varicella in immunocompromised children generally consists of intravenous administration of aciclovir, at least until all lesions are crusted.

Routine childhood vaccination should be completed whenever possible before transplantation, in addition to vaccination against HBV and varicella. Prophylaxis, comprising the administration of varicella-zoster immunoglobulin, is carried out in transplanted seronegative children on exposure. The administration of varicella vaccine before transplantation reduces the frequency and severity of the disease after transplantation.

Varicella vaccine may be used after transplantation, but there are fewer supporting data.

Hypertension

Hypertension is a particularly important complication in paediatric renal transplantation.

Up to 70–80% of paediatric patients required antihypertensive medication. This morbidity represents an extension of disease process prior to transplantation, but may also be due to steroid and CNI treatment. Transplant renal artery stenosis and dietary sodium loading are causative factors that should be considered. Hypertension and hyperlipidemia may contribute to cardiovascular dysfunction after renal transplantation [18], and cardiovascular disease is one of the principal causes of death in paediatric transplant recipients, as well as in adults.

Control of these cardiovascular risk factors is essential after renal transplantation in children.

Non-compliance with therapeutic regimen

Non-compliance after transplantation is a problem of great importance in the adolescent transplant population, accounting for 71% of cases of late graft loss in some series [19], and it is particularly often cited as a cause of graft failure in adolescents [20].

A major reason of non-compliance is thought to be the alteration in appearance that accompanies the use of immunosuppressive medication, including the cushingoid facies and growth retardation related to long-term daily corticosteroid administration, and the hypertrichosis and gingival hypertrophy associated with ciclosporin use. Non-compliance rates between 22 and 64% in adolescents have been reported. Some factors, such as young age, adolescence and poor socioeconomic status have been associated with increased levels of non-compliance.

Strategies such as educational programmes and family-based therapy have been proposed, but have not yet been universally successful in changing motivation, leading to improved compliance and outcomes. Transition from paediatric to adult services is a particularly difficult time that requires careful management.

References

1. EBPG Expert Group on Renal Transplantation. (2002) European best practice guidelines for renal transplantation. Section IV: Long-term management of the transplant recipient. IV.11 Paediatrics (specific problems). *Nephrol Dial Transplant* **17** (Suppl 4), 55–58.

2. Harmon WE. (2004) Pediatric renal transplantation. In: Avner ED, Harmon WE, Niaudet P (eds), *Pediatric Nephrology*, pp.1437–1468. Lippincott Williams & Wilkins, Philadelphia.
3. McDonald SP, Craig JC. (2004) Long-term survival of children with end-stage renal disease. *New Engl J Med* **350**, 2654–2662.
4. Rees L, Shroff R, Hutchinson C, *et al.* (2007) Long-term outcome of paediatric renal transplantation: Follow-up of 300 children from 1973 to 2000. *Nephron Clin Pract* **105**, 68–76.
5. Fine RN. (2007) Recurrence of nephrotic syndrome/focal segmental glomerulosclerosis following renal transplantation in children. *Pediatr Nephrol* **22**, 496–502.
6. Mohammad S, Alonso EM. (2010) Approach to optimizing growth, rehabilitation, and neurodevelopmental outcomes in children after solid-organ transplantation. *Pediatr Clin North Am* **57**, 539–557.
7. Becker T, Neipp M, Reichart B, *et al.* (2006) Paediatric kidney transplantation in small children: A single centre experience. *Transpl Int* **19**, 197–202.
8. Innocenti GR, Wadei HM, Prieto M, *et al.* (2007) Preemptive living donor kidney transplantation: Do the benefits extend to all recipients? *Transplantation* **83**, 144–149.
9. Feld LG, Stablein D, Fivush B, *et al.* (1997) Renal transplantation in children from 1987–1996. The 1996 Annual Report of the North American Pediatric Renal Transplant Cooperative Study. *Pediatr Transplant* **1**, 146–162.
10. Cecka JM. (1999) The UNOS Scientific Renal Transplant Registry. *Clin Transpl* 1–21.
11. Offner G, Toenshoff B, Höcker B, *et al.* (2008) Efficacy and safety of basiliximab in pediatric renal transplant patients receiving cyclosporine, mycophenolate mofetil, and steroids. *Transplantation* **86**, 1241–1248.
12. Sing A, Stablein D, Tejani A. (1997) Risk factors for vascular thrombosis in pediatric renal transplantation. A special report of the North American Pediatric Renal Transplant cooperative Study. *Transplantation* **63**, 1263–1267.
13. Bar-Dayan A, Bar-Nathan N, Shaharabani E, *et al.* (2008) Kidney transplantation from pediatric donors: Size-match-based allocation. *Pediatr Transplant* **12**, 469–473.
14. Bretan PN, Fiese C, Goldstein RB, *et al.* (1997) Immunologic and patient selection strategies for successful utilization of less than 15kg pediatric donor kidneys- long term experience with 40 transplants. *Transplantation* **63**, 233–237.
15. Satterthwaite R, Aswad S, Sunga V, *et al.* (1997) Outcome of en bloc and single kidney transplantation from very young cadaveric donors. *Transplantation* **63**, 1405–1410.
16. Sarwal MM, Pascual J. (2007) Immunosuppression minimization in pediatric transplantation. *Am J Transpl* **7**, 2227–2235.
17. Bhakta N, Marik J, Malekzadeh M, *et al.* (2008) Can pediatric steroid-free renal transplantation improve growth and metabolic complications? *Pediatr Transplant* **12**, 854–861.
18. Kim GB, Kwon BS, Kang HG, *et al.* (2009) Cardiac dysfunction after renal transplantation: Incomplete resolution in pediatric population. *Transplantation* **16**, 1737–1745.

19. Jarzembowski T, John E, Panaro F, *et al.* (2004) Impact of non-compliance on outcome after pediatric kidney transplantation: An analysis in racial subgroups. *Pediatr Transplant* **8**, 367–371.

20. Van Hearn E, de Vries EE. (2009) Kidney transplantation and duration in children. *Pediatr Surg Int* **25**, 385–393.

19 Post-transplant diagnostic imaging

Lakshmi Ratnam and Uday Patel

Although transplant longevity constantly improves, the graft is prone to many hazards along the way to established renal function. Graft rejection or recurrence of the original renal disease may occur. For these, the contribution of imaging is limited. However, imaging can contribute valuable and at times crucial information for impairment that is the result of morphologic or anatomical abnormalities. Furthermore, some of these can be dealt with by percutaneous or angiographic intervention, under radiological guidance.

The causes of renal dysfunction are many, but regarding radiological evaluation it is helpful to consider them in two broad categories: early and delayed (Table 19.1). These can then be further split into immediate (<48 h post-transplant) and occurring up to 6 weeks post-transplant. Such categorisation helps in planning and choosing the best imaging modality.

Postoperative complications are said to occur in 12–20% after grafting [1], although this is a historical figure, and modern figures are likely to be lower (Table 19.2). Regardless of the frequency, early recognition and remedy are paramount. Imaging, whether functional or anatomical, can help. The following paragraphs illustrate the value of each modality in the evaluation of transplant dysfunction. Before this discussion, the unique radiological anatomy of the transplanted kidney is briefly reviewed, as this is often key to identifying causes of transplant dysfunction on imaging.

Radiological anatomy of the renal transplant

Modern practice is to place the graft in an extra-peritoneal pocket within either iliac fossa, but inverted. So the right kidney is preferentially placed in the left iliac fossa, and vice versa. Thus the anatomical relations of the kidney are also changed – unlike the native kidney the collecting system is the most anterior relation. This has a bearing on interventional

Handbook of Renal and Pancreatic Transplantation, First Edition. Edited by Iain A. M. MacPhee and Jiří Froněk.
© 2012 John Wiley & Sons, Ltd. Published 2012 by John Wiley & Sons, Ltd.

Table 19.1 Imaging and the various complications that may occur after renal transplantation.

Early (<6 weeks)	Late
Acute or hyperacute rejection	Chronic rejection
Acute tubular necrosis	

Collections:
  Urinoma
  Lymphocele
  Haematoma
  Abscess	

Ureteral necrosis/stenosis/obstruction	Ureteral stricture
Vascular thrombosis (venous or arterial)	
Early vascular obstruction (other than thrombosis) Operative factors (e.g. kinking of the vascular pedicle)	Renal artery stenosis
Post-biopsy haemorrhage, arterio-venous fistula or pseudoaneurysm)	

Table 19.2 Frequency of the various post-renal transplant complications*.

Arterial stenosis	Up to 10%
Arterio-venous fistula/pseudo-aneurysm	1–18%
Renal vein thrombosis	0.3–3%
Renal arterial thrombosis	0.2–3.5%
Ureteral obstruction	2–10%
Urinary leak	1–5%
Postoperative peri-renal collections	Up to 14%

*These are figures quoted in the literature, and some are historical.

practice, with the upper pole being a safer entry point for percutaneous renal access.

The transplanted artery is now most commonly attached to the external iliac artery. Internal iliac anastomosis is less favoured although still used by some surgeons for living donor kidneys. External iliac artery anastomosis is generally carried out onto the anterior wall of the artery, but the exact orientation of the anastomosis may vary. This can have a bearing on the ease of imaging evaluation or intervention. Accessory arteries may be anastomosed onto the main renal artery, internal iliac artery or the inferior epigastric artery. Rarely, an interpositioned venous or synthetic graft may be necessary if the artery is too short. Venous anastomosis is almost always an end-to-side match to the external iliac vein. Accessory or small veins are usually ligated. Ureteral anastomosis is onto the antero-superior bladder wall, and an attempt at anti-reflux mechanism is made by creating a transverse tunnel through the bladder wall. The perinephric tissues can become fibrotic post-transplant, and this can make percutaneous access for intervention more difficult.

Ultrasound

Ultrasound is the mainstay of imaging evaluation of the post-transplant kidney. It is readily available, can be used at the bedside, and does not involve a radiation dose or the use of nephrotoxic contrast. Serial ultrasounds should be performed until function is established in the transplant kidney.

Normal appearances

Grey-scale ultrasound
The superficial nature of transplant kidneys enables good visualisation and accurate anatomical assessment, specifically to assess morphology of the renal transplant, presence of collections and dilatation of the collecting system. In particular, the renal pyramids are much more clearly visualised than in native kidneys and are hypoechoic. These are distinguished from a dilated pelvicalyceal system by the fact that they do not communicate with each other.

Colour Doppler ultrasound (CDU)
The use of CDU enables assessment of the overall perfusion of the transplant kidney as well as interrogation of the transplant and iliac arteries and veins. A normal spectral Doppler flow within transplant arteries shows a 'ski-slope' waveform with diastolic flow forming at least a third of the peak systolic velocity (PSV).

A PSV value of 2.5 m/s is taken as the upper limit of normal, with values above this representing significant transplant renal artery stenosis. Resistive (RI) and pulsatility (PI) indices, markers of peripheral vascular resistance, can be assessed. Normal values for RI should be <0.8 and PI <1.5 (Fig. 19.1).

$$\text{Pulsatility index (PI)} = \frac{(\text{Peak systolic velocity} - \text{End diastolic velocity})}{\text{Time-averaged mean velocity}}$$

$$\text{Resistive Index (RI)} = \frac{(\text{Peak systolic velocity} - \text{End diastolic velocity})}{\text{Peak systolic velocity}}$$

The main transplant renal artery is often tortuous due to anatomical considerations at anastomosis. This can cause difficulty during ultrasound assessment, as acceleration of flow around bends in the artery can mimic increased flow due to stenosis. Flow in the main renal veins may also be pulsatile owing to transmitted pulsation from adjacent renal artery or reverse flow from the right atrium into the inferior vena cava. Techniques to optimise flow assessment include the use of power Doppler, low pulse repetition frequency (PRF)/scale, high gain and low filters.

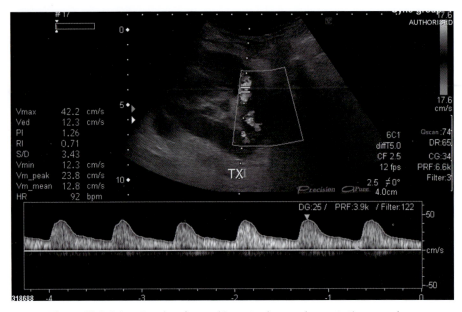

Figure 19.1 Colour Doppler of normal intra-renal artery demonstrating normal waveform.

Reversed or reduced diastolic flow

Causes of reversed or reduced diastolic flow are renal vein thrombosis or kinking, perinephric haematoma, severe acute tubular necrosis (ATN) (which can develop in hours) or severe acute rejection (which usually takes a few days).

Increased resistive or pulsatility index

Increased RI or PI can be caused by acute rejection or ATN, calcinuerin inhibitor toxicity, renal vein thrombosis, ureteric obstruction and infection [2]. Elevated RI at 3 months post-transplantation has been shown to have poor prognostic value with poor subsequent graft function and death [3,4].

Ultrasound evaluation of early complications

Acute rejection

Acute rejection may result in swelling of the kidney, causing it to have a more globular shape. Grey-scale ultrasound features include increased renal length and volume, increased corticomedullary differentiation and enlarged pyramids. Normal rate of growth of a healthy transplant kidney is approximately 0.1 cm/month in length [5].

Acute tubular necrosis

ATN is common in the early transplant period, with 10–30% of patients requiring dialysis during this time [4]. Ultrasound cannot differentiate between ATN and acute rejection. Renal biopsy is required for definitive diagnosis; colour Doppler is useful in monitoring clinical response.

Renal artery stenosis

Renal artery stenosis (RAS) ccurs in up to 10% of patients and may not be apparent clinically [6,7]. The majority of stenoses occur at or close to the surgical anastomosis. The clinical indications of a possible underlying RAS are hypertension resistant to standard therapy, deterioration in renal function, or reduced function after starting treatment with an angiotensin-converting enzyme inhibitor or angiotensin-II receptor blocker. Marked salt and water retention occasionally occurs. Predisposing factors are donor atherosclerosis and paediatric donor to adult patient.

The main renal artery should be assessed immediately downstream from the anastomosis. Increased velocity of greater than 2 m/s after angle correction with spectral broadening suggests significant stenosis (Fig. 19.2a). Within the intra-renal arteries, a tardus parvus waveform can be observed. A ratio of more than 2 for the PSV in the iliac artery compared with the PSV in the main renal artery also indicates a significant stenosis.

Renal artery thrombosis

Renal artery thrombosis is rare and usually occurs early. It can be asymptomatic. In a single vessel transplant, it is usually irreversible; in a multiple vessel transplant, a single vessel thrombosis may result in segmental infarction and preservation of function of the transplant. The use of ultrasound contrast can be useful in assessment of infarction.

Ultrasound findings are absent flow in the kidney and in the main renal artery. Confirmation of flow in the iliac vessels or other intra-abdominal vessels ensures this is a true finding rather than a result of technical factors.

Renal vein thrombosis

Renal vein thrombosis is more common than arterial thrombosis. It usually presents with acute pain and swelling and a drop in renal function and urine output, sometimes associated with visible haematuria. Early diagnosis and intervention may salvage the transplant.

Ultrasound findings are of thrombus in the main or intrarenal veins with dilatation of the renal vein, absent flow in the transplant vein and reversed/ absent (RI =1) diastolic flow in the main or intrarenal transplant artery. The absence of venous outflow causes high resistance to arterial inflow, resulting in raised RI values.

Ureteric complications

The ureter is the most vulnerable anastomosis post-transplant, as it has a precarious arterial supply. To overcome this vulnerability, the ureter is kept as short as possible; excessive dissection of the peri-ureteric fat is avoided to preserve small vessels, and the ureter is stented for up to 6 weeks post-transplant. Nevertheless, ureteric problems (ureteric necrosis,

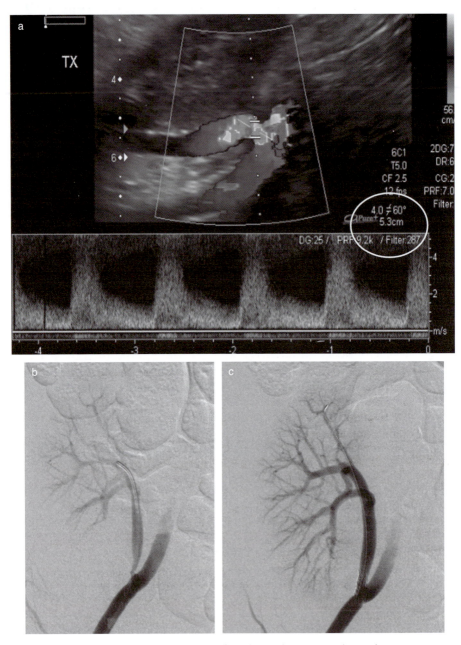

Figure 19.2 Montage of an example of renal transplant stenosis that underwent primary stent placement. (a) Doppler ultrasound images showing a suspected stenosis just above the anastamosis, with an elevated velocity measured at around 4m/s. (b) Angiogram confirming a tight stenosis, which has undergone stent placement with a good angiographic result (c). (A full colour version of this figure appears in the colour plate section.)

> **Box 19.1 Causes of ureteral obstruction in renal transplants.**
> * Ureteral ischaemia
> * Ureteral kinking
> * Previously unrecognised pelvi-ureteric junction obstruction
> * Extrinsic compression (lymphocele, urinoma, etc.)
> * Intrinsic obstruction (oedema, clot, tumour, calculus)
> * BK *Polyomavirus*

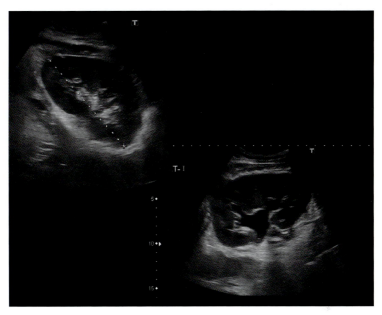

Figure 19.3 Ultrasound image of an initially undilated collecting system, which developed obstruction 2 weeks later.

leak and/or stricture) still occur in 3–6% of cases. In the early stage, ureteral necrosis/leak may be seen and later ureteric stricture can be a problem. Other causes of ureteral obstruction as listed in Box 19.1. Commonly the first sign is renal dysfunction or decreased urinary flow after the stent is removed, but a few cases present as late ureteric strictures.

Urinary obstruction

On ultrasound, renal dilatation and/or an urinoma are seen (Fig. 19.3). Renal dilatation is itself not always a sign of obstruction. It is common to see a mild degree of ureteric dilatation due to ureteral reflux and postoperative oedema. Raised RI and PIs may be present if there is external compression on the kidney, causing hydronephrosis. Although an attempt is made to create a non-refluxing ureteral anastomosis by creating an oblique tunnel, this is not always successful. Non-obstructive dilatation has also been described with acute rejection and ureteral oedema. If dilatation is seen with normal renal function/output the appearances should be kept under review or a MAG 3 study performed. Ureteral kinking is a rare cause of intermittent obstruction. Stones are said to occur in 1–2% of transplants. Other causes of ureteral obstruction are given below.

- Blood clot: post-biopsy or in the early post-transplant period, this may be due to blood clot in the pelvicalyceal system or bladder, which would be visible as echogenic debris within the system. Bladder irrigation may be all that is required to resolve this.
- Extrinsic compression: collection causing compression on the ureter.
- Ureteric stenosis: most commonly at the anastomotic site at the ureterovesical junction. Can be treated by balloon dilatation, ureteric stenting or surgical reanastomosis.
- Recently, BK polyomavirus infection has emerged as a factor in ureteric complications.

Urine leak

Urine leak may be due to breakdown of the ureterovesical anastomosis or ureteral necrosis. Clinical presentation may be with decreased urine output, urine leaking from the wound and abdominal pain. Occurs in up to 6% of patients [4]. Nephrostomy insertion is often used as a temporising measure and definitive treatment is usually surgical. Ultrasound may show a new collection.

Perinephric collections

Perinephric collections are usually seen in the first few weeks (Fig. 19.4).

- Haematoma – small haematomas are common and usually of no clinical significance. They appear as hypoechoic collections but may contain septae or debris within. A large haematoma can cause compression of the kidney, resulting in obstruction of the pelvicalyceal system or a Page kidney. If significant, percutaneous drainage is usually easily achieved.
- Abscess – uncommon. Usually results from an infected hematoma. If clinical indications suggest an infection, aspiration followed by drainage if infection is confirmed can be performed under ultrasound guidance.
- Urinoma – usually the result of a urine leak. This occurs most commonly at the ureterovesical anastomosis and therefore the collection is likely to be seen adjacent to the bladder. Occasionally urine can be seen to leak into the peritoneal cavity. If fluid is seen in the peritoneal cavity, this may be residual peritoneal dialysis fluid (confirm by the clinical history).
- Lymphocele – seen slightly later, several weeks after surgery. May be the result of damage to the lymphatics during surgery or incomplete dissection of the lymphatics in the peritoneal cavity. As with haematomas, these are usually of no consequence, in which case no treatment is required. When sufficiently large, although easily amenable to percutaneous drainage, this is often insufficient and carries a high

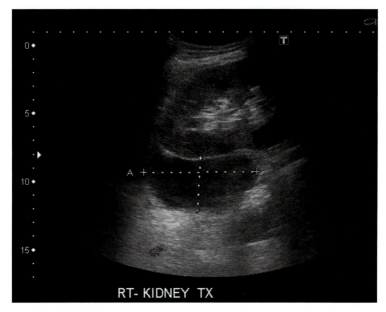

Figure 19.4 Ultrasound of a collection deep to the upper pole of a transplant kidney, which is not causing any hydronephrosis.

risk of introducing infection. Often definitive treatment requires surgical marsupialisation (see Chapter 22).

Infection

Infections usually have no signs on ultrasound. However, a focal hypoechoic area of pyelonephritis is sometimes seen with increased flow within. RIs and PIs can be raised. Occasionally, echogenic foci of fungal balls may be seen in the collecting system.

Drug toxicity

Drug toxicity has no effect on RI or PI. It is usually diagnosed by blood concentrations of drugs and/ or renal biopsy. Occasionally reduced blood flow is seen, but ultrasound is usually unhelpful.

Ultrasound evaluation of late complications

- Chronic rejection and drug toxicity – ultrasound cannot distinguish between rejection and toxicity from immunosuppressants. Previous episodes of acute rejection are the most consistent predisposing factors. Features of both include increased cortical echogenicity, raised RIs, prominent pyramids and loss of corticomedullary differentiation [8]. If there is clinical doubt, a biopsy must be performed for confirmation.
- Effects of primary disease – such as diabetes or glomerulonephritis.
- Causes of late complications cannot be distinguished on ultrasound. A failing kidney may shrink and become echogenic; however, a poorly

functioning kidney can continue to have normal ultrasound
appearance.

- Tumours – most common malignancies are skin related, cervical cancer
  and non-Hodgkin lymphoma. Tumours of the kidney itself are usually
  renal cell carcinomas, but there is an increased risk of lymphoma
  compared to native kidneys, presumed to be due to the
  immunosupression [9].
- Ureteric obstruction – late occurrence of ureteric obstruction from
  fibrosis at the ureterovesical junction or renal calculi can be detected on
  surveillance.
- Malignancy in native kidneys – acquired cystic disease in native kidneys
  following transplantation carries a small risk (1% lifetime risk) of
  increased malignancy [10].

Ultrasound-guided renal biopsy

There is easy access for ultrasound-guided renal biopsy, as the kidney lies
superficially. The biopsy site should either be marked with ultrasound or
preferably performed under direct ultrasound guidance. Relatively low
risk with complications requiring intervention or pain requiring opiate
analgesia in <5% [4]. (A detailed account of renal transplant biopsy
technique is provided in Chapter 22.)

Post-biopsy complications

- Pseudoaneurysm (PSA)
  - CDU demonstrates a typical swirling flow pattern within a cystic
    structure. Spectral waveforms have a characteristic 'to and fro' flow
    pattern.
- Arteriovenous fistula
  - Ultrasound findings are of an intense focus of fast turbulent flow,
    seen as a persistent multicoloured focus. The supplying artery and
    draining vein can sometimes be identified if sufficiently large.
    Spectral analysis shows high velocity, low-resistance flow in the
    supplying artery and highly pulsatile flow in the draining vein due to
    arterialisation of the vein. PI or RI ratio may be normal or reduced
    compared with surrounding vessels. Most arteriovenous fistulae and
    pseudoaneurysms resolve spontaneously and do not require
    treatment. The majority are asymptomatic, or transient haematuria
    may be seen. Intervention would only be required if there is active
    bleeding or sufficiently large to be producing a 'steal syndrome' from
    the kidney.
- Haemorrhage
  - Significant haemorrhage may require embolisation (see the section on
    catheter angiography below).

Future developments

The use of ultrasound contrast agents can be useful in the assessment of
renal perfusion. These agents are not nephrotoxic and are safe for use in
renal transplants. They are potentially useful in differentiating renal

artery stenosis from kinking and are able to provide qualitative and quantitative information about cortical capillary blood flow [6]. Elastography may have a role in assessment of focal and diffuse pathological processes in the transplant kidney but is yet to be validated.

Nuclear medicine

Of all the imaging modalities, nuclear medicine (NM) is the only one that allows ready functional evaluation of the transplant kidney [11]. Functional assessment based on computerised tomography (CT) and magnetic resonance imaging (MRI) is possible but technically more difficult. Radioactive tracers can be used to study the uptake (a direct correlate of the vascular inflow of the kidney and functional renal units) and also its excretory ability, and whether once excreted the tracer reaches the bladder promptly or not.

The usual indications for transplant renography are assessment of transplant dysfunction immediately, or soon after surgery. Of the renal-specific nuclear medicine studies, 99mTc-MAG is now favoured, as it can provide a 'one-stop' evaluation of renal perfusion, parenchymal uptake and excretion. Marked global decrease in perfusion will be seen with arterial occlusion, but lesser similar changes may also be seen with acute rejection, ATN, ureteric obstruction (Fig. 19.5) or compression of the kidney by collections, such as a lymphocele. Focal defects may be seen secondary to thrombosis of a branch or accessory artery. Global persistent retention of tracer within the parenchyma is a hallmark of acute tubular necrosis whilst focal absence of uptake is seen with focal infarcts. These are subjective assessments, but can be semi-quantified as a perfusion index although they are not in universal use.

Later images will evaluate excretion into the collecting system and highlight either ureteral stenosis (delayed bladder concentration with a dilated collecting system) or ureteral necrosis, in which case tracer will be seen to pool outside the ureter. It should be also be understood that with nuclear medicine studies changes on longitudinal studies are sometimes more informative, and equivocal findings warrant repeat studies. The value of nuclear medicine after the immediate transplant phase is now limited, having been usurped by the other imaging modalities, especially ultrasound. Its use with chronic rejection is also now limited. Lastly, NM has limited anatomical information. So, for example global poor perfusion may be diagnosed, but the location of the obstruction, if any, is not revealed. Most NM abnormalities will require further radiological, anatomical evaluation.

Computerised tomography

The role of CT in post-renal transplantation imaging is limited. In using CT, there is a radiation dose involved and usually a requirement for

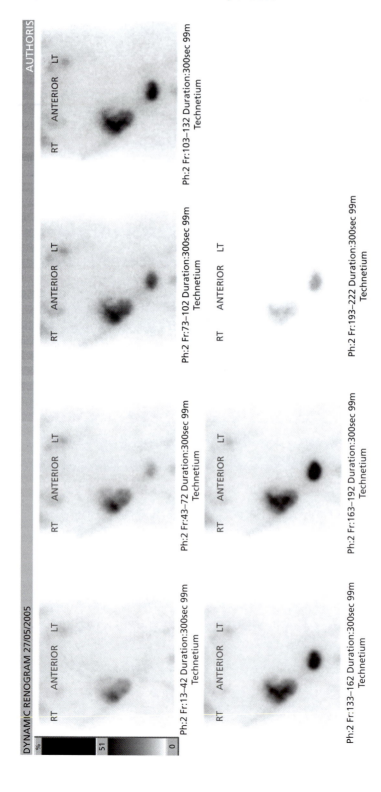

Figure 19.5 MAG 3 renogram of an obstructed kidney showing progressive concentration of tracer within the collecting system and no tracer activity within the ureter.

intravenous contrast, which can be nephrotoxic. CT is usually reserved for cases in which ultrasound imaging is inadequate or inconclusive. A standard CT examination would require injection of 100 mL of intravenous contrast, followed by a scan in the arterial phase (assess transplant and iliac vessels), venous phase (assess for parenchymal masses) and a delayed excretory scan (to assess the collecting system) [12]. The use of multi-slice CT also gives the capability of reformatting images in the coronal and sagittal planes, which can be very useful in the assessment of transplant vasculature and pyeloureteral structures, especially where they are tortuous.

Where there are complex collections, the anatomical delineation by CT is superior to that of ultrasound, both in defining the collection itself and it outlining its relationship to adjacent structures. This is particularly useful in obese patients. Once identified, CT can also be used for guidance if drainage is required. The presence of high attenuation in a hematoma can signify acute haemorrhage in a non-contrast CT, and active extravasation of contrast demonstrates ongoing haemorrhage. The presence of gas within a collection in a patient with clinical markers of infection is consistent with abscess formation. Focal, low-attenuation collections within the renal parenchyma are seen in focal pyelonephritis.

Although conventional digital subtraction angiography remains the gold standard for assessment of renal artery stenosis, CT angiography (CTA) is a useful non-invasive tool to visualise the vasculature. CTA is more accurate than ultrasound and is less prone to artefact from surgical clips than magnetic resonance angiography (MRA) [12]. Renal vein thrombosis is also demonstrable on CT. Where ultrasound does not clearly demonstrate an arteriovenous fistula or a pseudoaneurysm, the filling of these structures during arterial phase of CT acquisition confirms their nature and will outline the size clearly.

Renal graft torsion can be an early or late complication. Changes include altered axis of the transplant and vascular pedicle kinking, or secondary changes such as swelling or abnormal graft enhancement, hydronephrosis and sinus and peri-renal fat infiltration [12]. Where malignancy is detected, CT is useful both for confirming the primary tumour and for staging.

Magnetic resonance imaging and angiography

MRI is not ideally suited for transplant evaluation. In the early period, concerns about movement of surgical clips is a contraindication, and in all stages the recently recognised dangers of gadolinium-induced nephrogenic systemic fibrosis will be a concern, such that an estimated glomerular filtration (eGFR) <30 mL/min would be taken as an absolute contraindication [13] for contrast injection. For these reasons, its use is limited to evaluation of suspected vascular stenosis in the later transplant phase.

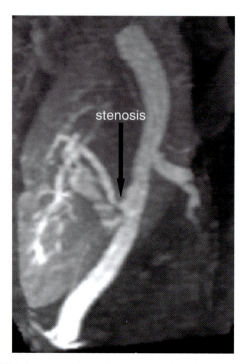

Figure 19.6 MRA demonstrating renal artery stenosis at the origin of the transplant renal artery.

If gadolinium-based contrast injection is feasible, then standard post-contrast MRI with 3D evaluation has a high accuracy for the identification of renal artery stenosis [14]. It can be used to confirm stenosis suspected either clinically or on an initial Doppler ultrasound (Fig. 19.6). It is of particular value in those with a borderline suspicion of stenosis on clinical grounds or after Doppler ultrasound. Regarding its accuracy, no firm comment is possible at the moment, as it has not yet been adequately investigated. Initial studies are promising, but its accuracy cannot be assumed to be perfect, and suspected stenosis should be confirmed with catheter angiography. More recently MRI without contrast has shown initial promise [15], and also requires further investigation; but if confirmed would increase the number of patients suitable for MRA.

Catheter angiography

Renal transplant angiography has been an established technique since the early 1960s. It has since been refined, with a higher safety margin; however, the indications have considerably narrowed. Originally it was the only method for intimate interrogation of the status and health of the transplant artery. Now its use is much more selective, as prior non-invasive investigations will select out a high-risk group.

Box 19.2 Indications for catheter angiography.
- Arterial thrombosis
- Venous thrombosis
- Arterial stenosis or kinking
- Venous stenosis
- Arteriovenous fistula
- Post-biopsy haemorrhage

Investigations such as Doppler ultrasound, CT or MRA will identify those with a high likelihood of arterial disease, and angiography is reserved as a second-line confirmatory investigation, and to plan and undertake endovascular therapy. The current indications for catheter angiography are given in Box 19.2. Iodinated contrast media are potentially nephrotoxic. The mechanism of renal toxicity has not yet been determined, and of the many attempts at reno-protection, only simple hydration has proven to be of benefit in studies. The current status has been reviewed [16] and recommendations can be viewed on the web site of the European Society of Urogenital Radiology (www.esur.org). Some patients are allergic to iodinated contrast media, in which case carbon dioxide can be used as a negative contrast medium, although the images are not as good.

Vascular thrombosis

Immediately post-transplant there is a small risk of either arterial or venous thrombosis. Reported incidence varies widely between 0.5 and 6.2%. Venous thrombosis is more common but it may be also associated with hyperacute rejection. Diagnosis is suggested by ultrasound, CT or MRI and confirmed if necessary by catheter venography. Treatment is surgical thrombectomy, but occasionally acute thrombolysis may be performed. There are only case reports of acute venous thrombolysis, with variable success and methods. Either intra-arterial injection of thrombolytic agents is performed or a catheter is advanced into the transplant vein for direct venous thrombolysis, enabling treatment of associated iliac vein thrombus also. Thrombolysis is usually chemical, but mechanical thrombectomy devices may be used. Some have suggested that a temporary inferior vena cava filter should be inserted when performing chemical thrombolysis, especially if there is a large volume of associated ilio-femoral thrombosis. Whichever method is used, success is not assured and surgery should not be delayed.

Surgical correction is usually performed for renal artery thrombosis. Successful catheter thrombolysis has occasionally been reported but is relatively hazardous, as arterial thrombosis usually occurs immediately post-transplant with risk of anastomotic haemorrhage.

Post-biopsy haemorrhage

The reported prevalence of post-biopsy haematuria is wide (0.06–13%) [1]. Most settle with expectant management. Persistent bleeding or that associated with haemodynamic upset is an indication for angiography and embolotherapy. Occasionally a large sub-capsular bleed may compress the kidney, resulting in the 'Page' phenomenon; in which case the blood pressure may be deceptively high. Prior ultrasound or CT may help to identify a post-biopsy arteriovenous fistula or pseudoaneurysm as the cause. On angiography, either of these will be readily seen, and immediate embolisation can be performed. This has a high success rate and is now the preferred option. However, studies have shown that most pseudoaneurysms will resolve without intervention (up to 70%) and embolisation should be reserved for those with severe or persistent bleeding, as even the most selective embolisation inevitably leads to some nephron loss.

Renal transplant artery stenosis

Suspected arterial stenosis is the most frequent indication for catheter angiography. In modern practice Doppler ultrasound (or CTA or MRA) will have raised a suspicion of stenosis, and thus the pre-test probability should be high. Nevertheless, it is common practice to not only confirm the stenosis on angiography, but also to grade its functional significance by measuring the pressure gradient across the narrowing. A greater than 10% drop in systolic pressure (or >10 mmHg) is taken as the threshold for intervention, and it is now the practice to follow with immediate angioplasty and/or stent insertion. Visible stenosis but without a pressure gradient would be considered non-flow limiting and does not require treatment. The stenosis is usually at the anastomosis, for a length of about 1 cm. Occasionally it may be long or in one of the branch arteries. Kinks may or may not be associated with a flow-limiting stenosis, and pressure measurement will solve the issue [17].

The cause of transplant renal artery stenosis is still unresolved, and some follow-up studies have suggested that they may be progressive in all cases but they can be sometimes very resistant to simple balloon dilatation (implying a significant fibrotic element), and increasingly primary stent insertion is chosen. However, the superiority of stenting over angioplasty has not been proven. The success of angioplasty or stenting is in the range 85–93% [18]; but restenosis (which can be within the stent) can occur in 5–30% [1], in which case repeat endovascular treatment can be performed. The occasional case may fail endovascular therapy and surgical correction will be necessary. Serious complications are seen in up to 4% of cases after angioplasty or stenting, of which the most feared is arterial rupture. Thus, the procedure is only performed if facilities for operative repair are immediately available within the hospital.

Antegrade pyelography, nephrostomy and antegrade ureteric stenting

Nephrostomy is the favoured immediate treatment for obstruction or a ureteric leak, as the transplant ureter is not easily stented by the retrograde route. The overall technical success rate of ultrasound or fluoroscopically guided nephrostomy is >97%, with a serious complication rate of 1–4% (major haemorrhage, septic shock, visceral injury) [19]. Technical success is lower in non-dilated kidneys, and possibly the complication rates may be higher. Performance figures for transplant nephrostomy are believed to be similar. Once the renal function has improved after nephrostomy insertion, any ureteric strictures may be treated by fluoroscopically guided dilatation or a stent may be inserted as definitive therapy, or prior to definitive surgical correction. Stents may also bypass a ureteral leak to allow natural healing.

Ureteric leaks occur in 1–5% due to ischaemia, necrosis or post-biopsy injury of the calyces/renal pelvis. With the use of stents post-transplant, they become clinically evident after stent removal. Decreased urine output is noted and on ultrasound a collection is seen. Aspiration of the collection will reveal a high creatinine content. Percutaneous treatment is external diversion with a nephrostomy, which has a reported success rate of 63–83% [17]. Once clinically stable, an antegrade ureteral stent may be inserted to await healing. The success rate of percutaneous balloon dilatation of strictures of the transplant ureter is around 73–100% in the early stage, but falls to 16–33% with late (>3 months) stricturing [1,19,20]. If dilatation is unsuccessful, and surgical revision is not an option, long-term stenting can be chosen. Plastic ureteral stents are exchanged every 6 months or a metal stent is inserted. Metal stents (Fig. 19.7a–b) are more durable, but some will obstruct due to urothelial hyperplasia and patients should be maintained on regular surveillance.

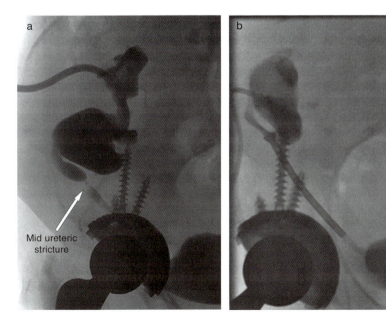

Figure 19.7 (a) Tight mid-ureteric stricture. (b) A metal stent has been placed, with good drainage seen.

References

1. Kobayashi K, Censullo ML, Rossman LL, *et al.* (2007) Interventional radiologic management of renal transplant dysfunction: Indications, limitations, and technical considerations. *Radiographics* **27**, 1109–1113.

2. Zimmerman P, Ragevendra N, Schiepers C. (2005) Diagnostic imaging in kidney transplantation. In: Danovitch GM (ed), *Handbook of Kidney Transplantation*, 4th edn, pp. 347–368. Lippincott Williams & Wilkins, Philadelphia.

3. Saracino A, Santarsia G, Latorraca A, *et al.* (2006) Early assessment of renal resistance index after kidney transplant can help predict long-term renal function. *Nephrol Dial Transplant* **21**, 2916.

4. Baxter GM. (2001) Ultrasound of renal transplantation. *Clin Rad* **56**, 802–818.

5. Lachance SL, Adamson D, Barry JM. (1988) Ultrasonically determined kidney transplant hypertrophy. *J Urol* **139**, 497.

6. Jimenez C, Lopez MO, Gonzalez E, *et al.* (2009) Ultrasonography in kidney transplantation: Values and new developments. *Transplantation Reviews* **23**, 1209–1213.

7. Fervenza FC, Lafayette RA, Alfrey EJ, *et al.* (1998) Renal artery stenosis in kidney transplants. *Am J Kidney Dis* **31**, 142–148.

8. Cosgrove DO, Chan KE. (2008) Renal transplants. What ultrasound can and cannot do. *Ultrasound Quarterly* **24**, 77–87.

9. Baccarani U, Adani GL, Montanaro D, *et al.* (2006) De novo malignancies after kidney and liver transplantations: Experience on 582 consecutive cases. *Transplant Proc* **38**, 1135.

10. Schwarz A, Vatandaslar S, Merkel S, *et al.* (2007) Renal cell carcinoma in transplant recipients with acquired cystic kidney disease. *Clin J Am Soc Nephrol* **2**, 750.

11. Jamar F, Barone R. (2005) Renal Imaging. In: Baert AL, Schiepers C (eds), *Diagnostic Nuclear Medicine*, 2nd edn, pp 83–100. Springer, London.

12. Sebastia C, Quiroga S, Boye R, *et al.* (2001) Helical CT in renal transplantation: Normal findings and early and late complications. *Radiographics* **21**, 1103–1117.

13. Royal College of Radiologists. (2007) *Gadolinium-based Contrast Media and Nephrogenic Systemic Fibrosis*. Available online from: www.rcr.ac.uk/docs/radiology/pdf/BFCR0714_Gadolinium_NSF_guidanceNOV07.pdf.

14. Hohenwalter MD, Skowlund CJ, Erickson SJ, *et al.* (2001) Renal transplant evaluation with MR angiography and MR imaging. *Radiographics* **21**, 1505–1517.

15. Liu X, Berg N, Sheehan J, *et al.* (2009) Renal transplant: Nonenhanced renal MR angiography with magnetization-prepared steady-state free precession. *Radiology* **251**, 535–542.

16. Solomon R. (2009) Contrast-induced acute kidney injury (CIAKI). *Radiol Clin North Am* **47**, 783–788.

17. Chua GC, Snowden S, Patel U. (2004) Kinks of the transplant renal artery without accompanying intraarterial pressure gradient do not require correction: Five-year outcome study. *Cardiovasc Intervent Radiol* **27**, 643–650.

18. Beecroft JR, Rajan DK, Clark TW, *et al.* (2004) Transplant renal artery stenosis: Outcome after percutaneous intervention. *J Vasc Interv Radiol* **15**, 1407–1413.

19. Ramchandani P, Cardella JF, Grassi CJ, *et al.* (2001) SCVIR Standards of Practice Committee Quality improvement guidelines for percutaneous nephrostomy. *J Vasc Interv Radiol* **12**, 1247–1251.
20. Juaneda B, Alcaraz A, Bujons A, *et al.* (2005) Endourological management is better in early-onset ureteral stenosis in kidney transplantation. *Transplant Proc* **37**, 3825–3827.

20 Transplant histopathology

Eva Honsová

Kidney

Introduction

The histological changes of rejection with mononuclear cell infiltration
of the graft were recognised very early on in the history of
transplantation. Antibodies are not seen in routine histological staining,
and antibody-mediated injury needed more complicated interpretation of
clinical laboratory and histological data. As a consequence, the cellular
theory dominated transplant medicine for almost 40 years, with therapy
concentrated on the suppression of T-lymphocyte-mediated rejection. As
data on the pathophysiologal and morphological changes of rejection
were generated, different centres were developing their own protocols and
their own definitions of the morphological features. The need for
internationally recognised standard definitions was identified as critical to
progress in this area. The first working meeting dealing with the
international standardisation of the nomenclature and criteria to be used
in the histological diagnosis of renal allograft rejection was held in Banff,
Canada in 1991. A group of nephropathologists, nephrologists and
transplant surgeons developed the first Banff standardised classification
of kidney transplant pathology. Their goal was to create a basis for
international uniformity in the reporting of the renal allograft pathology
and to devise a schema in which a given biopsy grading would imply
prognosis for a therapeutic response, which would ultimately lead to
improved management and treatment. The schema underwent
considerable evolution, and was repeatedly revised and modified in
follow-up meetings held every 2 years. The current Banff classification is
shown in Box 20.1 [1].

   Because of the large number of conditions that can affect the allograft,
sometimes in combination, renal biopsy provides critical information
enabling diagnosis, and leads to improvement in management and care
of renal transplant recipients. In one prospective clinical trial, the
pre-biopsy clinical diagnosis differed from the final diagnosis in 42% of
episodes of graft dysfunction, and the biopsy result often led to a
significant change in the clinical management [2].

Handbook of Renal and Pancreatic Transplantation, First Edition. Edited by
Iain A. M. MacPhee and Jiří Froněk.
© 2012 John Wiley & Sons, Ltd. Published 2012 by John Wiley & Sons, Ltd.

Box 20.1 The Banff Classification Scheme, 2007 update.
1. Normal
2. Antibody-mediated changes (may coincide with categories 3,4, 5, and 6) due to documentation of circulating anti-donor antibody, C4d, and allograft pathology
   Acute antibody-mediated rejection
   Chronic active antibody-mediated rejection
3. Borderline changes: suspicious for acute T-cell-mediated rejection (may coincide with categories 2, 5 and 6).
4. T-cell-mediated rejection (TCMR; may coincide with categories 2 and 5)
   Acute T-cell-mediated rejection (type/grade)
   IA: Significant interstitial inflammation and foci of moderate tubulitis
   IB: Significant interstitial inflammation and foci of severe tubulitis
   IIA: Mild to moderate intimal arteritis
   IIB: Severe intimal arteritis (comprising 25% of the luminal area)
   III: Transmural arteritis
   Chronic active T-cell-mediated rejection; 'chronic allograft arteriopathy' (arterial intimal fibrosis with mononuclear cell infiltration in fibrosis, formation of neointima)
5. Interstitial fibrosis and tubular atrophy, no evidence of any specific etiology (grade)
   I: Mild IF/TA (<25% of cortical area)
   II: Moderate IF/TA (26–50% of cortical area)
   III: Severe IF/TA (>50% of cortical area)
   IV: Other: changes not considered to be due to acute or chronic rejection

Handling of the renal transplant biopsy

The morphological features of rejection are focal in the early stages. Adequacy of the biopsy sample is therefore the first step in achieving a reliable diagnostic conclusion. According to the Banff criteria, an adequate light microscopy sample should contain 10 glomeruli and at least two interlobular arteries. It is important for the clinician to realise that the renal cortex represents a system of hollow structures (mainly tubules and vessels), and that any pressure on the unfixed tissue can cause irreversible changes, which can limit the possibility of diagnostic conclusions. Ideally, clinicians send two biopsy cores, which should by divided into samples for light microscopy and immunofluorescence (IF) or immunohistochemistry (IH), the largest proportion to be used for light microscopy examination. We routinely prepare eight slides comprising 28 tissue sections (2 to 3 μm thick), stained with haematoxylin and eosin (H&E), periodic acid Schiff (PAS), Sirius red with elastine, acid fuschin orange G (AFOG) and periodic sciff-methenamine (PASM). For IF/IH microscopy we cut off a part of the cortex. C4d is performed in all cases; IgG, IgA, IgM, C3, kappa, and lambda light chains are performed in cases with suspected glomerulonephritis/glomerulopathy (GN; that is cases with clinical evidence of proteinuria and/or haematuria), and in all cases 1 year or more after transplantation. Electron microscopy (EM) is required in cases of suspected GN or in situation where capillary remodelling (glomeruli or peritubular capillaries) should be evaluated (antibody-mediated rejection). Some centres recommend performing EM in all cases more than half a year after transplantation.

Donor organ and implantation biopsies

Almost all transplants have some pre-existing clinically undetected damage, most frequently arterionephrosclerosis of varying degrees. Although we can evaluate the number of sclerotic glomeruli and quantify the extent of interstitial fibrosis and the severity of the arterial and arteriolar luminal narrowing due to transfer of arterionephrosclerosis, the histopathologist's role in donor organ evaluation is limited. The process of arterionephrosclerosis is always focal with fibrotic scars under a capsule, which alternates with normal tissue. There is no study with conclusive criteria for glomerular, interstitial and arterial sclerosis beyond which a donor organ must not be used. However, implantation biopsies provide important data for subsequent comparative evaluation during the post-transplantation period.

Ischaemia-reperfusion injury

'Delayed graft function' is a clinical term describing a situation in which dialysis is required early after graft implantation, whereas the term 'primary non-function' is used when a graft has never produced urine. The main cause of delayed graft function is represented by ischaemia-reperfusion injury, which is related to the ischemia time and predisposing donor factors. The histological changes are similar to so-called acute tubular injury (formerly acute tubular necrosis) and include flattening of the epithelial cells, tubular dilatation, loss of the apical tubular brush border, and intratubular debris (Fig. 20.1). The average reported duration of delayed graft function was 10 to 15 days, and approximately 95–98% of the grafts functionally recovered [3].

Banff classification

The key structures that determine the fate of a graft are the vessels – mainly arteries. There are no collateral vessels in the kidney and, as a consequence, each occlusion or severe narrowing of the arterial lumen leads to ischaemic changes in the interstitial tissue, because the interstitium is supplied from vasa efferentia that start in the glomerular hilum.

According to the Banff classification, two main categories of rejection changes can cause kidney graft dysfunction: T-cell-mediated and antibody-mediated rejection. Both can be divided into acute or

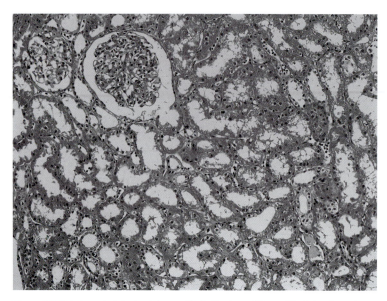

Figure 20.1 Ischaemic tubular injury with flattening of the epithelial cells and tubular dilatation (H&E). (A full colour version of this figure appears in the colour plate section.)

chronic processes. It is important to realise that the Banff classification we have been using is an evolving concept. In general, and also in graft tissues, the pathophysiological mechanisms of all parts of the immune system always work in cooperation, not only among components of the innate and adaptive immune response, but also between B and T cells. Therefore, strict discrimination between cell-mediated and antibody-mediated injury would not be appropriate. The terms 'acute' and 'chronic', which respect the clinical point of view on the cause of dysfunction, are rarely separate entities. There is a process of continuously developing changes in a complex situation in which previous diseases, transfer of vascular changes, residual changes after episodes of rejection, the influence of immunosuppressive drugs, etc. play a role. A good example of cooperation of various parts of the immune system represents so-called transplant arteriopathy (TA, rejection-induced changes, see below). TA, classified as mediated by T cells or antibodies, is characterised by progressive intimal sclerosis with narrowing of arterial lumina. Several authors showed that the development of TA requires a Th1 'cellular' response, which is dependent on presence of interferon-γ (INF-©). Animals with congenital absence or with antibody blockade of INF-© do not develop TA. INF-© secreted by T-cells and/or natural killer (NK) cells causes induction of class I and II antigens on endothelium, leading to increased binding of HLA antibody with antibody-mediated damage contributing to the inflammatory process.

Category 1: Normal
Normal morphology is sometimes seen in protocol biopsy samples.

Category 2: Antibody-mediated changes
It had been known from the beginning of the transplantation era that antibodies can mediate very severe graft injury in a process called hyperacute rejection (HR). This type of rejection can occur immediately after transplantation, sometimes during the operation when the clips on the vessels are removed and reperfusion starts. HR was observed when the kidney was transplanted into a recipient with pre-existing donor-specific antibodies (DSAs), and it can also be caused by antibodies against allogeneic blood groups A and B. HR is now rare due to careful pre-operative identification of potential DSA. HR is no longer included in the Banff classification. Although it is extremely rare it does still occur occasionally owing to the presence of anti-endothelial antibodies that are not detected by conventional approaches to antibody screening.

Light microscopic findings
The morphology of HR represents severe endothelial injury, which is followed by massive thrombosis of the blood vessels.

In the past two decades, several landmark observations enabled the definition of diagnostic criteria for antibody-mediated rejection (AMR). Halloran *et al.* identified acute kidney rejection associated with *de novo* anti-DSA production as a clinico-pathological entity with poor prognosis [4]. Secondly, Feucht *et al.* studied complement components and recognised the relationship of C4d deposition in peritubular capillaries (PTCs) in kidney grafts to graft dysfunction in recipients with high levels of panel-reactive antibodies (anti-HLA antibody) [5]. Feucht's observation represented a breakthrough and a great improvement in diagnosis of AMR. The rationale for the selection of C4d as a marker for AMR comes from its position in the complement cascade. The classical pathway of complement cascades is activated by antibodies and during this process C4 splits into several fragments – C4d is a terminal inactive split product. It is an attractive marker for detection, because it does not break spontaneously and is covalently bound in tissues. Positive C4d staining in PTC is a marker of AMR and provides evidence of a complement-fixing antibody bound to the endothelium. C4d can be detected by IF using commercially available monoclonal antibody (Fig. 20.2) and/or by IH. However, for IH only polyclonal antibody is available and formalin fixation and paraffin embedding result in decreasing sensitivity (Fig. 20.3).

Acute antibody-mediated rejection
Acute AMR can occur at any time after transplantation (from days to years), and has been observed in conjunction with all of the

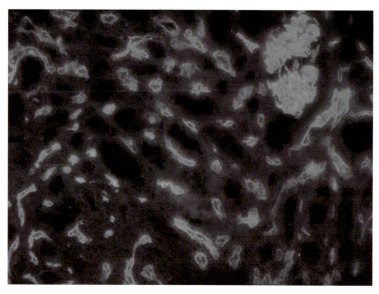

Figure 20.2 Diffuse positive staining of C4d along the peritubular capillaries (green) in immunofluorescence. (A full colour version of this figure appears in the colour plate section.)

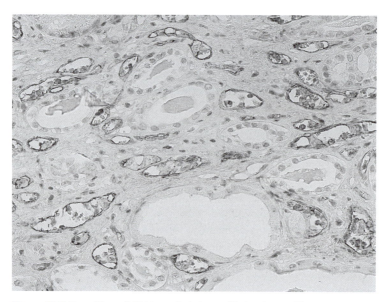

Figure 20.3 Deposition of C4d in peritubular capillaries detected by immunoperoxidase staining (brown) from paraffin-embedded tissue. (A full colour version of this figure appears in the colour plate section.)

immunosuppressive protocols that are currently used, even with depl
induction therapy. Antibodies to donor HLA class I or II antigens ar
present in 85–95% of patients with graft dysfunction and C4d-positive
PTC.

Light microscopic findings
Morphological features of AMR are non-specific and sometimes
unrecognisable without C4d staining. Early after transplantation the main
morphological findings can be features of acute tubular injury with
flattening of the epithelial cells, dilatation of PTC with leucocytes in their
lumina, and glomerulitis (mononuclear cells within the glomerular
capillary loops). More severe cases show endothelial injury followed by
thrombosis in the small vessels and features of thrombotic
microangiopathy (TMA). Severe cases of acute AMR overlap completely
with HR, including transmural arteritis with smooth muscle necrosis.
According to the Banff criteria, positive staining for C4d should be
bright, linear and diffuse (in >50% of PTC, excluding areas of interstitial
fibrosis). Our knowledge about the significance of focal C4d staining is
limited, and no guidelines exist for reporting weak staining or bright
staining in less than 50% PTC.

Differential diagnosis
Because C4d is only very rarely detected in the PTC in native kidney
biopsy samples, such as exceptional cases of systemic lupus
erythematosus, positive staining can be regarded as specific for 'transplant
antibody-mediated reaction'.

Chronic active antibody-mediated rejection
During the past 5 years evidence has been accumulating that anti-HLA
antibodies play a significant role in the pathogenesis of slowly progressive
graft damage and dysfunction. Several studies have reported that *de novo*
HLA class I and II antibodies represent a risk factor for premature graft
loss [6,7]. In 2005 the Banff consensus conference accepted chronic active
AMR as a distinct entity [8]. The diagnostic criteria combine morphology
(arterial intimal fibrosis without elastosis, duplication of glomerular
basement membrane (GBM), multi-laminated PTC basement membrane,
interstitial fibrosis), serology (anti-HLA or other anti-donor antibody),
and immunopathology (C4d in PTC). Colvin and his group proposed a
four-stage theory of the development of chronic AMR: 1) antibodies are
produced and bind to endothelium, 2) C4d is deposited in PTCs, 3) other
morphological signs of tissue injury occur, 4) finally graft dysfunction
appears [9].

Light microscopic findings
Histological features of graft injury are damage to endothelial cells with
tissue reaction to this injury. Long/term or repeated endothelial injury
leads to reduplication of GBMs, so-called transplant glomerulopathy. In
PTC, the basement membrane shows splitting. Intimal thickening and

luminal space reduction is a marker for very serious damage of arteries. This injury triggers a vicious circle combining rejection and ischaemic changes with progression to graft dysfunction and graft loss.

Category 3: Borderline changes

Biopsies with histopathological alterations insufficient for a firm diagnosis of acute T-cell-mediated rejection are regarded as showing borderline changes, and the decision as to whether such cases should be treated is based on clinical considerations.

Category 4: T-cell-mediated rejection
Acute T-cell-mediated rejection (acute cellular rejection)

Acute T-cell-mediated rejection (aTCMR) develops most commonly in the first several weeks after transplantation. The frequency of aTCMR episodes declines after the first 3 months, but it can occur at any time, especially when immunosuppression is inadequate.

Light microscopic findings and classification of aTCMR

In the Banff classification, tubulitis and intimal arteritis are lesions typical of aTCMR. Tubulitis (Fig. 20.4) is defined by the presence of mononuclear cells in non-atrophic tubules, whereas arteritis (Fig. 20.5) is diagnosed when mononuclear cells undermine the endothelial cells in the arterial intima ('endothelialitis' is a synonym for 'intimal arteritis'). TCMR has pleomorphic interstitial infiltrate of mononuclear cells, almost exclusively activated T cells (CD3-, CD4- and CD8-positive) and

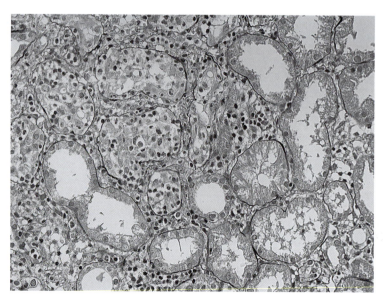

Figure 20.4 Interstitial inflammation with prominent tubulitis (mononuclear cells invade tubular epithelium, PASM). (A full colour version of this figure appears in the colour plate section.)

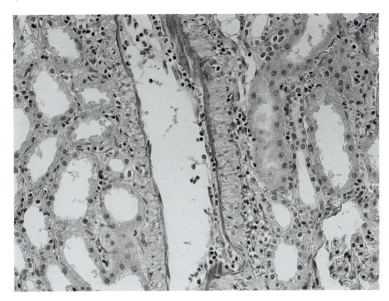

Figure 20.5 Intimal arteritis characterised by undermining of the endothelium by infiltrating lymphocytes (H&E with elastine). (A full colour version of this figure appears in the colour plate section.)

macrophages, associated with interstitial oedema. Infiltrating cells may be composed, for the most part, of macrophages/monocytes, especially when T-cell-depleting drugs (such as alemtuzumab) have been used as induction therapy. Scattered eosinophils and plasma cells are also common. The intensity of the inflammatory infiltrate together with the severity of tubulitis and intimal arteritis are used to classify rejection. Cases with interstitial inflammation and tubulitis represent Grade IA or B whereas intimal arteritis is the defining feature of Grade II. The presence of even a single vessel with endarteritis upgrades the rejection to Grade II. Grade II aTCMR (so-called vascular acute rejection) is often present in association with interstitial inflammation (Grade I), but it can occur in isolated form.

Grade III aTCMR is characterised by transmural arteritis with or without fibrinoid necrosis of the medial smooth muscle cells with accompanying lymphocytic infiltrate.

Differential diagnosis

Drug-induced allergic interstitial nephritis constitutes a diagnostic challenge. Both conditions have mixed inflammatory infiltrate in the cortex, and sometimes distinction between interstitial rejection (aTCMR Grade I) and allergic nephritis cannot be made. Fortunately both conditions respond to steroid therapy.

Various forms of infection, especially viral (polyomavirus nephropathy and cytomegalovirus (CMV)) cause interstitial inflammation and should be recognised as such. Their diagnostic features are described below. Some episodes of aTCMR can contain predominantly B cells in the inflammatory infiltrate, and these cases should be distinguished from post-transplant lymphoproliferative disorders (PTLDs).

Transplant arteritis is highly suggestive of rejection-induced damage. Similar vascular changes are seldom seen in native kidneys with vasculitis, systemic lupus erythematosus or accelerated hypertension.

Chronic active T-cell-mediated rejection: 'chronic allograft arteriopathy'

Chronic active T-cell-mediated rejection is defined by rejection-induced intimal thickening of arteries, which leads to occlusion of arterial lumina and chronic ischaemia of the graft.

Light microscopic findings
There are varying degrees of intimal sclerosis lacking elastic fibres with scattered or clustered mononuclear inflammatory cells (Fig. 20.6). Myofibroblasts with enlarged nuclei, occasional foamy cells, and enlargement of endothelial cells complete the picture. Transplant arteriopathy in active stage contains inflammatory cells but occasionally presents in the scarring stage as a 'burnt-out' process.

Differential diagnosis
The major differential diagnosis is arterionephrosclerosis. Both entities show intimal thickening with reduction of arterial luminal space, but intimal fibro-elastosis and lack of inflammatory cells are typical morphological features of arterionephrosclerosis (Fig. 20.7). Transplant

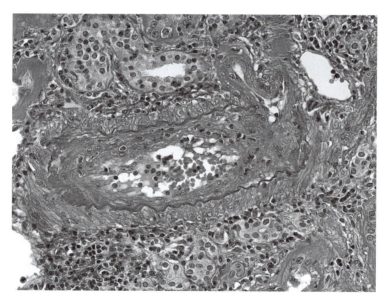

Figure 20.6 Advanced transplant arteritis with aggregates of mononuclear inflammatory cells and accumulation of fibrotic tissue in the intima (H&E with elastine). (A full colour version of this figure appears in the colour plate section.)

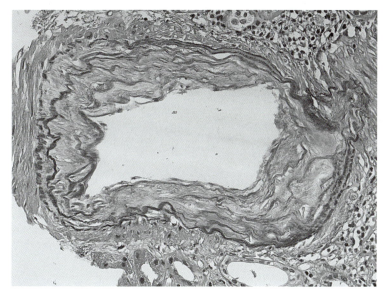

Figure 20.7 Donor arteriosclerosis with typical intimal fibroelastosis without inflammatory cells (H&E with elastine). (A full colour version of this figure appears in the colour plate section.)

arteriopathy can be superimposed on pre-existing arterionephrosclerotic vascular changes (Fig. 20.8).

Category 5: Interstitial fibrosis and tubular atrophy

Interstitial fibrosis and tubular atrophy (IF/TA) without any specific aetiology includes non-specific scarring, and is graded according its severity (Grade I–III).

Category 6: Other

Although Banff classification focuses on rejection-related changes, there are a lot of non-rejection causes that may involve the graft and must be considered in the differential diagnosis.

Drug-induced toxic changes

Calcineurin inhibitors (CNIs; ciclosporin and tacrolimus) are the cornerstone of most immunosuppressive regimens used for kidney and pancreas transplantation. Unfortunately, treatment with these drugs leads to two types of nephrotoxic side effects that are dose-dependent. The earlier change is functional toxicity due to vasospasm without morphological changes and is reversible. The other, developing later, is structural toxicity with changes in arterioles, glomeruli and tubules.

Light microscopic findings
CNI-induced arteriolar changes display swelling of the medial smooth muscle cells and occasional single endothelial and/or smooth muscle cell necrosis. The fully developed lesion shows PAS-positive hyaline nodules

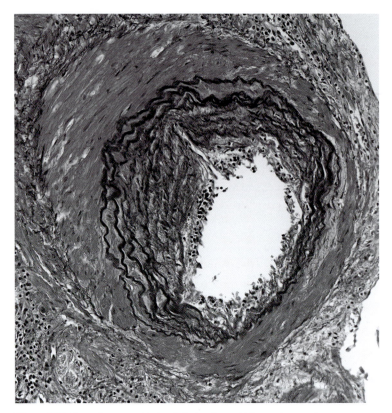

Figure 20.8 Transplant arteritis (early intimal arteritis) superimposed on pre-existing arteriosclerosis with intimal fibroelastosis (H&E with elastine). (A full colour version of this figure appears in the colour plate section.)

in the media and adventitia of the afferent arteriole with pearl-like patterns. In severe cases, CNIs induce TMA. Focal segmental sclerosis can be seen in glomeruli as a consequence of severe arteriolar injury. Interstitial fibrosis and tubular atrophy are regarded as non-specific secondary features caused by nephron loss.

Differential diagnosis
Arteriolopathy with hyaline nodules can also be a morphological feature of hypertensive arteriolopathy. Transplant recipients frequently suffer from arterial hypertension; even if CNI arteriolopathy more frequently involves advential parts of arterioles sometimes the same changes are seen in native biopsy samples of patients never treated with CNIs. I would report these lesions as arteriolopathy of combined aetiology (CNI toxicity and hypertensive).

Infection
Infections are a common cause of morbidity after renal transplantation. A variety of bacterial, viral, fungal and protozoal infections can affect

renal allografts. Acute pyelonephritis with morphological features identical with those seen in native kidneys can be diagnosed in grafts.

CMV infections with detectable inclusions involving renal allografts are rare. The diagnosis depends on the demonstration and diagnostic confirmation (which can easily be achieved by IH) of viral inclusions.

Polyomavirus nephropathy (PVN) has become the most frequent viral infection of kidney grafts in the past two decades. PVN is a serious complication because, unlike for CMV, specific and safe antiviral drugs are not available. Currently, PVN has a prevalence of 1–10% with a reported graft failure rate of more than 50% in some series. After a primary infection, which usually occurs in childhood and is asymptomatic, polyomaviruses remain in a dormant state in the epithelium of the reno-urinary tract with asymptomatic intermittent reactivation and low-level viruria. Under immunosuppression, polyomaviruses can not only reactivate but also cause viral nephropathy. During reactivation the cells containing viral inclusion slough off into the urine and can be detected in cytological preparations as decoy cells, but PVN is best diagnosed histologically.

Light microscopic findings
Typical morphological features are inclusions in the nuclei of the tubular epithelial cells. However, nuclear inclusions are not pathognomonic and diagnostic confirmation using IH with antibody to SV40 or *in situ* hybridisation is necessary to confirm the diagnosis (Figs 20.9, 20.10). Viral replication often causes necrosis of infected tubular cells with denudation of basement membranes. This virally induced acute tubular

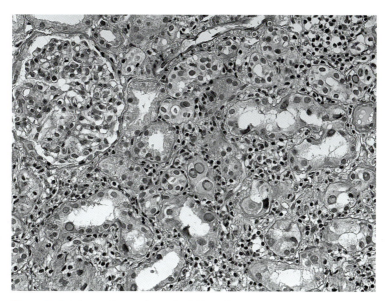

Figure 20.9 Polyomavirus nephropathy with nuclear inclusions in the epithelium and surrounding inflammation (H&E with elastine). (A full colour version of this figure appears in the colour plate section.)

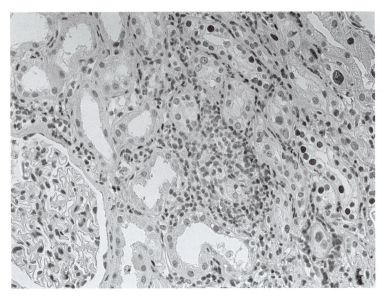

Figure 20.10 Confirmation of polyomavirus infection using immunostaining for SV40-T large antigen. Strong positive staining (brown) of the nuclei of infected tubular cells is demonstrated. (A full colour version of this figure appears in the colour plate section.)

necrosis represents a morphological correlate for allograft dysfunction. Later stages progress to irreversible interstitial fibrosis and can lead to graft loss.

Differential diagnosis
Other viruses must be ruled out, in practice by IH. The diagnosis of acute cellular rejection in cases of PVN remains a problem. We are currently unable to distinguish between inflammatory response to viral infection and inflammatory cells that represent Grade I of aTCMR. Both lesions have the morphology of interstitial nephritis.

Recurrent and *de novo* disease
Many primary glomerular diseases can recur in the allograft as well as systemic and metabolic illnesses with renal involvement. The morphological features are almost identical to those seen in native kidneys.

Post-transplant lymphoproliferative disorder
PTLD is defined as a lymphoid proliferation or lymphoma developing as a consequence of immunosuppression in recipients of a solid organ or bone marrow allograft. The Epstein–Barr virus (EBV) is thought to be an important co-factor in the majority of cases. PTLD may arise in lymphoid tissue and also in kidney grafts.

Light microscopic findings
The spectrum of morphological changes ranges from polyclonal proliferation (resembling infectious mononucleosis) to EBV-positive non-Hodgkin B-cell lymphoma. T-cell or NK-cell PTLD lymphomas are found in less than 15% of cases.

Differential diagnosis
When the renal graft is infiltrated by PTLD, the major differential diagnosis is aTCMR. Both conditions share a mononuclear infiltrate. Cases of PTLD often show dense, nodular formations of lymphoid cells without mixtures of polymorphonuclears, and without interstitial oedema. *In situ* hybridisation to detect EBV, and IH demonstrating B-cell lineage are helpful; tests for clonality help to confirm the presence of monomorphic PTLD.

Pancreas

As with the kidney, needle biopsy represents the gold standard for diagnosis of rejection.

Handling

An adequate biopsy should contain at least three lobular areas with their adjacent interlobular septa containing veins and pancreatic ducts. In general, H&E sections from three different levels, and staining for identification of fibrosis and pathology of vessel walls (Sirius red with elastine or Masson's trichrome) should be performed. IH for insulin and glucagon needs to be performed in patients with hyperglycaemia to look for the loss of beta cells, which indicates recurrence of autoimmune diabetes mellitus. C4d detection should be performed in all biopsy samples.

Banff classification

Early after transplantation, the majority of abnormalities are related to surgery. Both the exocrine and endocrine pancreatic tissue can be damaged during rejection. Several studies demonstrated that acinar lobules but not the islets are the target for cell-mediated rejection. However, patients suffering from AMR have hyperglycaemia.

The Banff classification follows similar principles to those for kidney grafts. There are categories of acute and chronic rejection, and also cell-mediated and antibody-mediated rejection (Box 20.2; details in reference [10]).

Category 1: Normal

Normal morphology is sometimes seen in protocol biopsy samples.

Light microscopic findings

Cases without inflammation or with inactive mononuclear cells without involvement of ducts or vessels.

> **Box 20.2 Banff pancreas allograft rejection working grading scheme.**
> 1. Normal
> 2. Indeterminate
> 3. Cell-mediated rejection, type (grade)
>   Acute cell-mediated rejection
>   Grade I/mild
>   Grade II/moderate
>   Grade III/severe
>   Chronic active cell-mediated rejection
> 4. Antibody-mediated rejection, type
>   Hyperacute AMR
>   Accelerated AMR
>   Acute AMR
>   Chronic active AMR
> 5. Chronic allograft rejection/graft sclerosis
>   Stage I (mild, <30% fibrosis)
>   Stage II (moderate, 31–60% fibrosis)
>   Stage III (severe, >61% fibrosis)
> 6. Other histological diagnosis
>
> The original schema includes more descriptive definitions [10].

Differential diagnosis

Recurrent autoimmune disease must be considered in patients with hyperglycaemia, and it can be diagnosed by IH staining for insulin and glucagon. In addition, the damage to islet cells can be caused by drug toxicity. Antibody-mediated rejection can have normal morphology in light microscopy, C4d detection is necessary for the diagnosis.

Category 2: Indeterminate for rejection

There is focal mild septal inflammation but the overall features do not fulfill the criteria for acute rejection.

Category 3: Cell-mediated rejection

Mild grade cell-mediated rejection is frequently associated with non-specific clinical signs, including laboratory data. In practice, monitoring of renal function is often used as a sign of rejection in both organs in patients with simultaneous kidney pancreas transplantation. However, this diagnostic test does not have absolute value, because isolated episodes of rejection in one of these organs may occur, in some studies in 30% of cases [11]. Acute rejection is earlier and more common after pancreas transplant alone [11].

Acute cell-mediated rejection
Light microscopic findings and classification of acute cell-mediated rejection
Acute cell-mediated rejection (ACMR) is characterised by active septal inflammation involving venules (venulitis, inflammatory cells under endothelium), ducts (ductitis, intra-epithelial inflammation), with neural or peri-neural inflammation. Morphology is completed by acinar inflammation and intimal arteritis (with inflammatory cells under endothelium). ACMR is graded as mild, moderate or severe.

Mild AMCR shows septal inflammation and/or mild acinar injury without arterial changes. Mild intimal arteritis or multifocal acinar inflammations characterise moderate ACMR. Severe ACMR shows moderate or necrotising arteritis or diffuse acinar inflammation.

Differential diagnosis
Mild rejection may resemble CMV pancreatitis. Infectious pancreatitis/peripancreatitis can mimic ACMR or CCMR. Clinical information is critically important.

Chronic active cell-mediated rejection
Chronic active cell-mediated rejection (CCMR) is characterised by arterial intimal fibrosis with mononuclear cells in newly formed intima (chronic allograft arteriopathy).

Category 4: Antibody-mediated rejection
AMR is poorly characterised. There are several types of AMR: hyperacute, accelerated, acute and chronic. Diagnostic criteria include C4d-positive interacinar and islet capillaries or small venules, presence of DSA in serum and graft dysfunction.

Light microscopic findings
The spectrum of morphological changes varies from normal histology in light microscopy, through inflammatory cells in capillaries to arterial wall necrosis.

Differential diagnosis
According to various morphological features, the differential diagnosis is also very variable. C4d detection is the key to diagnosis.

Category 5: Chronic allograft rejection/graft sclerosis
There are three grades of chronic allograft rejection/graft sclerosis (from mild to severe) according to percentage of fibrosis. Grading of fibrosis correlates with graft survival.

Category 6: Other
This category covers morphological changes that are not considered to be due to acute and/or chronic rejection (CMV, PTLD, etc.). Morphological features are similar to those described in the first part of this chapter, on kidney transplants.

References

1. Sis B, Mengel M, Haas M, *et al.* (2010) Banff '09 Meeting report: antibody mediated graft deterioration and implementation of Banff working groups. *Am J Transplant* **10**, 464–471.
2. Pascual M, Vallhonrat H, Cosimi AB, *et al.* (1999) The clinical usefulness of the renal allograft biopsy in the cyclosporine era: A prospective study. *Transplantation* **67**, 737–741.
3. Perico N, Cattaneo D, Sayegh MH, *et al.* (2004) Delayed graft function in kidney transplantation. *Lancet* **364**, 1814–1827.
4. Halloran PF, Schlaut J, Solez K, *et al.* (1992) The significance of the anti-class I response. II. Clinical and pathological features of renal transplants with anti-class I-like antibody. *Transplantation* **53**, 550–555.
5. Feucht HE, Schneeberger H, Hillebrand G, *et al.* (1993) Capillary deposition of C4d complement fragment and early renal graft loss. *Kidney Int* **43**, 1333–1338.
6. Terasaki P, Ozawa M. (2004) Predicting kidney graft failure by HLA antibodies: a prospective trial. *Am J Transplant* **4**, 438–443.
7. Worthington JE, Martin S, Al-Husseini DM, *et al.* (2003) Post transplantation production of donor HLA-specific antibodies as a predictor of renal transplant outcome. *Transplantation* **75**, 1034–1040.
8. Solez K, Colvin RB, Racusen LC, *et al.* (2007) Banff'05 meeting report: Differential diagnosis of chronic injury and elimination of chronic allograft nephropathy in the Banff schema. *Am J Transplant* **7**, 518–526.
9. Colvin RB. (2009) Pathology of chronic humoral rejection. *Contrib Nephrol* **162**, 75–86.
10. Drachenberg CB, Odorico J, Demetris AJ, *et al.* (2008) Banff schema for grading pancreas allograft rejection: Working proposal by a multi-disciplinary international consensus panel. *Am J Transplant* **8**, 1237–1249.
11. Bartlett ST, Schweitzer EJ, Johnson LB, *et al.* (1996) Equivalent success of simultaneous pancreas kidney and solitary pancreas transplantation. *Ann Surg* **224**, 440–449.

21 Infection

Rachel Hilton and Martin W. Drage

General principles

Solid-organ transplantation has expanded worldwide since the first successful human kidney transplant in 1954. As immunosuppressive agents and graft survival improve, infection and malignancy are now the main barriers to disease-free survival after organ transplantation. As the population of immunosuppressed patients grows, there is an increasing incidence and broader spectrum of opportunistic infections and of resistant infections. Much effort is therefore expended on the search for effective strategies for prevention, early and specific diagnosis and rapid and aggressive treatment of infection in transplant recipients.

Impaired inflammatory responses result in fewer symptoms, muted clinical findings and delayed clinical presentation, so diagnosis requires a high level of suspicion and an aggressive diagnostic approach. Improved microbiological diagnostic tools have been of great benefit in this respect. In addition, the presence of more than one pathogen within an infectious syndrome must be considered, for example the immunomodulatory effects of cytomegalovirus (CMV) facilitate concomitant infection with bacterial or fungal pathogens.

Among solid-organ transplantation, kidney transplantation carries the lowest risk of infection, due partly to the elective or semi-elective nature of the surgery. Sources of infection include the donated organ, reactivation of latent disease, common community-acquired infections and rarer opportunistic infections. It may be difficult to differentiate between these different sources.

A timeline for the major types of post-transplant infection is shown in Fig. 21.1. The peak risk of infection is during the early post-transplant period when the burden of immunosuppression is at its highest. However, opportunistic infections are rare during the initial month, as the full impact of immunosuppression requires prolonged exposure. Infections in this period may be nosocomial, may be associated with technical complications of surgery, or may be donor-derived. During months 1 to 6 after transplantation, prophylaxis with co-trimoxazole

Handbook of Renal and Pancreatic Transplantation, First Edition. Edited by Iain A. M. MacPhee and Jiří Froněk.
© 2012 John Wiley & Sons, Ltd. Published 2012 by John Wiley & Sons, Ltd.

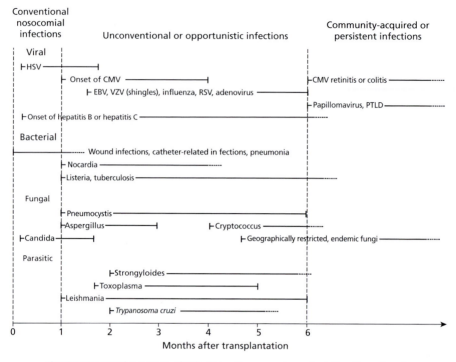

Figure 21.1 Usual sequence of infections after organ transplantation Reproduced from Fishman JA, Rubin RH. (1998) Infection in organ-transplant recipients. *N Engl J Med* **338**, 1741–1751. Copyright ©1998, Massachusetts Medical Society. All rights reserved.

should prevent most urinary tract infections (UTIs) and many opportunistic infections such as pneumocystis pneumonia, listeriosis, toxoplasmosis and nocardiasis. Viral pathogens and graft rejection are responsible for the majority of febrile episodes in this period. Herpesvirus infections are uncommon during this period if antiviral prophylaxis is used, but other viruses such as polyomavirus, adenovirus and recurrent hepatitis C virus (HCV) infection may emerge. The risk of infection in the late post-transplant period is potentiated by the high prevalence of diabetes mellitus, peripheral vascular disease and anatomical urological abnormalities in kidney transplant recipients. However, the overall risk of infection diminishes after 6 months post-transplant as immunosuppression is generally tapered beyond this period. Common community-acquired infections may be seen and may be more severe owing to immunosuppression, but the risk for most opportunistic infections is limited. Chronic viral infections may produce graft injury, such as cirrhosis from HCV infection in liver recipients, or malignancy, such as post-transplant lymphoproliferative disease (PTLD) from Epstein–Barr virus (EBV) infection. Patients who require augmented immunosuppression to treat rejection have an increased risk for late and often recurrent opportunistic infection. Such patients may benefit from prolonged or indefinite co-trimoxazole or antifungal prophylaxis.

Pre-transplant screening

Donors

It is important to ascertain the infectious history of the donor, particularly with respect to any pathogen that might be directly transmitted to the recipient along with the allograft. These include HIV, CMV, hepatitis B virus (HBV), HCV, tuberculosis, Creutzfeldt–Jakob disease and some fungi. Donor medical assessment should include enquiry about previous infections, vaccination, travel and occupational exposure, as well as asking about high-risk behaviour such as drug use, sexual practice and imprisonment.

There are differences in screening living and deceased donors owing to the different time frames available for evaluation. In living donors it is often possible to treat active infection and delay transplantation until the infection resolves. Living donors should be screened for syphilis, HIV, HBV and HCV and, where appropriate, tuberculosis via a tuberculin-purified protein derivative (PPD) skin test or whole blood interferon-gamma release assay (IGRA). In the event of a suspicious donor history, additional testing may be warranted. By contrast, the time frame for deceased donor evaluation is typically hours, and testing is often limited to serologic methods that are rapid and routinely available (Table 21.1). As a result, some infections, such as HIV and HCV, may be difficult to diagnose at an early stage before the development of specific antibody. A detailed social and medical history about the donor is required, and many centres would reject organs from high-risk donors for fear of failure to detect antibody during the seroconversion 'window' after infection. However, if the high-risk donor is found to be virus-negative using nucleic-acid amplification (NAT), the risk–benefit probably supports the use of these organs [1]. If a high-risk deceased donor is to be used, informed consent from the recipient should include counselling about the risk of transmitted infection.

In most cases where the donor has a confirmed bacterial infection, donation can still proceed, but the recipient may require prolonged (e.g. 2–4 weeks) treatment with appropriate antibiotics following transplantation. Most centres would be less likely to consider organ donation from a patient with widespread fungal or viral infection, due to the uncertainty of being able to offer adequate treatment to the recipient.

Recipients

Screening

Unrecognised or untreated infection in the recipient can reactivate or flare with post-transplant immunosuppression, so identification of pre-transplant latent infections or infectious exposure may lead to

Table 21.1 Requirements for microbiological testing of all organ donors (data from references [48,49]).

Infection	Test	Action on a positive result
HIV 1 and 2	HIV 1 and 2 antibody	Contraindication to donation
HTLVI/III	HTLVI/III antibody	Contraindication to donation. *Consider only in life-saving situations with informed consent*
Hepatitis B	HBsAg	Contraindication to donation. *Consider only in life-saving situations if the patient is already infected with or immune to Hepatitis B together with prophylaxis*
Hepatitis B	HBcAb	High risk of transmission to liver recipients; low risk of transmission for non-liver recipients. *Consider if the patient is already infected with or immune to hepatitis B together with prophylaxis*
Hepatitis C	HCV antibody	Contraindication to donation. *Consider only in life-saving situations or if the patient is already infected with Hepatitis C*
Syphilis	Treponemal-specific antibody	Donation acceptable. Recipient should receive three weekly doses of 2.4 million units of intramuscular benzathine penicillin
CMV	CMV antibody	Consideration should be given to risk of CMV-positive donation to CMV-negative recipients
Toxoplasma	Toxoplasma antibody	Give co-trimoxazole prophylaxis for at least 6 weeks to toxoplasma-antibody-negative recipients of positive donors
EBV	EBV antibody	Consideration should be given to risk of EBV-positive donation to EBV-negative recipients

reappraisal of transplant suitability or mandate changes in post-transplant management. The pre-transplant infectious history of the recipient must be ascertained, including exposure to tuberculosis and hepatitis viruses. It is important to enquire about pre-transplant immunisation, immune-altering conditions such as asplenia, prior exposure to immunosuppression, important co-morbidities such as diabetes mellitus, current or previous intravenous drug use, liver dysfunction, nutritional status and relevant geographic exposure to pathogens. Patients awaiting kidney transplants may have infective haemodialysis or peritoneal dialysis complications, or complex upper/

lower UTIs. All recipients should therefore have urine culture performed. Pre-operative serological testing helps identify at-risk candidates and this should include HIV, EBV, HBV, HCV, varicella zoster virus (VZV), CMV, syphilis and toxoplasmosis serology. Pre-transplant evaluation should also include a history of antibiotic allergies, a dental assessment and a chest X-ray for current infection and previous exposures. Any recurrent sources of infection must be minimised prior to transplantation, which might include dental extraction, or removal of infected polycystic kidneys.

Immunisation

Where possible patients should be immunised before transplantation, although the immune response to vaccination may be impaired in patients with long-standing kidney failure [2]. The vaccination history of the patient should be ascertained and any incomplete vaccinations should be corrected. Patients may particularly benefit from vaccination against influenza, pneumococcus, HBV and varicella, as well as diphtheria-pertussis-tetanus (DPT), inactivated polio and measles-mumps-rubella (MMR). Live vaccines should not be given to immunocompromised patients, so vaccination schedules against MMR and varicella should be completed several months prior to transplantation. Table 21.2 shows the vaccines that are recommended or contraindicated before and after transplantation.

Pathogenesis of post-transplant infection

The risk of infection is directly attributable to the overall immunosuppressive burden. Infection is therefore associated with the duration and dose of maintenance immunosuppression and augmentation of immunosuppression to treat rejection. Other general factors will also increase infection rates, such as neutropenia, the presence of open wounds or devitalised tissues, indwelling material such as catheters, lines and drains, metabolic abnormalities such as diabetes or uraemia or co-infection with immunomodulatory viruses such as CMV. Pre-existing latent infections such as herpesviruses, tuberculosis and toxoplasmosis may reactivate and cause morbidity. New infections may be acquired with the allograft or from post-transplant exposure.

Exposure to broad-spectrum antibiotics or to the hospital environment before or after transplantation can result in nosocomial colonisation, often with organisms displaying increased antimicrobial resistance. Such pathogens include methicillin-resistant *Staphylococcus aureus*, vancomycin-resistant enterococci, *Clostridium difficile* and certain fungi. Vancomycin-resistant *Enterococcus faecium* (VRE) infections are more likely in patients who have received pre-operative antibiotics, particularly vancomycin, and those who have been hospitalised in the intensive-care unit (ICU). *Clostridium difficile* infection should be suspected in all patients who have received antibiotics and subsequently develop diarrhoea or abdominal symptoms.

Table 21.2 Vaccination in transplant recipients [40].

Vaccines that may safely be administered to immunosuppressed patients	Vaccines that MUST NOT be given to immunosuppressed patients
Influenza vaccine	Oral polio vaccine
Pneumococcal vaccine	MMR vaccine (measle, mumps, rubella)
Inactivated polio vaccine	MR vaccine
Pertussis vaccine	Mumps vaccine
Adsorbed tetanus vaccine	Rubella vaccine
Adsorbed diphtheria vaccine	BCG (Bacillus Calmette-Guérin) vaccine
Haemophilus Influenzae type B vaccine	Yellow fever vaccine
Hepatitis A vaccine and hepatitis B vaccine	Smallpox vaccine
Cholera vaccine	Oral typhoid vaccine
Meningococcal polysaccharide vaccine	
Meningococcal C conjugate vaccine	
Typhoid vaccine	

Vaccine	Vaccinate before transplant?	Vaccinate after transplant?	Dose regimen and formulation	Monitor titres?	Comments
Influenza	Yes	Yes	Administer annually between October and January	No	
Hepatitis B	Yes	Yes	Four-dose schedule (0, 1, 2 and 12 months) of 20–40 µg intramuscular recombinant vaccine	Serial HBsAb titres should be assessed before and every 6–12 months after transplantation to assess ongoing immunity	When titres fall below protective levels, revaccinate with four-dose schedule of 40 µg
Pneumovax	Yes	Yes	PCV7 and PPV23 formulations both acceptable; both given intramuscularly; for dosing, follow manufacturer's recommendations	No	Readminister vaccine every 3–5 years after transplantation
Tetanus, diphtheria, acellular pertussis (DTP)	Safe	Safe	Follow manufacturer's recommendations	No	Insufficient evidence for or against revaccination
Varicella and zoster (both live attenuated virus)	Yes	Contraindicated	Follow manufacturer's recommendations	No	Live virus vaccines contraindicated in transplant recipients

Table 21.2 *Continued*

Vaccine	Vaccinate before transplant?	Vaccinate after transplant?	Dose regimen and formulation	Monitor titres?	Comments
Human papillomavirus	Yes, in women aged 11–26 years	Likely to be safe	Follow manufacturer's recommendations	No data available	Theoretically safe, but no safety or efficacy data in solid-organ transplant recipients

Approach to the transplant recipient with fever

Fever in a transplant recipient may indicate either infection, graft rejection, or less commonly a drug reaction or systemic inflammatory response. Acute rejection may present with mild flu-like symptoms, which rapidly resolve after treatment, although this presentation is less common using modern immunosuppressive drugs that modulate cytokine production. A tender and swollen graft in a febrile kidney transplant recipient may indicate severe rejection or graft pyelonephritis. Fever may occur during treatment of rejection using muromonab-CD3 (OKT3), alemtuzumab (anti-CD52) or polyclonal antibodies that trigger cytokine release. Febrile transplant recipients should be screened for chest and urine infection and for bacteraemia, and require close outpatient review, if not admission to hospital. Blood cultures should be drawn before initiation of antimicrobial therapy from the periphery and any central lines. Culture of fluid collections (e.g. subcutaneous, intra-abdominal, renal pelvis or pleural) may be necessary in patients who have unexplained fever or other evidence of infection in the postoperative period. Localisation and aspiration may be facilitated by ultrasound or computerised tomography (CT) guidance. Intravascular catheters and ureteric stents should be removed where possible and the tips cultured. For patients with suspected bacterial sepsis empirical therapy may be required, the choice of agent depending on the suspected site of infection, the likely pathogen and the centre-specific pattern of sensitivities. Initial therapy should be broad spectrum, and the duration of therapy guided by clinical signs and symptoms. Once a specific pathogen is identified the spectrum of therapy should be narrowed to avoid emergence of resistant organisms.

Bacterial infections

Infection during the first month is rarely due to opportunistic infection and usually results from bacterial pathogens in the wound, or the urinary or respiratory tract. The risk of infection correlates with the complexity of the surgery and particularly with complications such as urine leaks, wound haematomata and lymphocoeles. In addition, catheters and instrumentation provide portals of entry for endogenous and nosocomial agents. Pre-existing conditions unrelated to organ failure, such as diverticular disease or biliary disease, may become manifest in the post-transplant period with immunosuppression. The predominant pathogens are similar to those that infect non-transplant surgical patients and the pattern and antibiotic sensitivity usually reflect the centre's epidemiological patterns and antibiotic usage. Common organisms include Enterobacteriaceae and *Staphylococcus* and *Pseudomonas* species. More than half of all bacteraemias in kidney transplant recipients are due to Gram-negative bacilli [3], and the consequent mortality rate is high.

Urinary tract infection

Epidemiology and risk factors
UTI is the most common infection in kidney transplant recipients, mostly occurring during the first year and associated with higher rates of hospitalisation and death due to Gram-negative septicaemia in comparison with patients on the transplant waiting list. Late UTI (more than 6 months after transplantation) is associated with reduced allograft survival and increased mortality. *Escherichia coli* is the most common uropathogen, with *Enterococcus* species, *Pseudomonas*, coagulase-negative staphylococci, *Enterobacter* and other organisms also frequently occurring [4]. Candiduria is frequent but mostly asymptomatic. Risk factors for UTI include anatomical abnormalities, female gender, recipients of deceased donor kidneys, recipients of combined kidney and pancreas transplants, prolonged bladder catheterisation or vesico-ureteric stenting and net state of immunosuppression. Vesico-ureteric reflux is common in kidney transplant recipients and leads to an increased risk of acute pyelonephritis in children and allograft scarring in children and adults. Risk factors for candiduria include prior antibiotic use and ICU care.

Definitions and diagnosis
Bacteriuria may be defined as at least 105 colony-forming units of bacteria per mL of fresh unspun midstream urine and may be symptomatic or asymptomatic. Pyuria is defined as at least 10 white blood cells per high-power field of unspun midstream urine, and is indicative of an inflammatory response in the urothelium, usually to pathogenic invasion. Diagnosis of a symptomatic UTI requires greater than 105 bacteria per mL of urine together with typical symptoms or

signs. Some authorities propose a more sensitive definition and suggest that in a symptomatic transplant recipient at least 102 bacteria per mL of urine together with pyuria is diagnostic. 'Acute cystitis' describes symptomatic infection of the lower bladder with frequency, urgency, dysuria or suprapubic pain, sometimes accompanied by low-grade fever but without flank pain or allograft tenderness. 'Acute pyelonephritis' describes infection of the upper urinary tract or renal parenchyma, characterised by loin pain (if the native kidneys are affected) or allograft tenderness (if the transplanted kidney is affected) often with a high fever. 'Complicated UTI' describes infection in individuals with functional or structural abnormalities of the genitourinary tract, and by this definition all UTIs in kidney transplant recipients may be considered complicated due to functional (immunosuppression) and structural abnormalities (uretero-neocystostomy). The majority of kidney transplant recipients with bacteriuria have 'asymptomatic bacteriuria' but are more likely to develop future symptomatic UTI.

Treatment

Gram staining of urine should be performed to guide therapy, but review of previous uropathogens and local antibiotic susceptibility may enable early empirical treatment. There is no consensus as to whether asymptomatic bacteriuria should be treated, and there are data to suggest that treatment of late (beyond 1 year) asymptomatic bacteriuria does not prevent symptomatic UTI [5]. Transplant pyelonephritis can lead to life-threatening sepsis and should usually be treated with two empirical intravenous antibiotics, such as an aminoglycoside and a penicillin, while culture results are awaited. Treatment for 7 to 14 days is recommended, and imaging of the genitourinary tract should be undertaken if symptoms persistent despite appropriate therapy. Progression to kidney or perinephric abscess or emphysematous pyelonephritis may occur and requires a multidisciplinary approach to treatment, including percutaneous or surgical drainage of abscesses or removal of the graft. Broad-spectrum antimicrobial therapy should be initiated with a carbapenem, extended-spectrum penicillin, or third-generation cephalosporin. Duration of treatment should be at least 2 weeks or until adequate drainage of abscesses has been achieved. Anatomical abnormalities must be excluded in the case of relapsing UTI, the most common findings being vesico-ureteric reflux, vesico-ureteric stricture or neurogenic bladder. It is not clear whether asymptomatic candiduria warrants treatment in kidney transplant patients, although many are treated because of perceived risk to the allograft and the potential for involvement of the upper urinary tract. Treatment with oral fluconazole for 7 to 14 days and removal (or replacement) of urological stents and urethral catheters is recommended. Fluconazole increases exposure to the calcineurin inhibitors and mammalian target of rapamycin (mTOR) inhibitors and immunosuppressive drug dosing should be adjusted appropriately (see Chapter 16).

Prevention and prophylaxis

Prophylaxis with co-trimoxazole reduces the risk of UTI threefold, without encouraging resistant organisms, but the optimal dose and duration is unclear. Screening for UTI is not usually required, but is appropriate if there are signs of infection on urine dipstick analysis. The duration of urinary tract instrumentation, including catheters and ureteric stents, should be minimised where possible.

Wound infections and intra-abdominal infections

The incidence of surgical wound infections in kidney transplant recipients ranges from 2 to 25%, and infections typically present within the first month following transplantation, often due to bacterial infection of urine leaks and fistulas, wound haematomata and lymphocoeles [6]. The risk of infection is increased by the complexity of surgery and recipient factors such as obesity. Repeated percutaneous drainage of lymphocoeles may predispose to perinephric abscess formation. Fever, graft tenderness and a characteristic ultrasound appearance aid diagnosis. Diagnosis of wound infection or necrotic tissues should include aspiration of any drainable material, swab samples from the site and biopsy material where appropriate. Common organisms include staphylococci, streptococci, enteric Gram-negative bacteria, enterococci and, less frequently, anaerobic bacteria such as *Bacteroides fragilis*, or *Candida* species. An infected collection adjacent to the transplant renal pelvis is of great concern and demands close monitoring of the patient due to the risk of infection of the anastomoses leading to sudden severe blood loss. Percutaneous or open drainage is usually necessary for symptom resolution. Perioperative prophylactic antibiotics reduce the frequency of wound infections in the immediate postoperative period, and in general should be directed against skin pathogens (staphylococci and streptococci) and urinary tract pathogens (*E. coli*, *Klebsiella* and *Proteus* species). Choice of antimicrobial agent should depend on the centre's own susceptibility patterns, and duration of therapy should be minimised to reduce the risk of antibiotic resistance.

Pneumonia

Pulmonary bacterial infections in transplant recipients may be life-threatening and are more likely to occur in patients who require prolonged intubation, have underlying lung disease, increased risk of aspiration or impaired diaphragmatic function. Concurrent immunosuppression and the consequent attenuated inflammatory response means that radiological appearances of common lung infections may appear atypical. The differential diagnosis is wide and may include atelectasis, aspiration, infarction, haemorrhage or pulmonary oedema. Blood cultures are an important diagnostic tool, as a high proportion of patients with pneumonia have bacteraemia. Other diagnostic specimens include sputum, tracheal aspirates in ventilated patients, bronchoalveolar lavage (BAL) fluid, trans-thoracic fine-needle aspirates and occasionally lung biopsy. Chest CT scanning is very valuable in the diagnosis of pneumonia and to guide percutaneous or thorascopic biopsy of suspected lesions. Aerobic Gram-negative bacilli such as Enterobacteriaceae and *E. coli* account for many cases of pneumonia and there is a higher risk of nosocomial exposure to pathogens such as *Legionella* and *Pseudomonas*, which may be present in hospital water supplies. Additional pathogens include *S. aureus*, enterococci and *S. pneumoniae*.

Infective endocarditis

Most episodes of infective endocarditis in transplant recipients are associated with previous hospital-acquired infection, most notably central venous access and wound infections [7]. The spectrum of organisms is different to that in the general population, the most common being *Aspergillus fumigatus* or *S. aureus* with relatively few due to viridans streptococci. Fungal infections predominate within the first 30 days of transplantation, whereas bacterial infections predominate later. In the majority of cases there is no underlying valvular disease. The overall mortality is high, and many cases go unsuspected.

Listeriosis

In transplant recipients infection with *L. monocytogenes* most commonly manifests as meningitis or septicaemia, but may also cause febrile gastroenteritis [8]. Infection typically occurs some months after transplantation and may be associated with ingestion of contaminated foods such as unpasteurised dairy products and undercooked meat, or uncooked vegetables. Diabetes mellitus, CMV infection, and treatment with high-dose steroids are independent risk factors for this infection, whereas use of co-trimoxazole for prophylaxis is protective. Appropriate treatment includes high-dose intravenous amoxicillin and an aminoglycoside for 2 to 3 weeks, as *Listeria* has an innate resistance to cephalosporin antibiotics.

Nocardiosis

Prophylactic use of co-trimoxazole has greatly decreased the frequency of nocardial infection in organ transplant recipients to between 0.7 and 3.5% [9]. The highest risk is in lung transplant recipients. Other risk factors include augmentation of immunosuppression to treat rejection, neutropenia and uraemia. Nocardial infection in transplant recipients predominantly causes pneumonia, typically subacute or indolent with symptoms often present for weeks. Radiological manifestations are typically irregular nodular lesions, which may progress to cavitation, but also include diffuse pneumonic infiltrates or consolidation with pleural effusions. There may be both local and haematogenous spread to distant sites such as the brain, skin and subcutaneous tissues, bone and eye, and so a diagnosis of *Nocardia* pulmonary infection should prompt a search for disseminated disease, including magnetic resonance imaging (MRI) of the brain to exclude cerebral abscess. Definitive diagnosis requires demonstration of the organism on culture from a suspected site, but a presumptive diagnosis can be made if modified acid-fast staining reveals branching, Gram-positive, beaded filaments. Accurate identification generally requires molecular methodology. The treatment of choice is high-dose co-trimoxazole, although imipenem, amikacin, cephalosporins or quinolones may be used in combination. Linezolid has recently been shown to be effective as primary therapy. There is a high risk of relapse, so treatment should continue for up to 12 months, and some centres would continue prophylaxis once treatment is completed.

Clostridium difficile infection

Clostridium difficile infection is the most important cause of hospital-acquired diarrhoea. The incidence is increasing, estimated to be 3.5 to 16% in kidney recipients and 1.5 to 7.8% in pancreas–kidney recipients [10]. Antimicrobial therapy is the most significant risk factor, together with increasing age, non-surgical gastrointestinal procedures, presence of a nasogastric tube, use of anti-ulcer medications, stay on an ICU, duration of hospital admission, duration of antibiotic course and receipt of multiple antibiotics [11]. *Clostridium difficile*-associated syndromes include asymptomatic carriage, diarrhoea, intestinal perforation, pelvic abscess, pseudomembranous colitis and toxic megacolon. Immunosuppression is a risk factor for more fulminant disease. Diagnosis is made by enzyme-linked immunosorbant assay (ELISA) for toxin A or B (or both) in the stool rather than by culture. The negative predictive value of a negative toxin ELISA is greater than 95%. Nevertheless, cytotoxin may be absent in a small proportion of endoscopically proven cases, so a high index of suspicion should be maintained in all patients with abdominal symptoms or diarrhoea who have recently received antibiotics. Oral metronidazole is the standard first-line treatment, or oral vancomycin for more severe infection. The precipitating antibiotic should be removed. Resistance to metronidazole and vancomycin is not reported, but changing antibiotic is often tried empirically if symptoms persist. More than one-third of patients will suffer at least one recurrence. Adjunctive agents such as intravenous immunoglobulin (IVIG), probiotic agents, or toxin-binding resins such as cholestyramine have been used to treat initial or recurrent *C. difficile* infection, but there is insufficient evidence to recommend their routine use. Probiotics and toxin-binding resins may be harmful because of the risk of bacteraemia or the reduction in efficacy of antimicrobial therapy, respectively. In addition to infection-control measures, prevention must focus on reducing antimicrobial exposure, especially to broad-spectrum agents. There is no known effective prophylaxis against *C. difficile*. Pre-existing colonisation with *C. difficile* may be protective, so pre-emptive therapy in asymptomatic individuals is not indicated.

Legionella species infection

In the UK 95% of *Legionella* infections are due to *Legionella pneumophila*, principally serogroup 1 [12]. Risk factors for *Legionella* species infection include cigarette smoking, increasing age, multiple corticosteroid boluses, time spent on a ventilator, and contamination of water supplies or air-conditioning units. The usual manifestation is pneumonia, typically of abrupt onset with a high fever, headache, myalgia and a dry cough. Radiological manifestations are typically alveolar or interstitial infiltrates, but may also include cavitating lesions, pleural effusions or lobar consolidation. Culture requires charcoal media but is highly specific and more sensitive than direct fluorescent antibody microscopy of respiratory samples. Urinary antigen detection of *L. pneumophila* serogroup 1 is a very convenient and highly specific technique to aid rapid diagnosis and early treatment, and has largely replaced antibody detection, the traditional method of diagnosis. Intravenous erythromycin is the treatment of choice with the addition of rifampicin in severe cases. Alternative therapies include co-trimoxazole, fluoroquinolones, doxycycline and macrolide antibiotics such as azithromycin.

Mycobacterial infection

Epidemiology and risk factors
Mycobacterial and non-tuberculous mycobacterial (NTM) infections are common after transplantation, particularly among high-risk populations. Stratification of risk in transplant patients is difficult, as skin tests may be unreliable in patients with kidney failure, and newer tests (including whole-blood interferon-gamma assays, which are highly specific for *M. tuberculosis*) have not yet been validated in transplant recipients [13]. Patients at high risk include those who have had pulmonary or extrapulmonary TB in the past, or those from countries with increased mycobacterial exposure, including those from the Indian-subcontinent and those who are Black African.

Diagnosis and treatment
Pulmonary presentations of *M. tuberculosis* and NTM can appear as multilobar disease, focal infiltrates, nodular shadowing, empyema or a combination of findings. Disseminated disease is observed in a high proportion of transplant recipients, with involvement of skin, bone and central nervous system. Atypical presentation in transplant recipients may delay diagnosis, so a high degree of suspicion should be maintained in high-risk patients. Acid-fast staining of respiratory and biopsy specimens may reveal mycobacterial forms. Culture is necessary, however, for final speciation and specific mycobacterial probes aid species confirmation. The presence of granulomata in peripheral tissues is suggestive of disseminated disease.

Because of the increasing prevalence of multi-drug resistant strains it is recommended that treatment should include at least four antituberculous agents until sensitivities are known. Initial drug regimens should include 2 months of oral isoniazid, rifampicin, pyrazinamide and ethambutol, followed by an additional 4 months of isoniazid and rifampicin alone depending on sensitivities [14]. Adverse effects of antituberculous agents include liver toxicity and peripheral and optic neuropathy, and patients should be screened for the onset of these. Fluoroquinolones such as ofloxacin may be used as alternative components of multidrug regimens in patients with impaired liver function or who develop liver toxicity. Rifampicin is a powerful inducer of the cytochrome P450 enzyme system, leading to significant but predictable reductions in sirolimus and calcineurin inhibitor blood concentrations. Appropriate monitoring is required and doses of calcineurin inhibitors usually have to be increased two- to fivefold.

Prophylaxis

Tuberculosis prophylaxis should be given if the adjusted annual risk of tuberculosis is greater than the risk of hepatitis from tuberculosis chemoprophylaxis. These patients should receive isoniazid for 6 months following transplantation. The standard recommended dose of isonaizid is 300 mg once daily with concomitant administration of pyridoxine (vitamin B_6) 25 mg once daily to reduce the risk of neurotoxicity. No chemoprophylaxis regimen is wholly effective, and protective efficacies of 60% have been reported for a 6-month course of isoniazid alone [15]. A case can be made for longer-term prophylaxis, with some advocating life-long treatment. Patients should be monitored carefully with monthly recording of hepatic enzymes. Treatment should be withdrawn if plasma transaminases exceed three times the upper limit of normal or there is any increase in serum bilirubin.

Fungal infections

Risk factors for fungal infection include enhanced corticosteroid use to treat rejection, vascular, urinary or drainage catheters, total parenteral nutrition, gastrointestinal perforation and diabetes mellitus.

Candidiasis

Infections due to *Candida* species are the most common fungal infections in transplant recipients. Invasive candidiasis is typically seen in the first 3 months following transplantation, although later cases may occur among liver and small bowel recipients. *Candida albicans* is the dominant pathogen, accounting for approximately 50% of isolates [16]. *Candida* infection can manifest as mucosal candidiasis, urinary tract infections, wound infections and intra-abdominal infections. The risk relates to the nature of the surgery and particularly to the surgical anastomosis. For example, the risk is higher in bladder-drained than in enteric-drained pancreatic allografts. Other risk factors include acute kidney injury, CMV infection, primary graft failure, prolonged urinary catheterisation and need for surgical re-exploration. Definitive diagnosis requires identification of the organism in clinical samples such as blood, urine, drain fluid or abscess material, but the organism is difficult to culture and the overall sensitivity of blood cultures is only 70%. Newer non-culture-based methods of diagnosis, such as polymerase chain reaction (PCR)-based multiplex assays, are in development. Treatment is with antifungal agents such as amphotericin-B, triazoles such as fluconazole, itraconazole or voriconazole, or echinocandins such as caspofungin. Amphotericin-B is a well-recognised nephrotoxin, though less so in lipid formulation. The triazoles have significant drug–drug interactions, most notably with calcineurin inhibitors, so careful drug concentration monitoring is required. The echinocandins have few side effects or drug–drug interactions but must be given parenterally and require dose reduction in hepatic impairment. Optimal duration of therapy depends on the site and severity of infection, but is generally a minimum of 2 weeks. Removal of indwelling lines and catheters where possible is strongly recommended to aid fungal clearance. There are few data and no consensus regarding the optimal nature and duration of prophylaxis, although many centres give oral nystatin, amphotericin lozenges or fluconazole for the first month following transplantation.

Aspergillosis

Epidemiology and risk factors
Invasive aspergillosis remains a significant post-transplant complication, affecting between 1 and 4% of kidney transplant recipients [17]. Pneumonia and other tissue-invasive forms such as genitourinary, central nervous system (CNS), rhinocerebral, sinus, gastrointestinal, skin and musculoskeletal are recognised. Predisposing factors include the burden of immunosuppression, particularly high doses and prolonged duration of corticosteroids. Graft failure requiring haemodialysis is an additional risk factor. Mortality rates range from 65 to 75%.

Diagnosis and treatment
Delays in diagnosis are a major impediment to successful treatment of invasive aspergillosis. If intracerebral aspergillosis is suspected, a brain MRI scan should be performed along with a biopsy of any suspicious lesions. Cultures of respiratory tract secretions lack sensitivity, as fungus may only be detected in clinical samples in late stages of the disease, and culture of *Aspergillus* from respiratory tract samples does not always indicate invasive disease. Alternative tests such as antigen detection by galactomannan assay on serum, urine or cerebrospinal fluid, serum ®-D-glucan or nucleic acid detection by pan fungal PCR are under evaluation, and their precise role in the diagnosis and management of invasive aspergillosis in transplant recipients remains to be determined.

Prompt initiation of antifungal therapy is critical. Lipid formulations of amphotericin B have long been the mainstay of treatment, but newer triazole agents such as voriconazole and echinocandins such as caspofungin have potent anti-*Aspergillus* activity and better tolerability, and appear to be as effective with fewer severe drug-related adverse events. Voriconazole is now regarded as the drug of choice for primary treatment of invasive aspergillosis in all patients, including transplant recipients. Caspofungin has been used successfully as salvage therapy in invasive aspergillosis, alone and in combination with other drugs.

Liposomal amphotericin B is now reserved for patients developing treatment-limiting toxicity or where voriconazole is contraindicated; 3 mg/kg/day is as effective as 10 mg/kg/day and less toxic, so higher doses are no longer recommended [18]. Combination antifungal therapy with voriconazole and caspofungin may be appropriate for salvage therapy, for patients with more severe disseminated disease or with poor prognostic factors such as kidney failure. Triazole agents are potent inhibitors of cytochrome P450 and may significantly increase blood concentrations of calcineurin and mTOR inhibitors. A 50 to 60% reduction in calcineurin inhibitors dose may be necessary with the concurrent use of voriconazole and concurrent use of sirolimus is contraindicated. Caspofungin may reduce tacrolimus concentrations by up to 20% and may increase ciclosporin concentrations by 35%.

The optimal duration of therapy depends upon the response but is usually continued for 12 weeks, or until all clinical and radiographic abnormalities have resolved, and cultures, if they can be obtained, no longer yield *Aspergillus*. Reduction in immunosuppression including withdrawal of corticosteroids and reduction in calcineurin inhibitor dose is an important adjuvant measure. Surgical excision or debridement is indicated for persistent or life-threatening haemoptysis, for lesions close to great vessels or pericardium, for sino-nasal infections, for single cavity lung lesions, which progress despite adequate treatment, and for lesions invading pericardium, bone, subcutaneous or thoracic tissue. Surgical resection is also indicated for intracranial abscesses depending upon their location, accessibility and neurological effects.

Prophylaxis
Prophylaxis against invasive aspergillosis is not routinely recommended in kidney or pancreas transplant recipients.

Cryptococcosis
Cryptococcosis is the third most common invasive fungal infection in transplant recipients, with an overall incidence of 3% [19]. Cryptococcosis typically occurs late, around 16 to 21 months post-transplant. The onset may be earlier in lung recipients than in kidney recipients owing to the higher intensity of immunosuppression. Cryptococcal disease is generally due to reactivation of quiescent infection, as demonstrated by pre- and post-transplant serology. In rare cases there may be transmission from the donor allograft. Risk factors include use of corticosteroids and use of depleting antibodies, particularly alemtuzumab, for induction. Calcineurin-inhibitors appear to have anti-cryptococcocal activity, and use of these agents is associated with a reduced likelihood of disseminated disease. The majority of patients with cryptococcosis have disseminated disease or CNS involvement but in a third of cases disease is limited to the lungs. Cutaneous cryptococcosis may present with papular, nodular or ulcerative lesions or as cellulitis, and is often a consequence of haematogenous spread. Mortality rates are high, approaching 50% in

cases of CNS infection. All patients with suspected or documented cryptococcosis should have a lumbar puncture, blood and urine cultures and, in suspected pulmonary cases, bronchoalveolar lavage with or without biopsy. Cryptococcal antigen is the recommended test for cerebrospinal fluid or serum and can also serve as a marker of response to therapy. Brain MRI is more sensitive than CT for detecting cryptococcomas. Extraneural cryptococcal disease can occur in the skin, prostate gland, liver and kidney and can be diagnosed on biopsy of the involved site. Prostatic and kidney disease may present as yeast in the urine. Pulmonary disease may present as nodular opacities on chest X-ray and CT scan, and less often as effusions or consolidation. Treatment requires induction with a combination of amphotericin B and flucytosine for 2 to 4 weeks followed by consolidation with fluconazole for 6 to 12 months. There should be concomitant tapering of immunosuppression. Routine antifungal prophylaxis against cryptococcosis is not recommended as no specific high-risk group has been identified.

Pneumocystis pneumonia

Epidemiology and risk factors

Pneumocystis jiroveci, previously called *Pneumocystis carinii*, is a key opportunistic pathogen in organ transplantation. Before routine prophylaxis the overall incidence among liver and kidney transplant recipients was between 2 and 15% but is decreasing with reduction in the routine use of corticosteroids in organ transplantation and with the adoption of effective prophylaxis [20]. Risk factors for the development of *Pneumocystis* pneumonia (PCP) include immunosuppressive burden, particularly dose and duration of corticosteroids and use of depleting anti-lymphocyte antibodies, and co-infection with immunomodulatory viruses such as CMV.

Diagnosis and treatment

Symptoms of PCP often develop over the course of a few days, and are classically dominated by dyspnoea and hypoxaemia disproportionate to physical and radiographic findings. Fever and lymphadenopathy are uncommon. Chest radiography may be normal or reveal diffuse bilateral interstitial pulmonary infiltrates. CT scans are more sensitive than routine chest radiography, but although there is no diagnostic radiological pattern, certain patterns such as ground-glass opacification are suggestive (Fig. 21.2). Definitive diagnosis requires demonstration of organisms in lung tissue or respiratory tract secretions. The diagnostic yield from routine sputum is poor and patients should undergo initial screening via multiple induced sputum samples. All respiratory secretions should be stained using antibodies for PCP as well as routine tissue stains (Giemsa, silver and others). Samples should also be stained and cultured for routine bacterial, fungal, mycobacterial and other organisms to rule out other similar or concomitant infections. There should be a low threshold for bronchoscopy with BAL to obtain diagnostic samples and

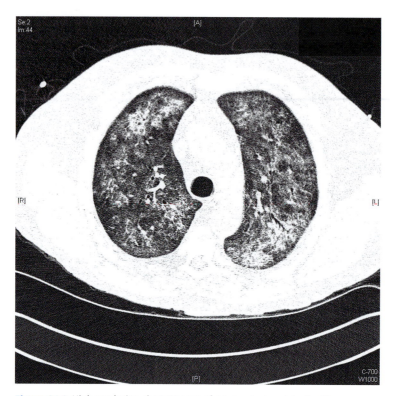

Figure 21.2 High-resolution chest CT scan of a transplant recipient with pneumocystis pneumonia showing characteristic ground-glass opacification.

expedite the diagnosis of concomitant infection. Co-infection with CMV is particularly common and may precede PCP.

Co-trimoxazole is the first-line agent and drug of choice. In severe infections, intravenous pentamidine may be used as a second-line agent, although it has numerous toxic side effects including pancreatitis, hypoglycemia, hyperglycemia, bone marrow suppression, kidney failure and electrolyte disturbances. Pentamidine should be avoided in pancreas transplant recipients because of the potential for islet cell necrosis. Hypoxic patients should receive adjunctive therapy with high-dose corticosteroids, ideally within 72 hours of starting antibiotic therapy for maximum benefit. The optimal dose of corticosteroids is not well established, but 40 to 60 mg of prednisone (or equivalent) given twice daily for 5 to 7 days before being tapered over a period of another 7 to 14 days is often recommended. Antimicrobial therapy should continue for a minimum of 14 days, or longer in severe infections. Immunosuppression should be reduced where feasible.

Prophylaxis

Routine anti-*Pneumocystis* prophylaxis is recommended for all patients for at least 6 months post-transplant. Co-trimoxazole is the drug of choice and may also have the advantage of preventing other opportunistic pathogens after transplantation, such as *Toxoplasma* and *Listeria* species, as well as more common respiratory, urinary and gastrointestinal pathogens. Side effects include bone marrow suppression, skin rash, hepatitis, interstitial nephritis, aseptic meningitis and pancreatitis. Trimethoprim inhibits creatinine secretion in the kidney tubules, resulting in an elevation of serum creatinine that does not necessarily reflect true kidney function. Dapsone is often used as a second-line agent for PCP prophylaxis but is contraindicated in patients with glucose-6-phosphate dehydrogenase (G6PD) deficiency. Side effects of dapsone include haemolytic anaemia and methaemoglobinaemia, classically in association with G6PD deficiency, although this is not a prerequisite. Other agents used for PCP prophylaxis include atovaquone and nebulised pentamidine.

Cocciodiomycosis and histoplasmosis

Patients who have resided in geographical areas with endemic mycoses should be screened before transplantation as reactivation can occur under immunosuppression. A patient with positive pre-transplant serology against *Coccidioides* or *Histoplasma* should be considered for prophylactic antifungal agents such as azoles.

Viral infections

Cytomegalovirus

Epidemiology, presentation and risk factors

CMV infection is the most common viral infection after transplantation and may vary in severity from asymptomatic infection to multiorgan involvement and death [21]. Fortunately, the availability of effective antiviral therapy has limited its lethal potential. The incidence of CMV seropositivity increases with age and the majority of adults in the UK have detectable anti-CMV IgG antibodies. After primary infection CMV establishes life-long latency. Without prophylaxis, CMV viraemia with or without symptoms occurs in at least 75% of patients between 1 and 6 months after transplantation and a high level of vigilance is required. Onset may be delayed in patients receiving CMV prophylaxis. The spectrum of CMV infection ranges from asymptomatic viral replication, through viral syndrome with fever and/or malaise, leucopenia or thrombocytopenia, to tissue invasive disease such as pneumonitis, hepatitis, retinitis or gastrointestinal disease. CMV also has an immunomodulatory effect, and is a risk factor for other infectious complications, such as bacteraemia, invasive fungal disease and EBV-related PTLD. CMV may cause both acute and chronic allograft injury, and is implicated in the development of chronic allograft nephropathy, bronchiolitis obliterans in lung transplant recipients and accelerated coronary artery disease in heart transplant recipients.

The risk of CMV disease is highest in donor-seropositive, recipient-seronegative (D+R−) recipients who lack cellular and humoral immunity to CMV. Pre-transplant screening should therefore be performed for both donor and recipient to enable stratification of risk. Other risk factors include overall immunosuppressive burden, particularly when lymphocyte-depleting antibodies are used for induction or anti-rejection therapy, and recipient factors such as age, co-morbidity and neutropenia. The risk of CMV also varies with the type of donated organ. Lung, heart–lung and small bowel recipients have the highest risk for CMV, whereas liver, pancreas and kidney recipients are at lower risk. This may be due to the intensity of immunosuppression, and/or the viral load present in the allograft.

Diagnosis

CMV diagnosis formerly relied upon tissue and shell-vial culture, but these methods are slow and relatively insensitive having now been superseded by more modern techniques. The pp65 antigenaemia assay is a semi-quantitative fluorescent assay based on detection of infected cells in peripheral blood and is more sensitive and specific than culture-based methods. Molecular tests to detect DNA or RNA are both qualitative and quantitative and very sensitive for detection of CMV. Measurement of quantitative CMV-DNA levels in plasma or whole blood is now widely used. In general, viral load correlates with the severity of infection, and, in addition to the absolute value, the rate of rise of viral load also predicts disease severity. Both the pp65 antigenemia assay and quantitative CMV viral load testing can be used in pre-emptive protocols to diagnose disease and guide therapy.

Prevention

The two commonly used strategies for CMV prevention are universal prophylaxis and pre-emptive therapy. Universal prophylaxis requires giving antiviral therapy either to all 'at-risk' patients or to a specified subset, beginning within 10 days of the transplant and continuing for a defined duration, usually 3 to 6 months. Using pre-emptive therapy, patients are monitored at regular intervals, generally weekly, for early evidence of CMV replication, and then treated with antiviral therapy to prevent symptomatic disease. Pre-emptive therapy may decrease drug costs and toxicity but requires a high level of coordination, frequent patient attendance and rapid access to test results. Prophylaxis theoretically prevents reactivation of other herpesviruses but is associated with higher drug costs, more drug toxicity and a higher risk of late-onset CMV disease, defined as disease occurring following discontinuation of prophylaxis. Late-onset disease may be missed due to late diagnosis in patients who are attending for less frequent follow-up, contributes to morbidity and has been shown to be associated with higher overall mortality. Both prophylactic and pre-emptive strategies are equally effective in preventing CMV disease but pre-emptive therapy may not reduce the indirect effects of CMV infection including bacterial and fungal infections and mortality. Prophylaxis reduces the incidence of opportunistic infection and CMV-related mortality, and may reduce the incidence of biopsy-proven acute rejection in kidney transplant recipients. It is not yet clear whether these benefits translate into better long-term graft survival.

Drugs that have been used for CMV prophylaxis include ganciclovir (oral and intravenous), valganciclovir, aciclovir, valaciclovir and immune globulin preparations. Valganciclovir is a valine ester pro-drug of ganciclovir with improved bioavailability compared with oral ganciclovir (60% versus 6%) and comparable efficacy for preventing CMV disease. Studies suggest that longer courses of prophylaxis (6 months or more) are associated with lower rates of viraemia and disease. In a trial comparing 200 versus 100 days of valganciclovir prophylaxis in over 300 D+/R− kidney transplant recipients, the incidence of confirmed CMV disease was 16% versus 37%, respectively [22]. Valaciclovir given for 90 days reduced the incidence of biopsy-proven acute rejection in CMV-seronegative kidney transplant recipients [23]. Aciclovir has less anti-CMV activity and is not recommended specifically for CMV prophylaxis. There are insufficient data to determine the benefit of adding immune globulin to current CMV prophylaxis regimens.

Treatment
Intravenous ganciclovir has long been regarded as the mainstay for CMV therapy, the typical treatment dose being 5 mg/kg twice daily. Optimal duration of therapy varies between 2 and 4 weeks. Oral valganciclovir (900 mg twice daily) achieves blood concentrations similar to intravenous ganciclovir and has similar efficacy for eradication of viraemia in patients with mild to moderate CMV infection. Intravenous ganciclovir is preferred for patients with severe infection or impaired gastrointestinal absorption. Due to its low bioavailability, oral ganciclovir is not recommended for CMV treatment because it is ineffective and may encourage the emergence of ganciclovir-resistant CMV strains. Molecular tests can be used to determine the optimal duration of antiviral therapy. There is a lower risk of relapse in patients without detectable CMV viraemia at the end of therapy, so treatment should generally continue until viraemia (measured either by antigenemia or nucleic acid testing) has dropped below the negative threshold value for a given test. With ultra-sensitive assays, this negative threshold value has not been well defined. After completion of treatment, a 1 to 3 month course of secondary prophylaxis may be considered depending on the clinical situation, although this approach lacks direct supportive evidence. Alternatively close clinical and/or virological follow-up after discontinuation of treatment is recommended.

Ganciclovir undergoes initial phosphorylation by a viral kinase encoded by the gene *UL97*, followed by tri-phosphorylation by cellular enzymes. The active drug inhibits CMV DNA polymerase encoded by the gene *UL54*. Mutations in *UL97* and less commonly in *UL54* can confer ganciclovir resistance and combined mutations often have high-level resistance. Alternative anti-CMV agents include foscarnet and cidofovir, both of which have significant nephrotoxicity. CMV isolates with *UL97* mutations may remain sensitive to foscarnet and cidofovir. The incidence of ganciclovir resistance is generally low, <3% with oral ganciclovir and <4% with valganciclovir [24]. Lung transplant recipients may have higher rates of resistance, and other risk factors include prolonged low-dose oral prophylaxis (e.g. with oral ganciclovir), D+/R− serostatus, and increased intensity of immunosuppression. Resistance should be suspected if the viral load fails to decrease or increases despite 2 weeks of adequately dosed antiviral therapy, particularly in the presence of other risk factors for resistance. Genetic resistance testing may aid recognition. Therapeutic options include increasing the dose of intravenous ganciclovir (up to 10 mg/kg twice daily), foscarnet (alone or in combination with low dose ganciclovir), or cidofovir. Immunosuppression should be reduced or discontinued if the infection is life-threatening.

Herpes simplex virus

Epidemiology, presentation and risk factors

Herpes simplex virus type-1 and -2 (HSV-1, HSV-2) are α-herpesviruses that establish latency in nerve root ganglia [25]. HSV-1 infection is acquired from early childhood and is highly seroprevalent in adults. HSV-2 is more often associated with genital herpes and has a lower seroprevalence, but nevertheless most transplant recipients are infected with HSV-1 or HSV-2, or both. Compared with immunocompetent individuals, transplant recipients have more frequent and more severe clinical manifestations of HSV. Mostly this is due to reactivation of previously acquired virus, particularly early after transplantation and in the setting of anti-rejection therapy. The most common clinical presentation is orolabial, genital or perianal disease. Lesions may be vesicular and/or ulcerative and may extend locally. Rarely, visceral or disseminated disease may occur, including disseminated cutaneous disease, oesophagitis, hepatitis and pneumonitis.

Diagnosis

The diagnosis of HSV is usually clinical, but laboratory confirmation may be required. Direct fluorescent antibody testing of mucocutaneous lesions, bronchoalveolar lavage and other samples provides rapid results. HSV grows well in tissue culture, but molecular tests such as PCR assays are more sensitive and are becoming the diagnostic test of choice particularly for identifying HSV in blood or other sterile fluids, as viral cultures rarely are positive from these samples. Serologic testing is rarely useful for diagnosing acute infections as most patients will be HSV seropositive.

Prevention and treatment

Antiviral prophylaxis to prevent CMV reactivation will also prevent HSV reactivation. For patients treated with anti-lymphocyte antibodies and not receiving anti-CMV prophylaxis some centres would adopt anti-human herpes virus prophylaxis with aciclovir or valaciclovir. In patients who experience frequent clinical recurrences antiviral therapy can safely be continued, even for many years, and is associated with less frequent aciclovir resistance than intermittent therapy. Disseminated, visceral or extensive cutaneous or mucosal HSV disease should be treated with intravenous aciclovir at a dose of 5–10 mg/kg every 8 hours. Reduction in immunosuppression should be considered for life-threatening HSV disease. More limited mucocutaneous disease can be treated with oral aciclovir or valaciclovir. Therapy should be continued until complete healing of the lesions.

Varicella zoster virus

Epidemiology, presentation and risk factors
VZV is a human α-herpesvirus that is ubiquitous and highly infectious [26]. Primary infection causes acute varicella or 'chickenpox', usually from direct contact with a skin lesion or through airborne spread from respiratory droplets. After initial infection, VZV establishes life-long latency in cranial nerve and dorsal root ganglia, and can reactivate years or decades later as herpes zoster or 'shingles'. Seroprevalance is almost universal, as most adults acquire the disease in childhood, and most children and young adults have been vaccinated with the live virus vaccine.

Primary varicella typically presents with fever, malaise and a vesicular rash across the trunk and face. Mucosal involvement can occur but there is relative sparing of the hands and soles of the feet. The illness is usually self-limiting and resolves within 7–10 days, but in rare cases progresses to more severe disease, visceral invasion, and rare but life-threatening complications, such as hepatitis, pancreatitis, pneumonitis and encephalitis. Varicella is rare in adult transplant recipients, but can be devastating, with visceral involvement, severe skin disease, and disseminated intravascular coagulation (Fig. 21.3). Herpes zoster presents with vesicular lesions in a characteristic dermatomal distribution. Pain is a common prodrome to the development of lesions. Herpes zoster is very common in the general population, and is estimated to occur in up to 20% of individuals during their lifetime. Secondary complications include bacterial superinfection and postherpetic neuralgia. Herpes zoster is also very common in transplant recipients, occurring in approximately 10% during the first 4 years. Invasive disease and dissemination similar to that seen in primary varicella infection has been reported and may be more likely with more intense immunosuppression.

Seronegative transplant recipients are at risk for primary varicella, which is almost always community-acquired rather than donor-derived. Patients with previous varicella disease or vaccination are at risk for the development of herpes zoster, and other risk factors include increasing age, heart and lung transplant recipients and the use of mycophenolate mofetil (MMF).

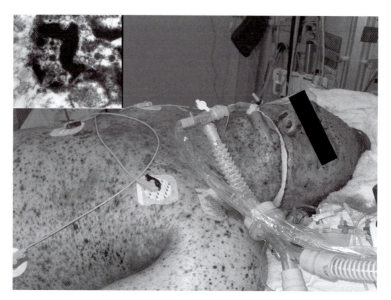

Figure 21.3 A transplant recipient with the severe primary varicella infection showing the characteristic skin eruption with associated respiratory failure, hepatic failure and disseminated intravascular coagulation. Insert: electron microscopy on liver tissue reveals viral nucleocapsids, typical of herpesviruses, associated with marginated chromatin. (A full colour version of this figure appears in the colour plate section.)

Diagnosis and treatment

The clinical presentations are so typical that diagnosis is generally clinical. Definitive laboratory testing can be used for atypical presentations and suspected disseminated or visceral disease. PCR is a sensitive test to detect VZV in vesicle fluid, serum, spinal fluid and other tissues. Other rapid and reliable methods for diagnosis include immunohistochemistry performed on scrapings taken from the base of skin lesions. Viral culture is slow and less sensitive and serologic testing can be unreliable and should not be used for diagnosis.

Patients with primary varicella are at risk of severe disease and should be treated early, within 24 hours of the onset of the rash, with intravenous aciclovir. Reduction in immunosuppression should be considered although steroid dosing should be maintained or even boosted to maintain an appropriate stress response. IVIG and VZV immunoglobulin are of no added value in established disease, although IVIG may be of use in severe early disease.

Patients with localised herpes zoster can be treated with oral aciclovir or valaciclovir as an outpatient with close monitoring. However, reactivation within the trigeminal ganglion (herpes zoster ophthalmicus) may be sight-threatening, and involvement of the geniculate ganglion (Ramsay Hunt syndrome) can lead to facial palsy, and these patients should preferably receive intravenous aciclovir therapy, and, in the case of trigeminal involvement, prompt ophthalmologic review. Disseminated or visceral disease should be treated as primary varicella with intravenous aciclovir.

Prevention

Many current prophylactic regimens against CMV will prevent VZV reactivation, but because the risk of reactivation is life-long for most transplant recipients, the use of routine or long-term VZV prophylaxis is not indicated. Seronegative patients should be offered varicella vaccination pre-transplantation provided there are no contraindications. Live vaccines are generally contraindicated in immunocompromised patients, so vaccination should be completed at least 2–4 weeks prior to transplant and is not recommended post-transplant.

Seronegative transplant recipients should receive post-exposure prophylaxis after significant contact with a person with active varicella or herpes zoster. Significant contact includes continuous household or social contact, hospital contact in adjacent beds or prolonged contact with an infectious patient. Options for post-exposure prophylaxis include passive immunoprophylaxis with varicella zoster immune globulin (VZIG) and/or antiviral therapy. VZIG should be given as soon as possible, within 96 hours of exposure, and does not prevent clinical varicella but lessens disease severity. Non-specific IVIG can be given as an alternative if VZIG is not available. Antiviral agents may be given as adjunctive therapy in patients receiving immunoprophylaxis or in patients who were unable to receive immunoprophylaxis within 96 hours of exposure. Oral aciclovir or valaciclovir should be given for 7 days beginning 7 to 10 days after exposure.

All patients admitted to hospital with varicella or herpes zoster should be placed in isolation, and seronegative close contacts that are immunocompetent should be immunised within 3 to 5 days of exposure or given appropriate VZV prophylaxis. Patients should be isolated until all lesions are crusted and patients with localised zoster should keep the lesions covered to decrease transmission risk.

Epstein–Barr virus and post-transplant lymphoproliferative disease

Epidemiology, presentation and risk factors

In developing countries infection with EBV is almost universal in early childhood, whereas in developed countries acquisition may be delayed until later life. In immunocompetent individuals, EBV is acquired through exposure to infected body fluids such as saliva, but in transplant recipients EBV may also be transmitted from the seropositive donor organ. The median onset of primary EBV infection is 6 weeks after transplantation and reactivation of latent EBV is most often seen in the first 2 to 3 months.

The spectrum of presentation of EBV infection ranges from uncomplicated infectious mononucleosis to aggressive PTLD, a much-feared and life-threatening complication of organ transplantation.

Infectious mononucleosis may present with fever, malaise, exudative pharyngitis, lymphadenopathy, hepatosplenomegaly and atypical lymphocytosis. Other non-PTLD manifestations of EBV infection include hepatitis, pneumonitis, gastrointestinal symptoms and haematological manifestations such as leucopenia, thrombocytopenia and haemolytic anaemia, some of which may be difficult to differentiate from PTLD. Patients with PTLD may be asymptomatic or may present with symptoms such as weight loss, fever, night sweats, sore throat, malaise, anorexia, gastrointestinal symptoms or headache. Clinical signs may include lymphadenopathy, hepatosplenomegaly, tonsillar enlargement, focal neurological signs or signs of bowel perforation. Disease may be nodal or extranodal, localised (often to the allograft) or widely disseminated. Some patients with PTLD may be anaemic, usually normochromic, normocytic but occasionally related to occult gastrointestinal bleeding causing iron-deficiency anaemia with hypochromia and microcytosis. Depending on organ involvement there may be disturbance in serum electrolytes, liver and kidney function tests. Elevations in serum uric acid and lactate dehydrogenase are relatively common.

The highest incidence of PTLD is seen in the first year post-transplant, but this represents only 20% of the total cumulative 10-year PTLD burden [27]. The overwhelming risk factor for PTLD is primary EBV infection; EBV genes are detectable in more than 90% of early (within the first year) PTLD cases. The underlying pathogenesis relates to the ability of EBV to transform and immortalise B lymphocytes, combined with the impact of immunosuppression on EBV-specific cytotoxic T lymphocytes (CTLs) that normally control the proliferative response. Another key risk factor is the type of transplant; small bowel transplant recipients are at the highest risk (up to 32%), recipients of pancreas, heart, lung and liver transplants are at moderate risk (3 to 12%) and kidney transplant recipients are at relatively low risk (1 to 2%) [28]. Younger recipient age, CMV infection and immunosuppression with depleting antibodies are additional risk factors for early PTLD, whereas risk factors for late PTLD are older donor age and longer duration of immunosuppression. A significant proportion (around one-third) of late-onset PTLD is EBV-negative, non-B-cell and phenotypically monomorphic.

Diagnosis, classification and staging

In immunocompetent patients, primary EBV infection or reactivation can be confirmed by measuring IgM and IgG antibody titres against viral capsid antigen (VCA), early antigen (EA) and Epstein–Barr nuclear antigen (EBNA). Anti-VCA and anti-EBNA IgG in the absence of IgM denotes latent EBV infection. Anti-VCA IgM followed by a rise in VCA-IgG denotes primary EBV infection. In a patient with previous latent infection, anti-VCA IgM denotes EBV reactivation. Persistence of anti-EA antibodies is more likely in PTLD, and previously seropositive patients with PTLD may have falling anti-EBNA titres in the setting of elevated EBV loads. However, serology is unreliable as a diagnostic tool in immunocompromised patients due to diminished humoral responses, and in patients receiving blood products due to passive transfer of antibody. The most important role for EBV serology in the context of transplantation is to determine pre-transplant donor and recipient EBV serostatus to assess PTLD risk.

EBV-DNA titres provide a guide to the net state of immunosuppression, and surveillance by PCR may be undertaken in high-risk individuals (children and seronegative adults). However, the sensitivity and specificity of quantitative EBV viral load for the diagnosis of early PTLD and symptomatic EBV infection remains unclear. In high-risk recipients, EBV viral load surveillance has good sensitivity for detecting EBV-positive PTLD but poor specificity, and might lead to significant unnecessary investigation. However, an elevated viral load would be of concern in patients with suggestive symptoms. In low-risk recipients with suggestive symptoms, EBV viral load lacks sensitivity, missing all cases of EBV-negative PTLD and some cases of localised EBV-positive PTLD, but is highly specific for EBV-positive PTLD. Measuring EBV-specific T-cell responses using Elispot and tetramer assays may improve the specificity of viral load to predict PTLD but is complex, costly and difficult to implement in a routine diagnostic laboratory.

Total body (head, neck, chest, abdomen and pelvis) CT is routinely used in the initial assessment of PTLD, but thereafter the choice of tests depends largely on the suspected site. Suspected intra-abdominal lesions may be evaluated with endoscopy, particularly where there are gastrointestinal symptoms such as bleeding, diarrhoea and weight loss. Positron emission tomography–CT (PET–CT) is emerging as a useful test in the evaluation of PTLD. Histopathology remains the gold standard for diagnosis but should be interpreted by a pathologist familiar with the histopathological features. Table 21.3 shows the World Health Organization (WHO) histopathological classification of PTLD [29]. Additional diagnostic tests may include a bone scan, bone marrow biopsy and a lumbar puncture to assist in ruling out bone, bone marrow and CNS disease, respectively. There is no current staging system for PTLD but, at the very minimum, staging should document the presence or absence of symptoms, the precise location of lesions, whether the allograft is involved and whether there is CNS involvement.

Treatment

Optimal management requires a multidisciplinary approach involving appropriately experienced transplant physicians, haemato-oncologists, histopathologists and radiologists. In most cases treatment requires a stepwise approach, starting with reduction in immunosuppression and introducing further therapeutic interventions based on clinical response and the histopathological characteristics of the PTLD (30). Reduction or cessation of immunosuppression may result in regression of PTLD lesions in up to 90% of low-risk cases, but there is considerable variation

Table 21.3 WHO histopathological classification of PTLD [29].

Categories of post-transplant lymphoproliferative disorder (PTLD)	
Early lesions	Plasmacytic hyperplasia
	Infectious mononucleosis-like lesion
Polymorphic PTLD	
Monomorphic PTLD	Classify according to lymphoma they resemble
B-cell neoplasms	Diffuse large B-cell lymphoma
	Burkitt lymphoma
	Plasma cell myeloma
	Plasmacytoma-like lesion
	Other
T-cell neoplasms	Peripheral T-cell lymphoma, not otherwise specified
	Hepatosplenic T-cell lymphoma
	Other
Classical Hodgkin lymphoma-type PTLD	

in the rate and degree of immunosuppressive dose reduction appropriate for each individual depending on the risk of rejection and the availability of alternative methods of support, nor is it clear how long to wait before escalating therapy. Nevertheless, in most cases there should be a clinical response to immunosuppressive dose reduction within 2 to 4 weeks. Complete or partial surgical resection and/or local radiotherapy may be adjuncts to immunosuppression reduction, and in localised disease may result in long-term remission. Surgery is essential for the management of specific complications such as gastrointestinal haemorrhage or perforation and local radiotherapy may be indicated in the treatment of CNS lesions. There is no evidence to support the use of antiviral agents such as aciclovir and ganciclovir in the absence of other interventions. There is increasing evidence to support the use of the anti-CD20 monoclonal antibody rituximab as the next step in treatment of PTLD after reduction in immunosuppression, although data from controlled clinical trials are lacking. The subset of patients most likely to benefit has not been clearly defined, although identification of CD20 markers in the PTLD tissue is necessary. In addition, the optimal timing and duration of rituximab therapy are unclear. Adverse events include tumor lysis syndrome and prolonged B-cell depletion. Bowel perforation at the PTLD site may occur during the recovery phase.

Anthracycline-based chemotherapy is not usually indicated as first-line treatment for early EBV-positive B-cell PTLD but should be considered in the setting of late-onset monomorphic PTLD, in EBV-negative, T-cell or CNS PTLD as well as in patients refractory to more conservative approaches. Initial response rates of approximately 70–80% have been observed, with relapse rates of approximately 20% [30]. Promising data are emerging on the use of chemotherapy with and without rituximab, with response rates between 65 and 100% [31]. In patients who achieve PTLD remission there is a risk of future allograft rejection, as the optimal management of immunosuppression during remission remains undefined.

Alternative treatment options include adoptive immunotherapy using EBV-specific CTL clones derived either from the donor or from a HLA-matched third-party. The utility of this approach is limited by the cost and time required to clone cell lines, and this strategy may not be feasible for transplant centres with low rates of PTLD.

Prevention

It is important to identify patients at high-risk for PTLD development by determining EBV serostatus prior to transplantation. Patients at risk of primary CMV infection or those receiving depleting anti-lymphocyte antibodies for induction or treatment of rejection represent a particularly vulnerable subgroup of recipients who should be monitored carefully for suggestive clinical symptoms or signs. Wherever appropriate, immunosuppression should be minimised and aggressive immunosuppression should be reserved for biopsy-proven acute rejection. Antiviral agents such as aciclovir and ganciclovir have been used as prophylactic agents to prevent PTLD, particularly in high-risk patients (EBV D+R−), but with limited supportive data. There may be indirect benefit by eliminating other viral infections that act as co-factors in the lymphoproliferative process. The role of the passive administration of EBV-neutralising antibodies (via IVIG) is unclear.

There are data to support quantitative EBV viral load surveillance for PTLD prevention in high-risk but not low-risk populations. High-risk patients require frequent sampling, ideally weekly during the high-risk period, because EBV viral load doubling times may be as short as 48 hours. However, the natural history of EBV viral load in transplant recipients in the absence of intervention is unknown and there are no clear thresholds at which pre-emptive intervention should be initiated. Pre-emptive strategies most commonly include reduction of immunosuppression, with or without addition of antiviral agents. More aggressive interventions involving low-dose rituximab and adoptive immunotherapy have been used in hematopoietic stem cell transplant recipients, but there are limited data regarding these interventions in the solid-organ transplant setting.

Other human herpesviruses: HHV-6 and HHV-7

Epidemiology, presentation and risk factors
Human herpesvirus 6 (HHV-6) and HHV-7 are lymphotropic β-herpesviruses that infect the majority of individuals during the first few years of life. Primary infection may be asymptomatic or present as a febrile illness associated with a rash, diarrhoea, respiratory symptoms

or seizures. Like other herpesviruses, HHV-6 and HHV-7 infections take up life-long latency in mononuclear cells, which may then be reservoirs for endogenous viral reactivation or transmission to organ recipients. As seropositivity for HHV-6 and HHV-7 is almost universal in adults, most post-transplant infections are due to reactivation of latent virus. Paediatric transplant recipients, especially those younger than 2 years of age, may be HHV-6 and HHV-7 seronegative and therefore are at risk of donor-allograft transmitted infection.

Estimated rates of post-transplant HHV-6 and HHV-7 infection vary between 20 and 55% [32]. Reactivation occurs within the first 2 to 4 weeks and is almost always subclinical. In less than 1% of cases, HHV-6 may manifest as a febrile syndrome accompanied by a degree of bone marrow suppression, an illness similar to CMV syndrome and often therefore attributed to CMV. Symptomatic disease due to HHV-7 is even less common. More importantly HHV-6 and HHV-7 may have indirect immunomodulatory effects and have been associated with CMV disease, fungal and other opportunistic infections.

Risk factors for HHV-6 and HHV-7 infection are not completely defined but intensity of immunosuppression is likely to be important, particularly when powerful lymphocyte-depleting agents such as muromunab-CD3 (OKT3) and alemtuzumab are used. Primary infections, presumably of donor origin, may occur in seronegative transplant recipients, and a few fatalities have been reported.

Diagnosis and treatment

The usefulness of serology as a diagnostic test is limited by the high seroprevalence of HHV-6 and HHV-7 in adults. The preferred method is detection by PCR in peripheral blood mononuclear cells, serum or plasma. Because of the low rate of clinical disease and the high rate of subclinical reactivation, routine monitoring is not recommended, nor is treatment usually required. In the setting of HHV-6 encephalitis or other clinical syndromes attributable to HHV-6 foscarnet, ganciclovir and cidofovir have been used clinically, based on in vitro data and anecdotal clinical reports, together with a reduction in immunosuppression.

Other human herpesviruses: HHV-8

Epidemiology, presentation and risk factors

Human herpesvirus 8 (HHV-8) is a γ-herpesvirus that infects CD19+ B cells and endothelial-derived spindle cells in Kaposi's sarcoma (KS) lesions. Unlike most herpes viruses HHV-8 is not ubiquitous. Seroprevalence is low (0 to 5%) in North America, northern Europe and Asia, moderate (5 to 20%) in the Mediterranean and Middle East and high (>50%) in parts of Africa [33]. The incidence of active post-transplant HHV-8, which may occur either as primary infection acquired from the allograft or as secondary reactivation of latent virus, reflects the geographic distribution. Hence, the incidence of KS after transplantation ranges from as low as 0.5% among transplant recipients in North America, Asia and northern Europe to as high as 28% among HHV-8-seropositive transplant recipients from the Middle East.

HHV-8 infection in immunocompetent individuals is associated with mild nonspecific symptoms of diarrhoea, fatigue, rash and lymphadenopathy, and results in the generation of CTLs that control HHV-8 replication and prevent its progression to neoplastic disease. In immunosuppressed individuals CTL activity is attenuated and HHV-8 may then be associated with neoplastic disease, particularly KS, a multicentric neoplasm of lymphatic endothelium-derived cells, which presents clinically as multifocal progressive mucocutaneous lesions which may disseminate to the viscera, including the allograft. Other less common neoplastic manifestations of HHV-8 include primary effusion lymphoma and Castleman's disease. HHV-8 may also cause fever, bone marrow suppression, and clonal gammopathy in transplant recipients. The median time to onset of KS is 30 months after transplantation, although it may occur as early as 3 months or as late as 10 years after transplantation. There may be earlier onset in liver (approximately 10 months) compared with kidney (34 months) recipients.

Risk factors for HHV-8-associated disease, specifically KS, include residence in an endemic area, intensity of immunosuppression, use of anti-lymphocyte antibodies and calcineurin inhibitors, older age and male gender.

Diagnosis, treatment and prevention

Serological methods have limited utility in diagnosing acute HHV-8 infection in transplant recipients, although pre-transplant donor and recipient screening may help stratify risk, especially in high-risk populations in areas where the virus is endemic. For high-risk individuals there may be benefit in using PCR to detect HHV-8 replication and predict the subsequent development of KS or to monitor patients with KS to assess response to therapy. Immunohistochemistry using monoclonal antibodies against HHV-8 is useful for the histopathological diagnosis of KS.

First-line therapy for the treatment of KS should be cautious reduction or cessation of immunosuppression. Conversion from calcineurin inhibitors to the mTOR inhibitor sirolimus should be considered, as sirolimus has antiproliferative properties that are useful in the treatment of KS, and conversion to sirolimus has been widely reported as leading to regression of KS lesions. Those patients whose lesions do not regress may require surgical excision, radiotherapy or cytotoxic chemotherapy. HHV-8 is sensitive to ganciclovir, foscarnet and cidofovir, but the added benefits of antiviral therapy for treatment or prophylaxis are unknown. Avoidance of over-immunosuppression in high-risk individuals and in those with detectable HHV-8 viraemia is recommended. Sirolimus use may confer a lower risk of KS, although KS has also been observed in sirolimus-treated patients.

Polyomavirus: BK and JC

Epidemiology, risk factors and presentation

Polyomaviruses are widespread among vertebrates and are species specific. It is likely that human polyomaviruses co-evolved with their hosts, accounting for their high prevalence, low morbidity, long latency and symptomless reactivation. Only two polyomavirus strains are known to be pathogenic in humans, polyomavirus hominis 1 (BK) and polyomavirus hominis 2 (JC), named with the initials of the patients from whom they were first isolated. These viruses cause disease only in immunocompromised patients, BK virus manifesting as a viral nephropathy, haemorrhagic cystitis or ureteral stenosis, and JC virus as a viral encephalopathy. Primary BK virus infection occurs during childhood, resulting in almost universal seropositivity worldwide. After infection, the virus persists in the genitourinary tract. Asymptomatic viral shedding into urine is relatively common, particularly in old age, pregnancy, diabetes mellitus or immunosuppression in association with transplantation or HIV infection.

During the past 15 years, polyomavirus-associated nephropathy (PVAN) has emerged as an important cause of allograft failure following kidney transplantation. BK is the most important virus associated with this condition, although rare cases of JC virus or SV40-associated nephropathy have been reported. The precise reason for the recent emergence of this condition is unclear, but may reflect increasing use of newer and more potent immunosuppressive agents. Additional risk factors for PVAN include donor BK virus seropositivity with recipient seronegativity (especially in children), HLA mismatch, allograft injury, acute rejection and to some extent, specific immunosuppressive medications (tacrolimus, mycophenolate mofetil, prednisone and polyclonal anti-lymphocyte induction). Although BK virus seronegativity is a risk factor for disease, the presence of BK-specific antibody does not appear to prevent or modify PVAN.

PVAN classically presents as allograft dysfunction with an asymptomatic rise in serum creatinine between 10 and 13 months post-transplant. The diagnosis of PVAN is difficult as there are no specific symptoms.

Diagnosis, treatment and prevention

Urinary shedding of 'decoy cells', tubuloepithelial cells with ground-glass intranuclear inclusions identified by Papanicolaou staining of urinary sediment, marks the onset of viral replication, and precedes the development of BK viraemia by a median of 4 weeks and biopsy-proven PVAN by a median of 12 weeks. DNA PCR quantification of viruria or viraemia may be used as alternative methods of screening [34]. All of these assays are highly sensitive (100%), but not highly specific (70–90%) for PVAN, as not all viruric or viraemic patients have biopsy-proven disease. It is not therefore possible to confirm the diagnosis of PVAN without a biopsy, but the absence of viruria or viraemia permit the diagnosis to be excluded with confidence. The 'gold standard' for diagnosing PVAN remains kidney biopsy, with demonstration of polyomavirus cytopathic changes, and the use of immunohistochemical staining to confirm the presence of the polyomavirus antigen. However, the histopathological changes are not pathognomonic, can be mistaken for allograft rejection, are focal and may be missed. A grading system has been proposed, which correlates biopsy findings with outcome [35].

The mainstay of therapy for PVAN is prompt immunosuppressive dose reduction, which, in conjunction with careful monitoring for BK viraemia, can forestall progression to overt PVAN and graft loss. There are very few systematic studies on the outcome of immunosuppressive dose reduction. It is not clear whether the reduction or elimination of antimetabolites is more effective than the reduction of calcineurin inhibitors. Tacrolimus trough concentrations are commonly targeted to <6 ng/mL, ciclosporin trough concentrations to <150 ng/mL, sirolimus trough concentrations to <6 ng/mL, and mycophenolate mofetil daily dose equivalents to ≤1000 mg. Even further reduction may be appropriate in individual patients. Recent studies suggest that even lower calcineurin inhibitor concentrations, targeting trough concentrations for tacrolimus of 3 ng/mL and ciclosporin of 100 ng/mL, may be considered as a first step [36]. Although early reduction of immunosuppression may be very effective, in all cases clinicians must balance the risk of graft injury due to recurrent rejection against that due to PVAN. As yet, no antiviral drug with proven efficacy against the BK virus has been licensed, but owing to strong clinical demand, a number of drugs such as low-dose cidofovir, leflunomide, intravenous immunoglobulin and fluoroquinolones have been explored in small case series [37]. However, there are no randomised controlled trials to show that adjunctive use of antiviral agents is superior to timely reduction in immunosuppression. Serial determinations of the level of viraemia have been shown to be effective in monitoring resolution of the disease.

The treatment of concurrent PVAN and allograft rejection is challenging. Some authorities will continue to taper immunosuppression notwithstanding rejection. Others recommend treating with a 'pulse' of corticosteroids followed by continued tapering of immunosuppression. Retransplantation after graft loss from PVAN is generally successful. It is unclear whether allograft nephrectomy is required, although this may be prudent if BK virus replication is ongoing.

Hepatitis B virus

Epidemiology and risk factors
With modern infection control practice and the implementation of widespread vaccination, the prevalence of chronic HBV infection in patients with dialysis-dependent kidney failure has declined in developed countries, ranging between 0 and 7% [38]. Although dialysis-associated outbreaks continue to be reported, acquisition of HBV through dialysis is now uncommon, and more likely to be attributed to standard risk factors

such as vertical transmission, intravenous drug use and sexual transmission. The prevalence of chronic HBV in kidney transplant candidates thus mirrors the population prevalence. Fewer than 5% of infected immunocompetent adults fail to clear HBV infection and become chronically infected, but this is more likely in uraemic patients, the very young and the elderly. With the introduction of effective antiviral agents such as nucleos(t)ide analogues, hepatitis B surface antigen (HBsAg)-positive kidney transplant recipients have demonstrated excellent outcomes, thus chronic hepatitis B infection is no longer a contraindication for transplantation. Patients with resolved HBV infection carry a low risk (<5%) of HBV reactivation, although when this does occur it may be rapidly fatal.

Diagnosis and treatment

The diagnosis of HBV relies on the same serological and virological assays used in the non-transplant population. HBsAg is detectable in serum during acute HBV infection and disappears when the infection resolves. Persistence for more than 6 months indicates chronic infection, with a low likelihood of spontaneous resolution. Hepatitis B core antigen (HBcAg) is a marker of viral replication found in hepatocytes that does not circulate in serum. Corresponding antibodies (HBcAb) appear during acute HBV infection, initially as an IgM antibody that indicates current or recent HBV infection. After 6 months this disappears, but anti-HBc IgG persists indefinitely as a marker of previous HBV exposure. Successful resolution of HBV infection is associated with protective antibody against HBsAg (HBsAb) and this signifies immunity against HBV. Additional markers that are of value are HBV DNA and hepatitis e antigen (HBeAg), both of which indicate active viral replication and potential infectivity.

Initial screening for HBV should be done at the time of transplant assessment and should include HBsAg, HBsAb and HBcAb. All patients with chronic HBV on antiviral therapy should undergo liver enzyme and HBV DNA monitoring every 3 to 6 months and HBsAg testing annually. As in the non-transplant population, HBsAg-positive patients should have an abdominal ultrasound (or CT/MRI if visualisation of the liver is inadequate) and alpha-fetoprotein for surveillance of hepatocellular carcinoma every 6 months.

HBV recurrence after transplantation is typically defined as the reappearance of HBsAg, generally in association with detectable HBV DNA in blood, although viraemia may occur in the absence of antigenaemia and both occur prior to biochemical or histopathological changes. If HBV recurs on appropriate prophylaxis, either noncompliance or drug resistance should be suspected. Pre-transplant treatment with antiviral therapy, particularly if HBV DNA can be rendered undetectable, reduces the risk of recurrence. For post-transplant recurrence despite prophylaxis, oral antiviral therapy should be adjusted based on the results of resistance testing. Lamivudine, telbivudine and adefovir are associated with higher long-term resistance rates and more potent antiviral agents such as entecavir and tenofovir are likely to replace these older agents.

Prevention and prophylaxis

HBV-uninfected transplant candidates who are non-immune should be vaccinated for HBV as early as possible, although in those with end-stage kidney disease only 55 to 65% develop a protective antibody response, even with double-dose regimens. Transplant recipients with chronic HBV who are not already on antiviral therapy should commence this at the time of transplantation to prevent reactivation, and this should continue indefinitely. The only well-studied agent in the setting of kidney transplantation is lamivudine. Given the high risk of resistance (approximately 70% at 5 years), the need for life-long therapy and the risk of a severe flare in an immunocompromised host if resistance develops, consideration should be given to choosing a more potent antiviral such as entecavir or tenofovir to limit the potential for resistance, particularly in those with high viral load or advanced fibrosis.

Patients with markers of previous HBV infection (HBcAb-positive and/or HBsAb-positive) carry a low risk of HBV reactivation, but antiviral prophylaxis may be offered in order to further limit this risk. Alternatively, recipients should undergo surveillance every 1 to 3 months for HBsAg, HBV DNA and liver enzyme transaminase levels, antiviral therapy being initiated at the onset of HBsAg positivity or if HBV DNA progressively rises.

Hepatitis-B-positive donors

HBV-uninfected non-immune transplant recipients may acquire HBV from the donor organ. HBsAg-positive donors confer a high risk of transmission, although satisfactory outcomes have been described with prophylaxis [39]. Recipients of an organ from such a donor, regardless of immune status, should receive combined prophylaxis with hepatitis B immune globulin (HBIG) and a nucleos(t)ide analogue. The optimal duration of prophylaxis is unknown, but it is recommended that the nucleos(t)ide analogue should continue indefinitely. Recipients of such organs should also undergo surveillance at least every 3 months with liver enzymes, HBsAg, and HBV DNA If these remain negative, consideration may be given to discontinuing HBIG 6 to 12 months post-transplant.

With efforts to expand the donor pool, HBcAb-positive, HBsAg-negative donors have been increasingly used. In liver transplantation, without prophylaxis the rate of HBV transmission from these donors is high, but in non-hepatic transplantation, HBcAb-positive donors confer a low (<5%) risk of transmission, and organs from these donors could be used with informed consent and appropriate prophylaxis. If the recipient is HBV-immune the risk of transmission is essentially eliminated and no prophylaxis is needed. Non-immune recipients should initially have prophylaxis with lamivudine or other antiviral therapy or HBIG. If the donor HBV DNA is positive or unknown, prophylaxis should be continued with HBIG for at least 3 to 6 months or lamivudine for at least

12 months. If the donor is HBV-DNA-negative, prophylaxis can be discontinued, but routine monitoring should continue with liver enzymes, HBsAg and HBV DNA every 3 months for at least 12 months post-transplant.

Infection control issues

The hepatitis B vaccine provides good protection against infection affording a 70% reduction in the risk of new hepatitis B infections in fully vaccinated patients [40]. All household and sexual contacts of HBV-infected recipients should be vaccinated and have documentation of seroconversion. HBV-infected recipients should not share razorblades, toothbrushes or other personal items that may be contaminated with even small amounts of blood.

Hepatitis C virus

Epidemiology and risk factors

HCV is now a far bigger problem in UK dialysis units than HBV since it is the most prevalent bloodborne virus in the community and there is currently no vaccine. Nevertheless, with scrupulous attention to infection control practices and screening of blood products, the transmission of HCV in dialysis units has declined, but the prevalence in UK dialysis units still ranges between 4 and 14% [41]. Among kidney transplant recipients the rate of progression of HCV-related liver fibrosis is accelerated in comparison to immunocompetent individuals, and this impacts adversely on both patient and graft survival. There is in addition an increased risk of post-transplant diabetes, graft dysfunction and proteinuria. Overall, however, survival is improved compared to remaining on dialysis and poor outcomes primarily occur in those with advanced fibrosis or cirrhosis at the time of transplant. Recipients with mild to moderate liver disease at baseline have a lower risk of progression.

Diagnosis and treatment

The diagnosis of HCV infection requires the same serological and virological investigations as in the non-transplant population. Initial screening for antibody to HCV should be performed pre-transplant and in seropositive patients qualitative HCV RNA should be measured to confirm current infection. The HCV genotype should be determined in any patient who is a potential candidate for HCV therapy. HCV viral load is an important factor in determining the probability of response to interferon-based therapy, but does not indicate disease severity nor the likelihood of disease progression. Abdominal ultrasound should be requested to identify complications of HCV-related liver disease such as ascites, portal hypertension and hepatocellular carcinoma. For chronic HCV infection, liver biopsy remains the 'gold standard' for assessing the degree of hepatic inflammation and fibrosis, in order to determine prognosis and to guide decisions about antiviral therapy and transplant eligibility. However, new dynamic tests such as liver fibroscan are currently undergoing evaluation.

Pre-transplant treatment of HCV has a beneficial effect on post-transplant outcomes but is associated with lower rates of sustained viral response and a higher rate of adverse events than in the general population. With standard interferon monotherapy the overall sustained viral response rate is 37% and ranges from 13 to 75% with pegylated-interferon [42]. Ribavirin remains contraindicated in patients with reduced kidney function (GFR <50 mL/min). It is currently recommended that patients with chronic HCV without advanced liver fibrosis may be listed for transplant but that interferon-based therapy should be considered prior to transplant. Those with bridging fibrosis or compensated cirrhosis should undergo interferon-based therapy and may be listed for transplant if a sustained viral response is achieved. Those with decompensated cirrhosis are generally not suitable for an isolated kidney transplant but may be considered for a combined liver and kidney transplant. HCV treatment after transplantation is generally contraindicated due to the risk of acute allograft rejection with interferon. However, this should be considered on a case-by-case basis in those with severe disease.

Transplantation of an HCV-positive organ into an HCV-negative recipient results in near universal transmission, and HCV thus acquired may have a particularly aggressive course with a high risk of death from infectious complications and fulminant hepatitis. Transplanting HCV-positive organs into HCV-negative recipients should therefore be avoided, with the possible exception of critically ill patients awaiting a life-sustaining transplant with informed consent.

Infection control issues
As with HBV, patients with HCV should not share personal items that may be contaminated with even small amounts of blood.

Human immunodeficiency virus

Epidemiology
Since the introduction of highly active antiretroviral therapy (HAART) in 1996, mortality in patients with HIV infection has decreased markedly. As a result, morbidity from other chronic conditions such as kidney, liver and heart disease is increasing. Patients with HIV are at particular risk for development of chronic kidney disease, most notably HIV-associated nephropathy (HIVAN), which is the third most common cause of end-stage kidney disease in Black individuals aged 20–64 years in the USA. The presence of HIV was historically regarded as a contraindication to transplantation because of concern regarding the potential worsening of HIV disease and increased risk of opportunistic infection by immunosuppression. However, current data suggest that transplant recipients with optimal control of HIV do as well in the short term as those without HIV, provided there is proper donor selection and

recipient management [43]. There have been no AIDS defining occurrences in transplant recipients with HIV using standard prophylaxis against opportunistic infections. As with non-HIV-infected individuals, survival for patients with end-stage kidney disease and HIV is better after transplantation than on maintenance haemodialysis.

Risk factors

All potential kidney transplant recipients should be tested for HIV regardless of risk factors. To limit the potential impact of HIV on transplant outcomes, patients should have well-controlled HIV infection before transplantation. Suggested criteria include a CD4+ T-cell count above 200 cells/μL for at least 6 months, and an undetectable viral load on a stable antiretroviral regimen for at least 3 months. A history of opportunistic infection or malignancy is no longer a contraindication to transplantation, other than in patients in whom the infection or malignancy is ongoing or untreatable (e.g. progressive multifocal leukoencephalopathy or chronic intestinal cryptosporidiosis). There remains ongoing prohibition of the use of HIV-infected organ donors.

Following kidney transplantation, inferior allograft survival is seen in recipients of older donor organs, those with delayed graft function and those with prolonged cold ischaemia [44]. Significantly increased rejection rates (two- to threefold) are seen, perhaps due to immune system dysregulation, or possibly to inadequate immunosuppression due to pharmacokinetic interactions with antiretroviral agents [45]. The administration of antithymocyte globulin either for induction or treatment of rejection has been associated with prolonged declines in CD4+ T-cell counts, loss of antiviral CTL responses and subsequent life-threatening bacterial infections. HIV viraemia is generally well controlled.

Monitoring and management

To assess ongoing virological control of HIV, quantitative HIV RNA and CD4+ T-cell counts should be measured regularly, within 1 month of transplantation and every 2 to 3 months thereafter. Transient HIV viraemia may be seen, but if this persists, resistance testing should be performed.

Several immunosuppressive agents may be useful adjuncts for controlling HIV. For example, ciclosporin binds cyclophilin A, a cytoplasmic protein required for HIV viral replication, and has been studied as part of a treatment regimen for HIV. Mycophenolate suppresses HIV replication, especially in combination with nucleoside reverse transcriptase inhibitors such as abacavir. There are, however, numerous drug interactions associated with antiretrovirals and immunosuppressive agents, and this is one of the most challenging treatment issues in HIV-infected transplant recipients [46]. Protease inhibitors significantly inhibit the metabolism of calcineurin inhibitors and sirolimus through potent inhibition of the cytochrome p450 system, which means that patients on these drugs require substantially lower doses of calcineurin inhibitors and sirolimus, and longer dosing intervals. Efavirenz increases the metabolism of calcineurin inhibitors, thereby necessitating higher doses. Consequently, very close monitoring of immunosuppressive drug concentrations is critical in patients with HIV and should begin on the first day post-transplant and continue daily until stable concentrations are achieved. Any subsequent change in drug therapy should take into account the potential for increased toxicity or diminished bioavailability both of the antiretroviral agents and of the immunosuppressive drugs, and specialist advice is recommended. Consideration should be given to replacement of potentially nephrotoxic drugs, in particular tenofovir, and use of raltegravir-based regimens to allow avoidance of ritonavir to minimise cytochrome P450 interactions. Approaches to ensure adequate immunosuppression at the time of transplantation include starting immunosuppression several weeks prior to a live donor transplant or a trial period of immuosuppressive therapy to establish the optimal drug regimen prior to listing for deceased donor transplantation.

Treatment of HBV before transplantation is essential in patients who are co-infected, and numerous agents such as lamivudine, adefovir, tenofovir and entecavir have been used successfully. Lamivudine resistance to HBV may be more common as a result of prolonged use of lamivudine as a component of HAART. Nevertheless, outcomes in these patients have been excellent. Treatment of HCV infection has been more difficult and, as with non-HIV-infected individuals, whenever possible should be attempted before transplant to diminish the risk of post-transplant recurrence.

Prophylaxis for opportunistic infections

Life-long prophylaxis against *Pneumocystis jiroveci* is recommended, preferably with co-trimoxazole. Additional prophylactic measures are determined by the CD4 count and by exposure risk. Secondary prophylaxis for patients with a history of opportunistic infections should be considered to prevent reactivation of latent infection. Vaccination should be assessed and updated before transplantation as for non-HIV-infected individuals, and annual re-immunisation against influenza and every 3 to 5 years against *Streptococcus pneumoniae* should be encouraged.

Respiratory viruses: adenovirus, respiratory syncytial virus, influenza, parainfluenza

Epidemiology and risk factors

Adenoviruses typically cause self-limited respiratory, gastrointestinal or conjunctival disease throughout the year without significant seasonal variation, and are most common among children, people living in close quarters (such as college students and military recruits) and immunocompromised patients. Adenovirus also has been associated with haemorrhagic cystitis and graft dysfunction in adult kidney transplant recipients. The seasonality of other respiratory viral infections among transplant recipients usually follows that of the general population. Respiratory syncytial virus causes seasonal annual epidemics worldwide. Influenza viruses are associated with substantial morbidity and mortality worldwide with epidemics during the winter months. Antigenic variability gives this virus a survival advantage enabling continued virulence during yearly epidemics. Parainfluenza circulates sporadically in the autumn and winter. Transmission of respiratory viruses occurs via person-to-person contact with infectious secretions or fomites. A range of disease is seen, from mild nasal congestion to more severe tracheobronchitis, bronchiolitis and pneumonia. Common symptoms include fever, rhinorrhoea, watery eyes, cough, sore throat, sputum production, wheezing, shortness of breath and fevers. Viral shedding is usually prolonged among transplant recipients, even with the use of antivirals, and this may contribute to an increased risk of resistant strains. Transplant recipients are at higher risk of infectious complications such as subsequent development of fungal and bacterial pneumonia.

Diagnosis and treatment

In general, all patients with presumed respiratory viral infection should have a nasopharyngeal swab, wash or aspirate performed and sent for rapid antigen detection using whichever technique is locally available, usually immunoassays to detect viral antigen. Rapid antigen testing can diagnose most adenovirus serotypes, influenza and respiratory syncitial virus (RSV). A negative rapid test does not rule out infection and should trigger additional testing with PCR, direct florescent antibody (DFA) or culture. Serology is generally not clinically useful. If upper tract samples fail to document the cause of the respiratory illness or if there is clinical or radiological evidence of lower tract involvement, bronchoalveolar lavage should be considered and sent for the range of available tests. Histologic evaluation remains the gold standard for the diagnosis of invasive adenoviral disease. Typical cytopathic inclusions ('smudge cells') may be seen and the presence of the adenovirus within tissue confirmed by histochemical staining.

There is no definitive treatment for adenoviral infection, and the most important component of therapy is supportive care along with a decrease in immunosuppression. Consultation with an infectious diseases expert is advisable when further treatment is considered. Agents that have activity against adenovirus include cidofovir, ribavirin and ganciclovir. The two classes of antiviral compounds that are approved for the treatment of influenza are M2 inhibitors (amantadine and rimantadine), which are effective against susceptible influenza A strains only, and neuraminidase inhibitors (zanamivir and oseltamivir), which are active against susceptible influenza A and B viruses. Treatment with these agents in transplant recipients is associated with a reduction in risk of lower respiratory tract complications, duration of symptoms and mortality. Transplant recipients may have prolonged viral replication and may require extended therapy beyond the standard 5 days. Likewise, immunocompromised transplant recipients may benefit from therapy even if they have had symptoms longer than 48 hours before presentation. Resistance to available antivirals complicates the routine management of influenza and recommendations about optimal management are updated based on real-time surveillance of circulating strains and their susceptibility. Current dosing recommendations from public health authorities should be consulted regularly. Supportive care is recommended for infection with RSV and parainfluenza, and reduction of immune suppression should be considered, particularly in those with severe disease. The role of specific antiviral treatment is controversial. A combination of aerosolised ribavirin and IVIg may be of benefit in severe RSV or parainfluenza infection.

Advice for travellers

Transplant recipients are less likely to respond to vaccines against routine and travel-related pathogens and more likely to have adverse effects from vaccines, yet are at increased risk of developing opportunistic and non-opportunistic infections. Advice from a travel medicine specialist familiar with their immunocompromised state and current medications is recommended. Patients should be discouraged from travelling to 'high-risk' areas within the first year after transplantation, when the immunosuppressive burden is at its highest, or following periods when they have been treated with higher levels of immunosuppression for allograft rejection. Pre-travel counselling should include advice about obtaining appropriate health insurance, including medical evacuation insurance. Where possible, pre-travel knowledge of the closest transplant centres may be helpful, and transplant recipients should be advised to seek medical care at these specialist centres, rather than obtaining local care.

Pre-travel vaccination

Vaccination for travel should be planned well in advance where possible. Live attenuated vaccines are generally contraindicated in transplant recipients, but routine immunisation is otherwise safe, although it may not be effective. Particular recommendations include a tetanus booster if this is not up to date, hepatitis A vaccine (preferably two doses 6 to 12 months apart), inactive parenteral vaccine against *Salmonella enterica* serovar Typhi, inactivated poliovirus vaccine (IPV or Salk), and meningococcal conjugate vaccine for travellers to endemic areas. The yellow fever vaccine contains a live attenuated viral strain and should not be given to transplant recipients. A doctor's letter confirming contraindication to vaccination is acceptable to most governments. Bacille Calmette-Guerin (BCG) is a live, attenuated strain of *Mycobacterium bovis* and is also contraindicated in transplant recipients because of the risk of disseminated infection. Some travellers may warrant vaccination against rabies or Japanese encephalitis, depending on the nature of travel and the level of risk.

Certain live attenuated vaccine strains, particularly oral polio, nasal influenza and smallpox vaccines, could be transmitted by close contacts of transplant recipients, and should be avoided. Other live vaccines such as measles, mumps, rubella, yellow fever, oral *Salmonella*, varicella and zoster vaccines are less likely to be transmitted by close contacts and may be given.

Non-vaccine precautions

Travellers' diarrhoea may be life-threatening to transplant recipients. Dehydration may compromise kidney function and markedly increase levels and toxicity of immunosuppressive agents, particularly tacrolimus. Patients should be advised to drink boiled or bottled water or other beverages, and to avoid ice, food sold by street vendors, raw or undercooked foods and unpasteurised dairy products. Travellers should be counselled on the importance of fluid replacement and should also carry appropriate self-treatment such as ciprofloxacin to take in the event of a diarrhoeal illness with fever, blood, pus or mucus in the stool. There is no evidence that malaria is more common or severe in transplant recipients. Travellers to malaria-endemic areas should be counselled about the importance of minimising insect bites, and should use prophylaxis against malaria based on their travel itinerary. Many antimalarial agents interact with calcineurin inhibitors, and dose adjustments may be required. The safest prophylactic regimen is doxycycline 100 mg once daily commenced 1 week before departure and continued for 2 weeks on return. Transplant recipients have a greatly increased risk of skin cancer, and it is important to recommend the use of hats, sunglasses, protective clothing and high-factor sun protection lotions.

References

1. Schweitzer EJ, Perencevich EN, Philosophe B, *et al.* (2007) Estimated benefits of transplantation of kidneys from donors at increased risk for HIV or hepatitis C infection. *Am J Transplant* **7**, 1515–1525.
2. Birdwell KA, Ikizler MR, Sannella EC, *et al.* (2009) Decreased antibody response to influenza vaccination in kidney transplant recipients: A prospective cohort study. *Am J Kidney Dis* **54**, 112–121.
3. Fortun J, Martin-Davila P, Pascual J, *et al.* (2010) Immunosuppressive therapy and infection after kidney transplantation. *Transpl Infect Dis* **12**, 397–405.
4. Rice JC, Safdar N, AST Infectious Diseases Community of Practice. (2009) Urinary tract infections in solid organ transplant recipients. *Am J Transplant* **9** (Suppl 4), S267–272.
5. Moradi M, Abbasi M, Moradi A, *et al.* (2005) Effect of antibiotic therapy on asymptomatic bacteriuria in kidney transplant recipients. *Urol J* **2**, 32–35.
6. Mehrabi A, Fonouni H, Wente M, *et al.* (2006) Wound complications following kidney and liver transplantation. *Clin Transplant* **20** (Suppl 17), 97–110.

7. Paterson DL, Dominguez EA, Chang FY, *et al.* (1998) Infective endocarditis in solid organ transplant recipients. *Clin Infect Dis* **26**, 689–694.

8. Fernandez-Sabe N, Cervera C, Lopez-Medrano F, *et al.* (2009) Risk factors, clinical features, and outcomes of listeriosis in solid-organ transplant recipients: A matched case-control study. *Clin Infect Dis* **49**, 1153–1159.

9. Clark NM, AST Infectious Diseases Community of Practice. (2009) Nocardia in solid organ transplant recipients. *Am J Transplant* **9** (Suppl 4), S70–77.

10. Riddle DJ, Dubberke ER. (2008) Clostridium difficile infection in solid organ transplant recipients. *Curr Opin Organ Transplant* **13**, 592–600.

11. Dubberke ER, Riddle DJ, AST Infectious Diseases Community of Practice. (2009) Clostridium difficile in solid organ transplant recipients. *Am J Transplant* **9** (Suppl 4), S35–40.

12. Gudiol C, Garcia-Vidal C, Fernandez-Sabe N, *et al.* (2009) Clinical features and outcomes of Legionnaires' disease in solid organ transplant recipients. *Transpl Infect Dis* **2009 11**, 78–82.

13. Ho TB, Hull JH. (2006) Tests for latent tuberculosis. *Nephrol Dial Transplant* **21**, 2029.

14. Subramanian A, Dorman S, AST Infectious Diseases Community of Practice. (2009) Mycobacterium tuberculosis in solid organ transplant recipients. *Am J Transplant* **9** (Suppl 4), S57–62.

15. British Thoracic Society Standards of Care Committee. (2005) BTS recommendations for assessing risk and for managing Mycobacterium tuberculosis infection and disease in patients due to start anti-TNF-alpha treatment. *Thorax* **60**, 800–805.

16. Pappas PG, Silveira FP, AST Infectious Diseases Community of Practice. (2009) Candida in solid organ transplant recipients. *Am J Transplant* **9** (Suppl 4), S173–179.

17. Singh N, Husain S, AST Infectious Diseases Community of Practice. (2009) Invasive aspergillosis in solid organ transplant recipients. *Am J Transplant* **9** (Suppl 4), S180–191.

18. Cornely OA, Maertens J, Bresnik M, *et al.* (2007) Liposomal amphotericin B as initial therapy for invasive mold infection: a randomized trial comparing a high-loading dose regimen with standard dosing (AmBiLoad trial). *Clin Infect Dis* **44**, 1289–1297.

19. Singh N, Forrest G, AST Infectious Diseases Community of Practice. (2009) Cryptococcosis in solid organ transplant recipients. *Am J Transplant* **9** (Suppl 4), S192–198.

20. Martin SI, Fishman JA, AST Infectious Diseases Community of Practice. (2009) Pneumocystis pneumonia in solid organ transplant recipients. *Am J Transplant* **9** (Suppl 4), S227–233.

21. Humar A, Snydman D, AST Infectious Diseases Community of Practice. (2009) Cytomegalovirus in solid organ transplant recipients. *Am J Transplant* **9** (Suppl 4), S78–86.

22. Humar A, Lebranchu Y, Vincenti F, *et al.* (2010) The efficacy and safety of 200 days valganciclovir cytomegalovirus prophylaxis in high-risk kidney transplant recipients. *Am J Transplant* **10**, 1228–1237.

23. Lowance D, Neumayer HH, Legendre CM, *et al.* (1999) Valacyclovir for the prevention of cytomegalovirus disease after renal transplantation. International Valacyclovir Cytomegalovirus Prophylaxis Transplantation Study Group. *N Engl J Med* **340**, 1462–1470.

24. Boivin G, Goyette N, Rollag H, *et al.* (2009) Cytomegalovirus resistance in solid organ transplant recipients treated with intravenous ganciclovir or oral valganciclovir. *Antivir Ther* **14**, 697–704.

25. Zuckerman R, Wald A, AST Infectious Diseases Community of Practice. (2009) Herpes simplex virus infections in solid organ transplant recipients. *Am J Transplant* **9** (Suppl 4), S104–107.

26. Pergam SA, Limaye AP, AST Infectious Diseases Community of Practice. (2009) Varicella zoster virus (VZV) in solid organ transplant recipients. *Am J Transplant* **9** (Suppl 4), S108–115.

27. Opelz G, Dohler B. (2004) Lymphomas after solid organ transplantation: A collaborative transplant study report. *Am J Transplant* **4**, 222–230.

28. Allen U, Preiksaitis J, AST Infectious Diseases Community of Practice. (2009) Epstein-barr virus and posttransplant lymphoproliferative disorder in solid organ transplant recipients. *Am J Transplant* **9** (Suppl 4), S87–96.

29. Swerdlow SH, Campo E, Harris NL, *et al.* (2008) Post-transplant lymphoproliferative disorders. In: Swerdlow SH, Campo E, Harris NL, *et al.* (eds), *World Health Organisation Classification of Tumors of Haematopoietic and Lymphoid Tissues*, 4th edn. International Agency for Research on Cancer Press, Lyon.

30. Lee JJ, Lam MS, Rosenberg A. (2007) Role of chemotherapy and rituximab for treatment of posttransplant lymphoproliferative disorder in solid organ transplantation. *Ann Pharmacother* **41**, 1648–1659.

31. Parker A, Bowles K, Bradley JA, *et al.* (2010) Management of post-transplant lymphoproliferative disorder in adult solid organ transplant recipients – BCSH and BTS guidelines. *Br J Haematol* **149**, 693–705.

32. Razonable RR, Zerr DM, AST Infectious Diseases Community of Practice. (2009) HHV-6, HHV-7 and HHV-8 in solid organ transplant recipients. *Am J Transplant* **9** (Suppl 4), S97–100.

33. Razonable RR, Zerr DM, AST Infectious Diseases Community of Practice. (2009) HHV-6, HHV-7 and HHV-8 in solid organ transplant recipients. *Am J Transplant* **9** (Suppl 4), S100–103.

34. Hirsch HH, Brennan DC, Drachenberg CB, *et al.* (2005) Polyomavirus-associated nephropathy in renal transplantation: Interdisciplinary analyses and recommendations. *Transplantation* **79**, 1277–1286.

35. Drachenberg CB, Papadimitriou JC, Hirsch HH, *et al.* (2004) Histological patterns of polyomavirus nephropathy: Correlation with graft outcome and viral load. *Am J Transplant* **4**, 2082–2092.

36. Egli A, Kohli S, Dickenmann M, *et al.* (2009) Inhibition of polyomavirus BK-specific T-Cell responses by immunosuppressive drugs. *Transplantation* **88**, 1161–1168.

37. Hirsch HH, Randhawa P, AST Infectious Diseases Community of Practice. (2009) BK virus in solid organ transplant recipients. *Am J Transplant* **9** (Suppl 4), S136–146.

38. Levitsky J, Doucette K, AST Infectious Diseases Community of Practice. (2009) Viral hepatitis in solid organ transplant recipients. *Am J Transplant* **9** (Suppl 4), S116–130.

39. Jiang H, Wu J, Zhang X, *et al.* (2009) Kidney transplantation from hepatitis B surface antigen positive donors into hepatitis B surface antibody positive recipients: A prospective nonrandomized controlled study from a single center. *Am J Transplant* **9**, 1853–1858.

40. Cohn J, Blumberg EA. (2009) Immunizations for renal transplant candidates and recipients. *Nat Clin Pract Nephrol* **5**, 46–53.

41. Wreghitt TG. (2004) Bloodborne virus infections in dialysis units: A mini-review. *Commun Dis Public Health* **7**, 92–93.

42. Berenguer M. (2008) Treatment of chronic hepatitis C in hemodialysis patients. *Hepatology* **48**, 1690–1699.

43. Blumberg EA, Stock P, AST Infectious Diseases Community of Practice. (2009) Solid organ transplantation in the HIV-infected patient. *Am J Transplant* **9** (Suppl 4), S131–135.

44. Locke JE, Montgomery RA, Warren DS, *et al.* (2009) Renal transplant in HIV-positive patients: Long-term outcomes and risk factors for graft loss. *Arch Surg* **144**, 83–86.

45. Roland ME, Barin B, Carlson L, *et al.* (2008) HIV-infected liver and kidney transplant recipients: 1- and 3-year outcomes. *Am J Transplant* **8**, 355–365.

46. Frassetto LA, Browne M, Cheng A, *et al.* (2007) Immunosuppressant pharmacokinetics and dosing modifications in HIV-1 infected liver and kidney transplant recipients. *Am J Transplant* **7**, 2816–2820.

47. Fishman JA, Rubin RH. (1998) Infection in organ-transplant recipients. *N Engl J Med* **338**, 1741–1751.

48. Department of Health. (2000) Guidance on the Microbiological Safety of Human Organs, Tissues and Cells used in Transplantation.

49. Fischer SA, Avery RK, AST Infectious Disease Community of Practice. (2009) Screening of donor and recipient prior to solid organ transplantation. *Am J Transplant* **9** (Suppl 4), S7–18.

22 Management during the first three months after renal transplantation

Iain A.M. MacPhee, Joyce Popoola and Daniel Jones

Introduction

This chapter brings together the process of management during the first 3 months after transplantation with detail on each component provided in other chapters. The first 3 months after transplantation is a critical period, which has considerable influence on long-term transplant outcomes.

The patient journey

From the operating theatre recovery area to the ward

Transplant recipients require close monitoring from the moment they arrive in recovery. At this stage the patients have a variable level of consciousness and are unable to take fluids orally. They always have intravenous access, a urinary catheter and not infrequently a wound drain *in situ* and in some cases a central venous cannula. The interval during which they are held in recovery not only allows for time to recover from the effect of anaesthesia but also enables a prompt return to theatre should there be any immediate surgical problems that can be corrected readily: bleeding, vascular thrombosis and ureteric obstruction. Doppler ultrasound before transfer to the ward can be used to diagnose early graft thrombosis or poor perfusion in time to allow surgical rescue. Being alert to pain and its control is crucial at this point, as severe pain can be an indicator of an underlying complication. Analgesia is addressed below.

The underlying principles of management of the transplant patient in the immediate postoperative period are those of the management of acute kidney injury. The single most important task is to optimise haemodynamics to ensure perfusion of the transplanted organ(s).

Handbook of Renal and Pancreatic Transplantation, First Edition. Edited by Iain A. M. MacPhee and Jiří Froněk.
© 2012 John Wiley & Sons, Ltd. Published 2012 by John Wiley & Sons, Ltd.

Table 22.1 Monitoring based on physical examination and investigations.

Physical examination	Vital signs – pulse, blood pressure, temperature, respiratory rate
	Systemic examination – abdomen, chest
	Daily weights
	Jugular venous pressure
	Urine output
	Drain sites/wound
Investigations	Daily FBC and biochemical profile
	Drug trough concentrations of immunosuppressants alternate days
	Pre-operative culture results from donor kidneys and recipients should be reviewed
	Urinalysis and urine cultures at least once weekly
	Doppler ultrasound/MAG3 scan
	Renal transplant biopsy if indicated

In monitoring patients, there is no substitute for careful clinical assessment, including pulse and blood pressure, jugular venous pulse or central venous pressure, evidence of peripheral vasoconstriction and auscultation of the chest for signs of pulmonary oedema (Table 22.1). The fluid balance needs to take into account output from all sources (i.e. urine, wound drains and blood loss). Fluid correction in the early postoperative period should normally be with 0.9% saline, although this may need to be varied depending on the results from other electrolytes. In some instances fluid replacement needs to be with whole blood or colloids, particularly if there was significant blood loss intraoperatively or in the presence of ongoing bleeding.

The full blood count (FBC), creatinine and electrolytes should be checked immediately postoperatively. The haemoglobin is important not only in order to take account of intraoperative blood loss but also to help quantify bleeding at a later time point. Hyperkalaemia is a common problem in the early postoperative phase, particularly in patients with delayed graft function. It should be corrected urgently, particularly if associated with electrocardiogram changes consistent with hyperkalaemia. Consideration should be given to dialysis in an oliguric patient with serum potassium >5.5 mmol/L. Blood glucose concentrations need to be monitored, particularly in diabetic patients, as hyperglycaemia may lead to osmotic diuresis and polyuria. High-dose intravenous steroid administered perioperatively occasionally results in hyperglycaemia in patients not known to be diabetic previously. Calcium and phosphate concentrations are also important, as there is often a tendency to hypophosphataemia in polyuric patients. Serum magnesium should be checked in polyuric patients with replacement if severe depletion develops, <0.4 mmol/L, due to risk of arrhythmia.

The following algorithm for immediate post-transplant monitoring is suggested.

- Vital signs – heart rate, blood pressure, temperature and respiratory rate initially every 15 minutes then hourly after 4 hours if stable.
- Wound and operation site – checking of wound site for pain, swelling and volume and colour and nature of fluid emerging from drain site.
- Urine output – monitor hourly for volume and appearance.
- Medications – the immediate pre-operative, peri-operative and postoperative medications should be reviewed on chart and confirmation to be given, particularly the update of immunosuppressants for the patient's timeline.
- Fluid Input – this needs to be monitored closely immediately postoperatively in order to optimise fluid balance. For the most part input should equate with output to keep the patient euvolaemic, but if the patient is anuric or oliguric and volume depleted on assessment then administration of a fluid bolus may be required. In our centre post-transplant patients are given 0.9% NaCl intravenously at an hourly rate equal to the previous hour's urine output plus 50 mL. Polyuria may be driven by excessive fluid input. Reduction in volume of replacement to about 75% of output may be necessary in extreme cases of polyuria. However, if polyuria continues in spite of reduced fluid input, it may be necessary to continue to replace urine output to avoid the patient becoming fluid depleted.

Patients are usually kept in recovery until they regain consciousness and may require further monitoring in recovery to ensure stability and that no intervention is required prior to transfer.

Management on the ward

The transplant recipient is subsequently transferred to the ward, usually within 24 hours unless problems arise in the recovery unit. In most European centres the length of hospital admission ranges between 5 and 14 days unless there are associated complications warranting a longer stay. Early discharge requires frequent availability of outpatient follow-up with easy direct access for patients. Capacity for same-day ultrasound scanning and renal biopsy are essential.

Close monitoring of patients (see Table 22.1) remains essential; however, at this stage it is required less frequently (about 4 hourly unless complications have developed). Blood sampling is required at a minimum on a daily basis. Avoidance of arteriovenous fistula sites and arms with an intravenous infusion running may pose a challenge to the phlebotomist, who should be well trained in taking blood from these patients. Owing to the complexity of the monitoring of the transplant patient by a multidisciplinary team, it is essential to have readily available, regularly updated charts for entry of data in addition to patient clinical notes. These charts need to incorporate not only aspects of clinical monitoring and investigations but also immunosuppressant regimens and check-offs once they have been administered for review on ward rounds.

Patients are usually able to take oral fluids on the first day postoperatively then gradually be introduced to an oral diet once their bowels are moving. Constipation is a common problem, with potentially serious consequences if the patient develops faecal impaction. Early mobilisation usually helps, with the addition of suppositories or enemas if the bowels have not opened by day 2 or 3 postoperatively. Physiotherapy should be started early for breathing exercises and general mobilisation. All plastic tubes should be removed as soon as possible to reduce the risk of infection and aid in mobilisation. Wound drains are usually removed within 48 hours and the urinary catheter is usually removed between 2 and 5 days postoperatively, although in cases of anuria they may be removed earlier. Patients should be weighed every day to aid in the assessment of fluid status.

Outpatient follow-up from days 8–90 after transplant

The first outpatient appointment should entail a thorough assessment of the patient's past medical history, medication history and history of the transplant operation, associated complications and progress since discharge. The main driver to frequency of review in the early post-transplant period is the fact that acute rejection in the context of modern immunosuppressive regimens is asymptomatic, and delay in treatment reduces the rate of response. Acute rejection is commonest during the first month after the transplant and is rare beyond 2 months, with the exception of some regimens based on alemtuzumab. In the first 2 weeks patients are often seen as frequently as three times a week. In the absence of complications they may then be seen twice weekly for the next 2 weeks, weekly for the second month then between weekly and biweekly for the third month. At each appointment it is essential to assess the patient's well-being, keep a monitor on the rate of creatinine fall, assessment of immunosuppressive drug blood concentrations and to initiate investigations and management accordingly. Some units adopt a practice of all transplants being followed up in the transplant centre long term. Although this concentrates transplant expertise, transfer back to referral centres allows patients to obtain their care closer to home and is the model most widely employed in the UK now. Comprehensive and accurate information transfer is required to optimise the transition process. A timeline of early post-transplant events is shown in Table 22.2.

Specific management issues

Diagnosis and management of transplant dysfunction

The traditional diagnostic structure for renal impairment of pre-renal, renal and post-renal causes serves as a good template for the investigation of renal transplant dysfunction. The investigation of delayed graft function or a fall in glomerular filtration rate (GFR) in a graft is essentially the same. Transplants where serum creatinine concentration has plateaued at above the expected range should also be investigated for graft dysfunction. The diagnostic algorithm should start with simple non-invasive tests, proceeding to invasive tests only if necessary. In general, pre-renal and post-renal causes are investigated first, followed by

Table 22.2 Timeline for early post-transplant events.

Event	Weeks after transplantation											
	1	2	3	4	5	6	7	8	9	10	11	12
Removal of bladder catheter												
Discharge from hospital												
Removal of ureteric stent and peritoneal dialysis catheters												
Early protocol biopsy												
Ligation of proximal arterio-venous fistulae												

progression to renal biopsy to diagnose renal causes if no diagnosis is reached. A flow chart for diagnosis of transplant dysfunction is shown in Fig. 22.1.

Pre-renal

History and examination should determine whether the patient is intravascularly deplete, hypotensive or septic. Renal transplant ultrasound scan with Doppler measurement can confirm renal perfusion with demonstration of flow in the main renal arteries and veins and Doppler signal in the renal parenchyma. Thrombosis of the renal artery or vein may be identified. An important differential diagnosis for an apparently thrombosed graft is hyperacute rejection due to the presence of pre-formed anti-donor antibodies. With the use of crossmatch testing (see Chapter 4) this should be an extremely rare event. Increased peak systolic velocity in the transplant artery may indicate renal artery stenosis but is not diagnostic and would indicate angiography. Increased resistance index indicates interstitial oedema, which can be a marker of rejection. In a non-functioning transplant a renogram can be used to confirm perfusion of the kidney and identify perfusion defects. Demonstration of tracer uptake by the kidney without excretion into the collecting system is most likely to represent acute tubular necrosis. Detailed information on radiological investigation of the transplant is provided in Chapter 19.

Post-renal

The simplest cause for apparent anuria is a blocked urinary catheter, most often due to blood clots in a patient with haematuria. This can be confirmed by flushing the catheter to test patency.

Ureteric obstruction

Ureteric obstruction is uncommon in the presence of a ureteric stent but not impossible. It is usually asymptomatic and presents with deteriorating graft function with demonstration of hydronephrosis on

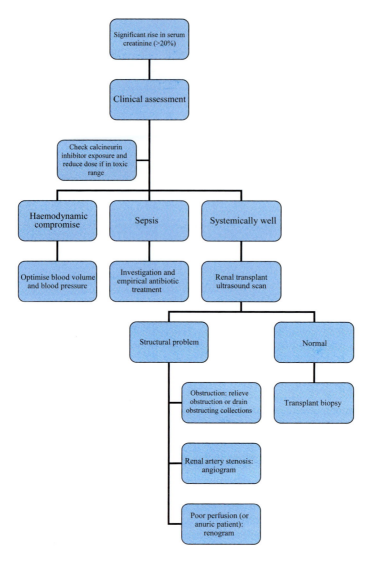

Figure 22.1 Investigation of transplant dysfunction.

ultrasound scanning (see Chapter 19). Ultrasound scan can demonstrate the presence of fluid collections such as lymphoceles that may be causing obstruction. It is essential to have confirmation that the bladder was empty at the time of scanning, as it is usual to have reflux into the collecting system with a full bladder. It is usual to have a mild degree of hydronephrosis in the immediate post-transplant period owing to oedema at the utero-vesical anastomosis. Insertion of a percutaneous nephrostomy under radiological guidance both relieves the obstruction and allows antegrade pyelography to define the anatomical lesion. Early causes of obstruction include blood clots, extrinsic compression and technical problems with the anastomoses. Later stenoses are most often due to ischaemia, but immunological rejection and BK polyomavirus may be aetiological factors. If an anatomical lesion is identified, it may be amenable to balloon dilatation with refinements including use of cutting balloons or thermo expandable stents. A retrograde approach to the ureter by cystoscopy is rarely successful, as identification of the ureteric orifice is technically difficult. Where no anatomical lesion is identified, reintroduction of a JJ ureteric stent with a further attempt at removal after approximately 6 weeks is often effective. Where the above measures have failed the options are either a long-tem JJ stent changed every 6 months or open surgery with reimplantation of the ureter or formation of a Boari flap. The latter can be technically challenging, particularly if the kidney has been implanted with the collecting system posterior to the vessels.

Lower urinary tract obstruction

Lower urinary tract obstruction may be a problem, particularly in older males who were oliguric before transplantation and may have had chronic lower urinary tract obstruction due to prostatic hypertrophy that had not been apparent previously. Signs and symptoms of urinary tract infection should be sought with urine stick testing for blood, protein or nitrite and urine microscopy followed by culture with determination of antibiotic sensitivities.

Urine leak

Urine leaks are usually due to breakdown of the ureterovesical anastomosis or ureteral necrosis. Clinical presentation may be with decreased urine output, urine leaking from the wound and abdominal pain, a rise in serum creatinine concentration or apparent delayed graft function when a well-functioning kidney is discharging urine into the retroperitoneal or peritoneal cavity. Reabsorption of serum creatinine into the blood may prevent a fall in the serum creatinine concentration. Aspiration of any collection identified by ultrasound can allow the biochemical identification of yellow fluid as urine or serum. Samples should be sent for measurement of potassium and creatinine in urine (if the patient is not anuric), serum and the aspirated fluid. If potassium and creatinine concentrations are significantly higher in the fluid than in serum the fluid is likely to be urine. The concentrations may be lower than those in any urine sampled due to some reabsorption into blood. Fluid from lymphoceles has a high triglyceride concentration. Options for management include decompression of the urinary tract using a catheter for bladder drainage or where ureteric obstruction is a factor, insertion of a percutaneous nephrostomy.

Renal

The differential diagnosis in the early period is broad and includes acute tubular necrosis (ATN), acute rejection, calcineurin inhibitor (CNI) nephrotoxicity, recurrent primary renal disease, viral nephropathy (most commonly BK polyomavirus or cytomegalovirus (CMV)) and transplant pyelonephritis. Having excluded pre- and post-renal causes of graft dysfunction, with the exception of transplant pyelonephritis, diagnosis of renal causes requires a renal biopsy (see below for method). This is the only way of making a definitive diagnosis of ATN or acute rejection.

Acute tubular necrosis

The typical pattern for ATN due to ischaemia-reperfusion injury is an initial diuresis for several hours after transplantation followed by anuria. Donor factors are the dominant predictors of ATN with increased incidence with donation after circulatory death, older donors and longer cold ischaemia time. In an anuric patient on the day after transplantation with Doppler ultrasound scan indicating perfusion of the kidney and a renogram demonstrating uptake of the tracer by the renal parenchyma without excretion into the bladder, the most likely diagnosis is ATN. After 1 week, there may be coexistent rejection and delayed graft function is a risk factor for acute rejection. Weekly protocol biopsies should be used to screen for acute rejection in non-functioning transplants.

Acute rejection/CNI toxicity

Acute rejection is most common during the first 2 months after transplantation, with the exception of immunosuppressive regimens based on alemtuzumab, in which late rejection is more common. In the event of acute rejection and in HLA-antibody-incompatible transplants, donor-specific antibody should be measured. ABO antibody titres should be determined in blood-group-incompatible transplants. Blood concentration measurement of the CNIs may indicate potential toxicity. However, there are several problems with relying on this measurement to make a diagnosis. The first is operational, in that in many centres the result may not be available until late in the day, and certainly beyond the time when a renal biopsy could be taken and processed for a same-day result. A second issue is that acute rejection can occur in the presence of apparently toxic concentrations of CNI. CNI-induced vasospasm may cause graft dysfunction in the absence of any histological changes. A normal biopsy allows safe reduction in CNI dose with monitoring of serum creatinine concentration for improvement.

Early recurrent disease

Focal and segmental glomerulosclerosis

The most common recurrent disease in the early period after transplantation is focal and segmental glomerulosclerosis (FSGS), which is usually manifest by development of nephrotic syndrome (proteinuria, hypoalbuminaemia and oedema). In the early stage of recurrence the biopsy tends to be normal by light microscopy, but foot process fusion may be seen with electron microscopy. Idiopathic primary FSGS recurs in

20–50% of renal transplants and up to 80% if there was recurrence in a previous transplant [1]. Recurrence is more likely with early age at onset and rapid progression to end-stage renal failure. Eighty percent of recurrences occur within the first month after transplantation. Patients with primary FSGS should have measurement of proteinuria daily for 1 week, weekly for 4 weeks, every 3 months for the first year and then annually thereafter [2]. FSGS may respond to plasma exchange with the addition of cyclophosphamide in place of mycophenolate/azathioprine or rituximab to routine immunosuppression, but the supporting evidence base is sparse [3].

Haemolytic uraemic syndrome (HUS)

Any patient with haemolytic uraemic syndrome (HUS) as their primary renal disease who has graft dysfunction should be investigated for evidence of microangiopathy: platelet count, blood film for evidence of erythrocyte fragmentation, and plasma haptoglobin and serum lactate dehydrogenase as evidence of haemolysis. In general, HUS due to *E. coli* 0157 toxin, also known as diarrhoea associated or D+, although diarrhoea is not always a feature, does not recur after transplantation. Inherited HUS, due to mutations in the circulating complement regulatory proteins factor H and factor I, has a high rate of recurrence, with 80% of patients losing their grafts within 2 years. Patients with these mutations should not be offered renal transplantation alone, with consideration of a combined liver/kidney transplant. Data for recurrence in individuals with anti-factor H autoantibodies are sparse but suggest a high rate of recurrence. Antibody removal with rituximab has been reported to allow safe transplantation. Mutations in membrane co-factor protein (MCP) do not result in recurrence, presumably owing to expression on donor endothelium. Recurrence usually occurs within the first month after transplantation. Plasmapheresis replacing with fresh frozen plasma or cryo-supernatant can be effective and has been employed pre-emptively at the time of transplantation. Eculizumab, which inhibits the formation of the complement membrane attack complex is a potential therapy [4,5].

De novo HUS, also known as post-transplant microangiopathy, has been associated with treatment with ciclosporin, tacrolimus and sirolimus. Viral infection, such as with CMV, can also be a trigger. Management is based on attempts to withdraw the offending drug and treatment as for recurrent HUS [5].

Other diagnoses

Viral inclusion bodies may be present with viral identification by immunohistochemistry. Appropriate investigations to confirm systemic infection should be requested. Rarely, transplant pyelonephritis is diagnosed in the absence of other evidence of urinary tract infection. Transplant pyelonephritis presents with fever, sometimes rigor, and a painful tender transplant. Inflammatory markers are raised and there is pyuria with infected urine.

Early protocol biopsy

The role of protocol biopsies is an evolving area. Most centres perform implantation biopsies routinely to identify pre-existing donor pathology, which can be invaluable in interpreting subsequent diagnostic biopsies. All physicians being trained to perform percutaneous renal biopsies should witness an open biopsy on at least one occasion to see the extent of bleeding and engender an appropriate perception of risk. Many units now undertake biopsies 2–3 months after transplantation to screen for subclinical rejection, in particular where a step down in intensity of immunosuppression is planned. In our experience, the main finding, as reported in the published literature, is that approximately 10% of patients have at least Banff grade 1 acute cellular rejection [6]. There is some debate as to whether early protocol biopsies improve outcomes, with the widely quoted negative study published by Rush *et al.* [7]. This was in the context of patients continuing on a potent three-agent regimen comprising tacrolimus, mycophenolate and steroids throughout the first year after transplantation. For regimens based on reduction in intensity of immunosuppression after the first year, early biopsies prevent an inappropriate reduction in immunosuppression in patients with ongoing low-grade rejection. The presence of histological evidence of CNI nephrotoxicity in the absence of acute rejection would prompt a switch from the CNI to an alternative agent such as sirolimus or reduction in blood CNI concentrations. In the Mayo clinic protocol biopsy series [8], fibrosis with inflammation at 1 year after transplantation predicted subsequent deterioration in transplant function and may identify patients requiring more immunosuppression.

Renal transplant biopsy: procedure

In general, renal transplant biopsies can be undertaken as an outpatient procedure, although it is prudent to admit patients at high risk of bleeding for overnight observation after the biopsy. The following are the criteria that we use locally for patients suitable for day case biopsy:
- eGFR >20 mL/min
- urea <30 mmol/L
- body mass index (BMI) <30 kg/m^2
- aspirin or warfarin can be stopped as outpatient
- suitable responsible person at home overnight after biopsy
- no serious co-morbid disease.

Pre-biopsy considerations

For elective biopsies aspirin/clopidogrel should be stopped 1 week in advance. However, this will not be possible for urgent biopsies. In patients with an absolute indication for aspirin (e.g. coronary artery or stroke disease), this will need to be continued during the early post-transplant period. For patients without an absolute indication for aspirin, discontinuation at the time of the transplant with reinstitution at 3 months after transplantation reduces the risk of bleeding from biopsies during the time when they are likely to be required urgently to diagnose graft dysfunction. For patients taking aspirin, there is an increased bleeding risk but not to the extent of contraindicating biopsy. Although withholding aspirin on the day of the biopsy will not reduce bleeding risk substantially, it may make subsequent management of any bleeding easier. Percutaneous biopsy in patients on clopidogrel is excessively hazardous, and an open procedure with haemostasis is probably safer in this situation. Warfarin should be stopped at least 2 days in advance if indication allows. The need for intravenous heparin until the day of the biopsy will depend on the indication for anticoagulation.

Haematological and clotting factors should be checked within 24 hours of the biopsy for inpatients and no longer than 3 days prior to day case patients (unless previously anticoagulated and then haematological and clotting parameters should be performed on the day of the biopsy before proceeding). We use the following criteria as safe limits for biopsy. A review of management and prevention of uraemic bleeding is provided in reference [9]. A low haemoglobin/haematocrit not only reduces the patient's margin to survive bleeding but also actually increases the risk of bleeding. In a patient with delayed graft function, dialysis on the day before the biopsy may improve platelet function.

- haemoglobin >10 g/dL (+ haematocrit >0.3)
- platelet count >100 × 10^9/L
- international normalised ratio (INR) <1.2
- activated partial thromboplastin time (APTT) ratio <1.15
- group and save for blood transfusion should be sent prior to any biopsy

Desmopressin acetate (1-deamino-8-D-arginine vasopressin, DDAVP) can be administered to uraemic patients to improve platelet function by increasing the amount of factor VIII on the platelet surface. Our local policy is to administer desmopressin to patients with GFR <25 mL/min/1.73 m^2 or urea >30 mmol/L and in any patient who has not stopped aspirin prior to biopsy. A dose of 0.3–0.4 μg/kg (maximum dose 20 μg) is given intravenously over 30 min in 50 mL 0.9% saline administered 1 hour before the biopsy. Blood pressure should be no greater than 160/90 on the day of biopsy. If there is evidence of transplant pyelonephritis, this should be treated with antibiotics prior to biopsy. A 16-gauge core-cutting needle achieves the best compromise between adequacy of sample and safety. There is no evidence that reducing the core size to 18-gauge improves safety, but there is the risk of reduced biopsy adequacy [10].

The following complication rate was found in a recent audit of transplant biopsies in London transplant centres:

- visible haematuria in 10% (1 in 10) biopsies that settles spontaneously
- bleeding requiring blood transfusion <2% (1 in 50)
- requirement for interventional radiology or surgery to control haemorrhage in <0.07% (1 in 1500)
- nephrectomy to control haemorrhage in <0.03% (1 in 3000) biopsies (the kidney may have to be removed to stop the bleeding).

Although deaths have occurred following complications of biopsies, this is extremely rare.

Biopsy technique

Ultrasound should be performed to ensure that adequate views can be obtained before starting. The aim is to obtain tissue from the renal cortex. Real-time ultrasound guidance of the biopsy is the safest approach, ensuring that the anticipated projection of the needle avoids vessels and the urine-collecting system. A sterile plastic sheath may be used to cover the ultrasound probe to avoid the risk of infection. Ultrasound jelly should be applied to the probe before applying the sheath, which is held in place with rubber bands. Sedation is not normally required. Real-time ultrasound should be used to anaesthetise the route to the kidney. Lidocaine 1 or 2% should be used. Care should be taken not to exceed the maximum recommended dose of 200 mg (i.e. 20 mL of 1% lidocaine or 10 mL of 2% lidocaine). A small cut in the skin should be made with a scalpel to allow easy passage of the biopsy needle.

The upper outer pole is usually the easiest area to biopsy safely. A review of the surgical operation note before biopsy is advised to check for any abnormal anatomy. If an area of kidney is known not to be perfused, for example based on renogram evidence, this site should be avoided. A biopsy from the lower pole of a transplant is acceptable if views suggest this is more accessible, but care needs to be taken not to transect the inferior epigastric artery (which runs in the rectus sheath and may even have been used to revascularise part of the transplant). In biopsying the upper outer pole, care must be taken to avoid crossing the peritoneum with the risk of bowel perforation. It is best to avoid biopsy across a fluid collection, as this reduces the likelihood of tamponade in the event of bleeding. Doppler views should be reviewed to avoid areas of increased vascularity. Standard practice is to take two cores of kidney to ensure adequate sampling (see Chapter 20). However, where the risk of bleeding is perceived as particularly high, it is reasonable to collect a single adequate core, while accepting the potential limitations in terms of the Banff criteria. In general, no more than three passes should be attempted. Following the biopsy, pressure (approximately 3 minutes) should be applied to the biopsy site to achieve local haemostasis and a dressing applied. The adequacy of local pressure can be assessed by pressing with the probe while set to a Doppler view (adequate pressure should significantly reduce the Doppler signal).

Post-biopsy monitoring

Signs of bleeding include visible blood in the urine, abdominal pain more than a dull ache after biopsy, or a significant fall in blood pressure or tachycardia. Day-case biopsies require bed rest for 6 hours with monitoring of pulse and blood pressure every 15 min for the first 2 hours, every 30 min for the next 2 hours followed by hourly observations for the final 2 hours. The biopsy site should be inspected at each observation point for signs of bleeding. Any urine passed should be collected and inspected for visible blood. Patients who do not meet day-case criteria should remain as inpatients and receive standard 4 hourly observations after the initial 6 hours of observation unless the clinical situation determines otherwise. Day-case patients can be discharged home if they have been haemodynamically stable for 6 hours after biopsy, have passed urine that does not contain visible blood, are pain-free and able to mobilise at their usual level. They should be advised to avoid heavy manual activities for 5 days and that usually 1 or 2 days away from work is sufficient.

Management of biopsy complications

In the event of post-biopsy bleeding, this often settles spontaneously with bed rest and blood transfusion. In the event of bleeding that has not settled, or a haemodynamically compromised patient, the first approach to stopping bleeding is interventional radiology with angiography to identify the bleeding point and embolisation (Chapter 19). Nephrectomy to control bleeding is a last resort that is rarely required. Bleeding into the collecting system may result in clot retention of urine requiring passage of an irrigating bladder catheter.

Specific early surgical complications

Lymphocele

Small lymphoceles picked up as an incidental finding on ultrasound scanning that are not compressing the transplant will usually resolve spontaneously without intervention. If there is compression of the transplant with functional obstruction, the first step is radiologically guided percutaneous drainage. This may be either a single procedure, which may be repeated, or a drain may be left *in situ*. The main risk of drainage is the introduction of infection. Instillation of sclerosants including povidone iodine into the lymphocele has been reported to increase the rate of resolution but may take several weeks [11]. If lymphoceles fail to resolve, the definitive procedure is drainage of the lymphocele into the peritoneal cavity. This can be performed as an open or laparoscopic procedure. A procedure that has been recently demonstrated to reduce the incidence of lymphoceles is prophylactic peritoneal fenestration at the time of transplant surgery [12].

Wound complications: dehiscence and infection

There is an increased incidence of wound complications in obese transplant recipients and those treated with mammalian target of rapamycin (mTOR) inhibitors, which inhibit wound healing. Conventional management of wound infections includes radiological characterisation of any collections with drainage either percutaneously or by surgery with appropriate antibiotic treatment.

Specific Issues requiring attention in the transplant recipient

Analgesia

Analgesia in the early period, especially for the first 24 hours, is best delivered through a patient self-operated parenteral system. An issue that is often overlooked is the reduced elimination of glucuronide-conjugated opiate metabolites in patients with renal failure leading to toxicity. If morphine is to be used, a longer than conventional lock-out period should be employed, but it is preferable to avoid morphine, using an alternative such as fentanyl. Regular paracetamol can provide useful background analgesia. In the ensuing 48 hours, parenteral analgesia should be discontinued and replaced with oral substitutes such as tramadol or other opiates. It is not uncommon for patients to continue to require analgesia 1 to 2 weeks after discharge; however, every effort should be made to wean patients as soon as possible. These agents may lead to constipation and so should be given with regular stimulant laxatives such as senna. Pain control is often very individual and may require consultation with pain-relief experts and anaesthetists. Increased pain levels after surgery should always be explored thoroughly as it may herald significant pathology. Non-steroidal anti-inflammatory drugs (NSAIDS) should not be used owing to their adverse effect on intrarenal haemodynamics.

Thromboprophylaxis

In patients not on pre-existing anticoagulant or antiplatelet treatment, heparin should be given as prophylaxis against deep venous thrombosis and renal transplant vein thrombosis. It is best to avoid low-molecular-weight heparin owing to accumulation with renal impairment, and a conventional regimen would be 5000 units of unfractionated heparin given subcutaneously twice daily until discharge from hospital. A combination of aspirin and heparin increases the incidence of bleeding and it is probably best to avoid heparin in patients with an absolute indication for aspirin unless there are specific complications requiring systemic anticoagulation. Patients with an absolute indication for long-term anticoagulant therapy such as valve replacements, thrombophilia or atrial fibrillation, should be converted to intravenous heparin peri-operatively with careful monitoring using the APTT. Anticoagulation with heparin in the early post-transplant period (first 48 hours) may reduce the incidence of transplant artery thrombosis in the presence of multiple small arteries.

Erythropoiesis-stimulating agents

It is not uncommon for transplant recipients to be anaemic after surgery, partly as a result of peri-operative blood loss. Haemoglobin usually falls to a nadir at around 1 month after transplantation, with a return to pre-transplant levels by around 3 months. Administration of erythropoietin during this period has little, if any, impact on this pattern, suggesting an erythropoietin-resistant state superimposed on erythropoietin deficiency. This probably reflects the use of the antiproliferative drugs causing myelosuppression, the acute inflammatory response to the transplant procedure with relatively poor graft function as a contributor. Although the transplant provides a new source of natural erythropoietin, making the use of recombinant erythropoietin redundant, this may take several months. The impact of administration of exogenous erythropoietin on recovery of erythropoietin production by the transplant has not been defined. Iron, folate and vitamin B_{12} concentrations should always be checked in anaemic patients and deficiency treated. Resistant anaemia may be the result of gastrointestinal bleeding. Persistent anaemia should be corrected where possible, as it contributes to morbidity (for instance by delayed wound healing) and has a substantial impact on patient well-being.

Blood transfusions

Transfusion of blood or other human products should be avoided where possible because of attendant risks associated with it, such as anaphylaxis, sensitisation and transmission of infection. However, in some situations transfusions are unavoidable, such as in severe symptomatic anaemia or in cases of rapid blood loss leading to haemodynamic compromise. Patients with CMV-negative serology who received a transplant from a CMV-seronegative donor should always be given CMV-negative blood. Patients who are unwilling to accept blood transfusion because of religious convictions may be willing to allow the use of a cell-saver peri-operatively to minimise the impact of peri-operative blood loss.

Post-transplant erythrocytosis

Post-transplant erythrocytosis is an intriguing condition affecting 10–20% of transplant recipients, usually in association with normal plasma concentrations of erythropoietin. The risk of thrombotic problems is minimised by reduction of the haematocrit to less than 45%. Angiotensin-converting enzyme (ACE) inhibitors and angiotensin-II receptor blockers are often effective in achieving this, but venesection may be required [13].

Calcium-phosphate product, hyperparathyroidism and the use of cinacalcet

Patients carry their CKD-related calcium- and phosphate-related problems into the post-transplant period. Although the functioning transplant enables 1-hydroxylation of vitamin D, converting the hormone to its active form, tertiary hyperparathyroidism persists in many patients. Alfacalcidol may not be required for vitamin-D replacement, but it may still be useful in controlling the hyperparathyroidism. If hypercalcaemia develops, the alfacalcidol should be discontinued. With restoration of renal function the chemical abnormalities of hyperparathyroidism revert to the physiological pattern of an elevated serum calcium concentration and reduced serum phosphate with restoration of one of the target organs for parathyroid hormone rather than the phosphate retaining state in renal failure. As a consequence, hypophosphataemia frequently occurs in the early post-transplant period, with CNI-induced tubular toxicity as a likely co-factor, which appears to be more of an issue with tacrolimus than ciclosporin. When serum phosphate falls to below 0.32 mmol/L the potentially serious complications of muscle weakness and rhabdomyolysis, which may involve the myocardium, ensue [14]. This may be corrected by increasing intake of phosphate-containing foods, such as oily fish and dairy products and/or the use of phosphate supplements such as sandozPhos and Neutra-Phos when severe. It is important that cinacalcet is not discontinued in the peri-transplant period to avoid loss of control of hyperparathyroidism. Phosphate binders should be discontinued at the time of transplantation. If hyperparathyroidism fails to resolve after the transplant, parathyroidectomy may be required, although treatment with cinacalcet may be sufficient.

Gout

Gout is a not uncommon problem in the early transplant period with the stress associated with the peri-operative period and dietary changes as likely contributory factors. Additionally the use of CNIs, particularly ciclosporin, loop or thiazide diuretics and co-trimoxazole are among the medications that seem to contribute. It can be readily treated with simple analgesia such as paracetamol, prednisolone or colchicine (0.5 mg three times daily). NSAIDs should not be given. Allopurinol is used for prophylaxis in those with a strong predilection to episodes. Allopurinol should not be given to patients treated with azathioprine, owing to the risk for severe myelosuppression through inhibition of the metabolism of azathioprine.

New-onset diabetes after transplantation

Approximately 25% of newly transplanted patients develop new glucose intolerance or overt diabetes mellitus in the early post-transplant period. Of these, approximately half return to normoglycaemia with modification in immunosuppressive drug exposure, with the remainder requiring lifelong treatment for diabetes. Those with pre-existing diabetes often develop difficult-to-control diabetes, requiring an escalation of their diabetic therapy, including the introduction of insulin in those already on oral hypoglycaemic drugs. This is largely as a result of the immunosuppressant regimens based on diabetogenic drugs: steroids, CNIs (particularly tacrolimus) and sirolimus. The risk factors for new-onset diabetes after transplantation (NODAT) are essentially the same as those for type-2 diabetes mellitus and include increasing age, obesity, family history of type-2 diabetes and ethnic group (commoner in individuals who are ethnically African, South Asian or Hispanic). Hepatitis C virus infection increases risk [15]. Attempts to use less diabetogenic regimens in those patients at highest risk are warranted. It is important to manage this complication early on because of its effect on cardiovascular outcome. Given that transplantation is a therapy that hopes to prolong survival, inflicting NODAT on a patient probably actually reduces their life expectancy, and as such is one of the most serious complications of transplantation. Management in the first instance includes tailoring of immunosuppressant regimens such as early withdrawal of steroids, use of lower CNI blood concentrations, dietary manipulation and discouraging excessive weight gain. Tacrolimus blood concentrations of greater than 15 ng/mL were associated with increased incidence of NODAT [16]. In cases where conservative measures are inadequate, oral hypoglycaemics may need to be introduced followed by insulin if required. In terms of choice of oral hypoglycaemic agent, metformin would be a logical choice but is difficult to use in patients with renal impairment. Conventional guidance is to use a reduced dose in patients with GFR <45 mL/min/1.73 m^2 and to avoid in patients with GFR <30 mL/min/1.73 m^2 due to risk of the potentially serious complication, lactic acidosis. The more straightforward option is to use a sulfonylurea, but this comes at the expense of weight gain.

Proteinuria

Patients with end-stage renal failure as a result of proteinuric disease such as FSGS and IgA nephropathy should always have their urinary protein leak quantified before transplantation. This enables an objective assessment of increased urinary protein leak in the recipient, allowing identification of early recurrent disease. ACE inhibitors, angiotensin-II receptor blockers and statins should be given to proteinuric patients to reduce protein leak.

Hypertension

In general, hypertension is less well controlled after transplantation than before, owing to a combination of CNIs and steroids and probably mediators released from the transplant in response to ischaemia. Target blood pressure is addressed in detail in Chapter 23. There is no need to attain optimal blood pressure of <130/80 in the very early period, when drug doses are likely to be tapered and fluid overload resolves. A pragmatic target of <140/85 during the first few weeks after transplantation to enable safe biopsy is probably acceptable, with adherence to more stringent targets in the longer term.

Most clinicians would discontinue ACE inhibitors or angiotensin-II receptor blockers at the time of transplantation, owing to their potential adverse effect on GFR. However, there is no evidence that this is detrimental to transplant outcome and, in spite of standard practice, early use of ACE inhibitors is not an unreasonable strategy. Introduction of these drugs during the first 3 months has potential to cause diagnostic problems because of a fall in GFR leading to increased need for investigations, including biopsy. After the first 2–3 months when acute rejection is uncommon, introduction of ACE inhibitors/angiotensin-II receptor blockers can be undertaken with more confidence and a step-up in serum creatinine of 10–20% with stabilisation need not be investigated. Although there is no direct evidence of benefit in the long term over other classes of drugs, extrapolation from the data on progressive chronic renal failure due to other causes makes them an attractive choice for long-term management of hypertension in transplant recipients, particularly those with proteinuria.

In the early period after the transplant the dihydropyridine calcium channel blockers (e.g. nifedipine as a sustained release preparation, amlodipine) are the easiest drugs to use. They do not reduce GFR and attenuate the vasospastic effect of the CNIs [17]. In the peri-operative period there may be an advantage to the use of drugs with a shorter half-life, such as nifedipine-LA in the event of excessive fall in blood pressure. The non-dihydropyridine calcium channel blockers (diltiazem and verapamil) significantly inhibit cytochrome P450 and P-glycoprotein, resulting in increased oral bioavailability of the CNIs and mTOR inhibitors. They should be introduced with cautious monitoring and dose adjustment of the immunosuppressive drugs. This should also be taken into account when discontinuing diltiazem or verapamil, as there is a risk of the patient becoming under-immunosuppressed.

Beta-blockers should not be discontinued in the peri-operative period, as this increases the risk of intraoperative cardiac events.

Prescribing

Polypharmacy in the early post-transplant period is a major issue, with a number of narrow therapeutic index drugs with the potential for significant drug interactions. It is essential that all prescribing decisions are made or discussed with a transplant clinician. Key interactions to be aware of are drugs with an influence on cytochrome P450 and P-glycoprotein that affect the oral bioavailability of the CNIs and mTOR inhibitors (discussed in detail in Chapter 16). The most common inhibitors that increase immunosuppressive drug exposure are the imidazole antifungals (e.g. fluconazole, ketoconazole) and the macrolide antibiotics (e.g. erythromycin, clarithromycin). The commonest inducers that reduce immunosuppressive drug exposure are rifampicin and the anticonvulsants, carbamazepine and phenytoin. Some would advocate adjusting anticonvulsant regimens before transplantation to avoid these drugs. However, if seizures are well controlled, it is reasonable to continue but to use twofold higher initial doses of CNI than in standard practice.

GFR is in a state of change in the early post-transplant period and renally eliminated drugs require dose adjustment. This is particularly important for the synthetic nucleoside antivirals (e.g. valganciclovir, aciclovir) where doses must be increased as renal function improves to avoid subtherapeutic blood concentrations and reduced if renal function deteriorates to avoid toxicity. An important influence of renal function on drug metabolism that is often overlooked is the increased elimination of mycophenolic acid in patients with renal impairment. Higher doses are required in patients to achieve therapeutic blood concentrations in the early period after transplantation than later, when good renal function is established.

Prophylactic treatments

Most patients will be prescribed some anti-infection prophylaxis including co-trimoxazole to prevent *Pneumocystis jiroveci* infection, and many patients will be given antifungal treatment (see Chapter 21 for a detailed discussion). Patients treated with steroids are usually given a gastric acid suppressant, either a proton pump inhibitor or an H_2 receptor blocker to reduce the risk of steroid-induced peptic ulceration.

Lifestyle and dietary advice

One of the key benefits of transplantation is a return to a normal healthy diet rather than the very restrictive diet of patients with advanced renal failure. Excessive weight gain is a common problem owing to resolution of uraemia, with improved appetite and the appetite-boosting effect of steroids. Cardiovascular co-morbidity, in particular hypertension, is common. Patients should be advised to avoid excessive calorie intake and to minimise intake of animal fats and sodium. Smoking cessation should be encouraged. An appropriate level of exercise should also be encouraged [18]. A detailed account of cardiovascular risk factor management including hyperlipidaemia is provided in Chapter 23.

Contraceptive advice

Pregnancy should be avoided during the first year after transplantation. Restoration of fertility, which will not have been a major consideration for most female dialysis patients, requires contraceptive advice. Recent comprehensive guidance, issued by the Centers for Disease Control (CDC) in the USA, on contraceptive use across the full range of medical conditions including solid organ transplantation can be found at http://www.cdc.gov/mmwr/preview/mmwrhtml/rr59e0528a1.htm.

Oestrogen-containing combined oral contraceptives are often avoided because of the potential for increased risk of vascular complications. The CDC guidance suggests that combined preparations are acceptable for 'uncomplicated' transplant recipients but not for 'complicated' patients. Progesterone-only preparations are probably safer but come with a slightly higher failure rate. There has been concern over the incidence of infection associated with use of intrauterine devices (IUD), although with modern devices this is probably not a major issue. Progesterone-coated IUDs are particularly useful for control of menorrhagia.

Dialysis access

Central venous catheters used for dialysis access should be removed as soon as the patient is independent of dialysis. Peritoneal dialysis catheters can be removed at the time of ureteric stent removal, 4–6 weeks after transplantation. With live donor transplantation, where there is a high chance of immediate graft function, it is reasonable to remove peritoneal dialysis catheters at the transplant operation.

Proximal arteriovenous fistulae, particularly those that have become aneurysmal can increase cardiac output significantly with increased cardiac workload. When good graft function is established, 3 to 6 months after transplantation, brachiocephalic arteriovenous fistulae should be ligated. This is less of an issue for radial fistulae, which can be left unless they have become aneurysmal, in which case they should be ligated.

References

1. Vincenti F, Ghiggeri GM. (2005) New insights into the pathogenesis and the therapy of recurrent focal glomerulosclerosis. *Am J Transplant* **5**, 1179–1185.
2. KDIGO. (2009) KDIGO Clinical Practice Guideline for the care of kidney transplant recipients. *Am J Transplant* **9** (Suppl 3), S1–S155.
3. Hickson LJ, Gera M, Amer H, *et al.* (2009) Kidney transplantation for primary focal segmental glomerulosclerosis: outcomes and response to therapy for recurrence. *Transplantation* **87**, 1232–1239.
4. Taylor CM, Machin S, Wigmore SJ, *et al.* (2010) Clinical practice guidelines for the management of atypical haemolytic uraemic syndrome in the United Kingdom. *Br J Haematol* **148**, 37–47.
5. Zuber J, Le Quintrec M, Sberro-Soussan R, *et al.* (2011) New insights into postrenal transplant hemolytic uremic syndrome. *Nat Rev Nephrol* **7**, 23–35.
6. Naesens M, Lerut E, Damme BV, *et al.* (2007) Tacrolimus exposure and evolution of renal allograft histology in the first year after transplantation. *Am J Transplant* **7**, 2114–2123.
7. Rush D, Arlen D, Boucher A, *et al.* (2007) Lack of benefit of early protocol biopsies in renal transplant patients receiving TAC and MMF: A randomized study. *Am J Transplant* **7**, 2538–2545.
8. Park WD, Griffin MD, Cornell LD, *et al.* (2010) Fibrosis with inflammation at one year predicts transplant functional decline. *J Am Soc Nephrol* **21**, 1987–1997.
9. Hedges SJ, Dehoney SB, Hooper JS, *et al.* (2007) Evidence-based treatment recommendations for uremic bleeding. *Nat Clin Pract Nephrol* **3**, 138–153.
10. Nicholson ML, Wheatley TJ, Doughman TM, *et al.* (2000) A prospective randomized trial of three different sizes of core-cutting needle for renal transplant biopsy. *Kidney Int* **58**, 390–395.
11. Montalvo BM, Yrizarry JM, Casillas VJ, *et al.* (1996) Percutaneous sclerotherapy of lymphoceles related to renal transplantation. *J Vasc Interv Radiol* **7**, 117–123.
12. Syversveen T, Midtvedt K, Brabrand K, *et al.* (2011) Prophylactic peritoneal fenestration to prevent morbidity after kidney transplantation: a randomized study. *Transplantation* **92**, 196–202.
13. Yildiz A, Cine N, Akkaya V, *et al.* (2001) Comparison of the effects of enalapril and losartan on posttransplantation erythrocytosis in renal transplant recipients: prospective randomized study. *Transplantation* **72**, 542–544.
14. Halevy J, Bulvik S. (1988) Severe hypophosphatemia in hospitalized patients. *Arch Intern Med* **148**, 153–155.
15. Kasiske BL, Snyder JJ, Gilbertson D, *et al.* (2003) Diabetes mellitus after kidney transplantation in the United States. *Am J Transplant* **3**, 178–185.
16. Maes BD, Kuypers D, Messiaen T, *et al.* (2001) Posttransplantation diabetes mellitus in FK-506-treated renal transplant recipients: Analysis of incidence and risk factors. *Transplantation* **72**, 1655–1661.

17. Ruggenenti P, Perico N, Mosconi L, *et al.* (1993) Calcium channel blockers protect transplant patients from cyclosporine-induced daily renal hypoperfusion. *Kidney Int* **43**, 706–711.
18. Painter PL, Hector L, Ray K, *et al.* (2003) Effects of exercise training on coronary heart disease risk factors in renal transplant recipients. *Am J Kidney Dis* **42**, 362–369.

23 Management of long-term complications

Paul N. Harden, Richard Haynes, Iain A.M. MacPhee and Jiří Froněk

Part 1: Cardiovascular disease

Burden of disease

The principal focus of management of the transplant recipient has been for many years to protect the graft from immunological rejection. However, as acute rejection rates have fallen, increasing attention has been paid to the causes of late graft loss [1]. It has become apparent that death with a functioning graft is a major cause of graft loss – and that cardiovascular death and malignancy are the leading causes of death – in transplant recipients after the first year post-transplantation [2]. Cardiovascular disease accounts for more than 50% of all deaths after the first year, although the relative contribution of malignancy to post-transplantation mortality is increasing and has overtaken cardiovascular disease in Australasia in recent years [3]. In this chapter we will overview the aetiology, clinical presentations and management options of cardiovascular disease and malignancy post-transplantation.

The rate of cardiovascular mortality is more than 20 times higher in renal transplant recipients aged 25–34 years compared with the age- and sex-matched general population [3]. The disparity between the renal transplant and general populations declines with age, but the risk of cardiovascular death only become similar after the age of 65. This may be because older potential transplant recipients are investigated more thoroughly for underlying cardiovascular disease (and patients with it are not offered transplantation), or because of incomplete ascertainment of causes of death in older people.

Cardiovascular morbidity is also more common in renal transplant recipients than the general population: in one study of 403 renal transplant recipients who had no clinical evidence of atherosclerotic disease at the time of transplantation, over 15% went on to develop atherosclerotic complications during the follow-up period (average of 46 months). Registry data from the USA show an annual incidence of 10%

Handbook of Renal and Pancreatic Transplantation, First Edition. Edited by Iain A. M. MacPhee and Jiří Froněk.
© 2012 John Wiley & Sons, Ltd. Published 2012 by John Wiley & Sons, Ltd.

of hospitalisation for cardiovascular problems in the transplant population [4].

Nature of cardiovascular disease in renal transplant recipients

In the general population most cardiovascular disease is caused by atherosclerosis, which manifests as myocardial infarction, angina, ischaemic stroke, transient ischaemic attack and peripheral arterial disease. It is increasingly recognised that patients with advanced kidney disease (including those on dialysis) are at much higher risk of cardiovascular disease, but the nature of the cardiovascular disease is different. Whereas coronary disease accounts for over half of cardiovascular mortality in the general population, it accounted for less than one-fifth of cardiovascular mortality in a population of diabetic haemodialysis patients. It is becoming increasingly clear that as renal function falls although the risk of cardiovascular disease increases, the type of cardiovascular disease also changes. This is consistent with pathological observations that demonstrate an increasing burden of arterial stiffness and structural heart disease as renal function falls. These predispose to heart failure, arrhythmias and sudden cardiac death (SCD) [5]. As an example, the annual incidence of SCD in the chronic kidney disease (CDK) population is 2.8%, which is five times that in the general population. In the US dialysis population, SCD accounts for two-thirds of all cardiac mortality [4,6].

Renal transplantation improves renal function significantly, although it rarely restores normal renal function. However, a typical patient with CKD progresses to end-stage renal failure (ESRF) over many years and accumulates cardiovascular damage (e.g. vascular calcification, left ventricular structural changes, atherosclerosisis) during this time and these structural changes and the risks they confer are not reversed – at least not rapidly – by transplantation. For example, admission for heart failure is three times more common in the transplant population compared with the general population. Risk scores based on traditional cardiovascular risk factors (e.g. the Framingham risk score) underestimate the cardiovascular risk, suggesting that additional factors are involved [6]. Renal transplant recipients therefore continue to be at risk of the cardiovascular disease typical of advanced kidney disease (especially as their graft function declines), but the precise nature (and the effect of graft function on it) has not been well studied.

Effect of transplantation on cardiovascular disease

Although transplantation increases survival compared to remaining on the waiting list considerably [7], the effect of transplantation on cardiovascular disease is less clear. Transplantation – and the associated immunosuppression – have variable effects on cardiovascular risk markers, some of which are favourable and some of which are not (see Table 23.1).

Table 23.1 Effects of transplantation on various cardiovascular risk markers.

Favourable	Neutral/uncertain	Unfavourable
Blood pressure	Left ventricular hypertrophy	Dyslipidaemia
Cigarette smoking		Body mass index
		Glucose tolerance

Blood pressure

Three-quarters of renal transplant recipients remain classified as hypertensive according to current definitions [8], but blood pressure control is often improved by transplantation [9]. Immunosuppressant medications are involved in the aetiology of post-transplant hypertension. Although corticosteroids increase blood pressure (via mineralocorticoid sodium retention effects and weight gain) at high doses, chronic low-dose corticosteroid therapy probably has little effect on blood pressure. Calcineurin inhibitors (CNIs) also increase blood pressure by activating the renin-angiotensin and endothelin systems [10].

The increase in body mass index (BMI) following transplantation also raises blood pressure (see below). Transplant renal artery stenosis may also raise blood pressure, but the prevalence of this is uncertain, with estimates ranging from 1 to 23% depending on definition.

Cigarette smoking

Although transplantation does not have a direct effect on tobacco consumption, the enforced abstinence around the time of surgery does afford an opportunity to permanently cease tobacco consumption. One small study in Turkey found that although 42% of renal transplant recipients smoked cigarettes before transplantation, only 12% continued to do so postoperatively [11].

Left ventricular hypertrophy

Left ventricular hypertrophy is the predominant feature of 'uraemic' cardiomyopathy and is present in over 70% of patients with ESRF. Echocardiographic studies have suggested that left ventricular mass reduces after successful transplantation, but these may be confounded by the restorative effects of transplantation on intravascular (and hence intraventricular) volume and the assumptions made in calculating left ventricular mass by echocardiography. Cardiac magnetic resonance imaging provides a more precise method of measuring left ventricular mass, and a study using this method showed no change in left ventricular mass after transplantation [12].

Dyslipidaemia

The dyslipidaemia observed in CKD is characterised by raised triglyceride concentrations, low high-density lipoprotein cholesterol (HDL-C) concentrations and normal concentrations of low-density lipoprotein cholesterol (LDL-C), although the LDL particles may be smaller. Following transplantation, concentrations of HDL-C tend to rise and – more ominously – so do LDL-C concentrations. It is difficult to disentangle what the effects are of transplantation (and improved kidney function) are and what are side effects of immunosuppression.

Corticosteroids have multiple effects on lipid metabolism, including hyperinsulinaemia-mediated stimulation of hepatic very-low-density lipoprotein (VLDL, the precursor to LDL) hepatic synthesis and downregulation of LDL receptors [13]. Randomised trials of steroid withdrawal suggest that steroids may increase total cholesterol, although they do not appear to alter the total:HDL cholesterol ratio [14].

CNIs also contribute to dyslipidaemia post-transplantation, although tacrolimus appears to have smaller effects than ciclosporin. Ciclosporin increases LDL-C and reduces HDL-C in a dose-dependent manner independently of concurrent corticosteroid use [15]. Conversion from ciclosporin (target C0 50–200 ng/mL) to tacrolimus (target C0 5–8 ng/mL) reduced LDL-C from 3.48 to 3.11 mmol/L [16]. Sirolimus has well-described effects on lipids and increases both cholesterol and triglycerides. Although early studies targeted relatively high trough concentrations (and hence may have exaggerated the effects of sirolimus), more recent studies confirm that sirolimus use is associated with higher concentrations of cholesterol despite more common use of lipid-lowering therapies.

Body mass index

Many patients with ESRF and on dialysis are malnourished, so weight gain following transplantation may be a sign of improving health. However, in many patients the weight gain continues, and the average weight gain in the first year after transplantation is over 10 kg. More than 30% of kidney transplant recipients are obese (BMI >30 kg/m^2) after 1 year compared with 10% at the time of transplantation. One single-centre observational study has shown that the risk of cardiac disease (especially heart failure and atrial fibrillation) rises from 9 to 30% from the lowest to highest quartile of BMI [17].

Homocysteine

Increased concentrations of homocysteine have been identified in the general population as a risk marker for cardiovascular disease, and genetic 'Mendelian randomisation' studies have supported the hypothesis that it may be causal. Although transplantation frequently reduces homocysteine concentrations, they remain elevated compared with healthy controls and indeed patients with CKD (possibly due to an effect of ciclosporin) [18].

Glucose tolerance

New-onset diabetes mellitus after transplantation (NODAT) is not uncommon, affecting up to half of all kidney transplant recipients (depending on the definition used and population studied) [19].

Non-modifiable risk factors for development of NODAT previously have been reported as ethnic group, genetic background, older age, family history of diabetes, and previous glucose intolerance. Modifiable risk factors are obesity, hepatitis C virus and cytomegalovirus infections, and immunosuppressive drugs. Again, CNIs and corticosteroids are the major culprits, although in randomised trials tacrolimus is more diabetogenic than ciclosporin [20]. Recent data suggest that sirolimus is as diabetogenic as tacrolimus. Whereas steroids and sirolimus cause insulin resistance, CNIs are also toxic to pancreatic beta cells.

NODAT appears to confer a similar risk of cardiovascular disease as pre-existing (i.e. prior to transplantation) diabetes. The risk of cardiovascular mortality is increased about 1.5–3 times in patients with NODAT compared with normoglycaemic controls. Importantly, even impaired fasting glucose or impaired glucose tolerance ('pre-diabetic' states) are associated with an increased cardiovascular risk. The high prevalence and prognostic implications of glucose intolerance after transplantation justify the recommendation for screening in the post-transplant period.

Chronic kidney disease

Successful transplantation causes a substantial improvement in renal function, but the glomerular filtration rate (GFR) remains moderately reduced in most recipients. A recent meta-analysis of observational studies in the general population has reliably demonstrated an inverse relationship between estimated GFR and cardiovascular risk. Observational studies of renal transplant recipients have confirmed that the same association is observed after renal transplantation. In the Assessment on Lescol in Renal Transplantation (ALERT) study, each 100 µmol/L increase in serum creatinine was associated with a 90% increased risk of a major adverse cardiac event (HR 1.89; 95% CI 1.42–2.55) after adjustment for other risk factors.

Interventions to reduce cardiovascular risk

The burden of cardiovascular disease is therefore very great in the transplant population. Transplantation itself – although having a favourable effect on overall patient survival and quality of life – has some adverse effects on cardiovascular risk markers. It is therefore imperative to manage cardiovascular risk factors as aggressively as possible to reduce the risk of cardiovascular disease. Ideally such management would be based on high-quality evidence from randomised trials and meta-analyses of such trials. Unfortunately, there are very few high-quality trials of cardiovascular interventions in transplant recipients. It is therefore frequently necessary to extrapolate from trial evidence in the general population until more direct evidence becomes available. Observational data in the transplant population will be confounded both by disease (i.e. reverse causality) and treatment, so such studies may give misleading results.

Lifestyle modification

Although pharmacological interventions will be required in the majority, lifestyle modification is applicable to all transplant recipients.

Smoking cessation

Smoking cessation substantially reduces the risk of cardiovascular disease and death in the general population. Unsurprisingly, smoking also increases the risk of cancer, cardiovascular disease and death in the renal transplant population, and such risks are mitigated by stopping [21]. It may take up to 5 years for the benefits of cessation to become apparent, highlighting the need to encourage this as early as possible with patients (ideally before they require transplantation).

Exercise, diet and weight control

Exercise, diet and weight control are an interrelated triad. Regular aerobic exercise increases HDL-C by 3–9% in healthy sedentary people, with greater increases occurring with frequent low-intensity exercise. HDL-C has an inverse association with cardiovascular disease, so raising it may be worthwhile (although there is no randomised trial data to support this yet). Walking, however, is probably not sufficient alone to increase HDL-C but does reduce LDL-C. If exercise does not lead to weight loss it does not appear to increase HDL-C. Obesity is associated with poor outcomes in both the general population, presumably at least in part mediated through its effects on lipids, blood pressure and insulin resistance. Similar associations have also been observed in the transplant population, so it is reasonable to advocate normalisation of weight [22]. In addition, salt intake should be minimised, especially in patients with hypertension. A low-salt diet contains only 2 g salt per day, although most patients find this hard to achieve.

Immunosuppression modulation

As noted above, many immunosuppressants have potentially deleterious effects on cardiovascular risk factors. Therefore cardiovascular risk needs to be taken into account when deciding on an immunosuppressant regimen for a given patient (e.g. if they are at particularly high-risk for NODAT then it may be desirable to avoid tacrolimus and steroids – or wean them rapidly). However, although there are often conflicting priorities, it is important not to underestimate the importance of cardiovascular disease in renal transplant recipients and therefore give it due weight in the decision-making process. No trials to date comparing different immunosuppression regimens have reported cardiovascular end points, so inferences must be drawn from the effects on intermediate variables such as blood pressure and LDL-C.

Reducing blood pressure

Observational data in the general population shows a continuous log-linear positive association between systolic blood pressure and cardiovascular disease. For every 20 mmHg increase in systolic blood pressure (or 10 mmHg increase in diastolic blood pressure) the risk of stroke death more than doubles and the risk of coronary or other vascular death doubles. The causal nature of this association is confirmed by large-scale randomised trials, which have reliably demonstrated that lowering blood pressure reduces the risk of cardiovascular events and mortality [23]. A 5/2 mmHg reduction in blood pressure (typical of that achieved by standard antihypertensive agents) reduces the risk of major cardiovascular events by about one-fifth (HR 0.78; 95% CI 0.73–0.83). Although there may be some subtle differences in the efficacy of various antihypertensive agents, the most important factor is the degree of blood pressure reduction achieved [24].

Patients with mild CKD (e.g. CKD stages 1–3) have been included in these trials, and some have reported the outcome in this subgroup. For example, the Perindopril Protection Against Recurrent Stroke (PROGRESS) study included 1757 participants with stage 3 or greater CKD among the 6105 participants with prior cerebrovascular disease who had been enrolled [25]. Assignment to active therapy was associated with a one-third reduction in the risk of stroke in these CKD patients (HR 0.65; 95% CI 0.50–0.83), which was similar to that observed in the whole study population. Similarly, in a post-hoc analysis of the Heart Outcomes and Prevention Evaluation (HOPE) study, patients with impaired kidney function (serum creatinine >124 μmol/L or 1.4 mg/dL) benefited from a similar reduction to patients with normal renal function in cardiovascular events with ramipril 10 mg daily compared to placebo with no increase in the risk of adverse events.

There have been a number of small trials of various antihypertensive agents in kidney transplantation, but these trials have focused on graft-related outcomes and have been too small or too short to collect any useful data on cardiovascular outcomes [26]. Therefore, the best data on which to assess the effects of blood pressure reduction are those from the general population, as discussed above. Because transplant recipients are younger on average than those patients in the trials, the benefits of blood pressure reduction may be even greater because the association between blood pressure and risk is stronger at younger ages. In the absence of direct randomised trial data, it would seem reasonable to apply data from the general population, as there is no reason to think that kidney transplant recipients will differ significantly. Current international guidelines recommend that adult transplant recipients should have blood pressure maintained at <130/<80 mmHg [27]. No specific class of antihypertensive is recommended unless urinary protein excretion is ≥1 g/day, in which case either an angiotensin-converting enzyme (ACE) inhibitor or angiotensin II receptor blocker (ARB) are recommended.

Reducing LDL cholesterol

LDL-C also has a log-linear association with coronary disease in the general population, with a 1 mmol/L increase in non-HDL-C (a surrogate for LDL-C, which is expensive to measure directly) being associated with a 50% increase in the risk of coronary disease (HR 1.50; 95% CI 1.39–1.61) and a 10% increase in the risk of ischaemic stroke (HR 1.12; 95% CI 1.04–1.20). Randomised trials of lowering LDL-C with HMG-CoA reductase inhibitors ('statins') have shown very clearly that at 1 mmol/L reduction in LDL-C leads to a one-fifth reduction in major coronary events (HR 0.77; 95% CI 0.74–0.80) and stroke (HR 0.83; 95% CI 0.78–0.88).

Subgroup analyses of some of these large statin trials have confirmed that the relative risk reduction is similar in patients with mild CKD to that in the general population. For example, pooling data from the three pravastatin studies, of 19,700 participants, 4491 (28%) had CKD stage 3. Randomisation to pravastatin was associated with a reduction in the risk of the primary outcome (myocardial infarction, coronary death or percutaneous/surgical coronary revascularisation). The hazard ratio of 0.77 (95% CI 0.68–0.86) was similar to the effect of the statin on the primary outcome in participants with normal kidney function. The Study of Heart and Renal Protection (SHARP) trial showed a clear benefit of reducing LDL-C in patients with both advanced CKD and those on dialysis. The observed benefits were very similar to those seen in previous trials conducted in the general population.

There has been one large study of statin in the kidney transplant population. In the ALERT study, 2102 patients receiving ciclosporin-based immunosuppression were assigned to receive fluvastatin 40 to 80 mg or placebo [28]. After a mean follow-up of 5.1 years there was a 17% reduction in the combined primary end point of cardiac death, non-fatal myocardial infarction and coronary intervention procedures in the fluvastatin-treated group, which did not reach statistical significance (RR 0.83; 95% 0.64–1.06) [28]. A post-hoc analysis excluding interventional procedures from the primary end point demonstrated a reduction associated with statin therapy (RR 0.65, 95% CI 0.48–0.88), as did a follow-up analysis based on the primary end point but including an additional 2-year extended period during which all participants were offered open-label treatment (RR 0.79, 95% CI 0.63–0.99). Although ciclosporin is known to increase blood concentrations of statins, no safety issues were encountered during the ALERT study. The results of ALERT are completely consistent with the effects of a similar LDL-C reduction in the general population, and therefore suggest that the only reason the initial result failed to meet a conventionally significant result was the size of the study (which although large in transplant medicine is small in the field of cardiovascular disease).

There is therefore good evidence to support reducing LDL-C in kidney transplant recipients. This is supported by the SHARP study, which demonstrated that reducing LDL-C is as effective in patients with CKD as the general population [29]. Although it excluded transplant recipients, it seems unlikely that they would differ substantially to other patients with CKD. In the general population more intensive LDL-C reduction is superior to standard LDL-C reduction. Therefore, intensive LDL-C reduction should be used, and the trial data show that benefit will accrue regardless of the starting LDL-C concentration [30] (although the absolute benefits will be smaller at lower LDL-C concentrations because of the smaller absolute reduction in LDL-C induced by treatment). Current guidelines recommend that transplant recipients are treated if LDL-C is ≥2.59 mmol/L, aiming to reduce LDL-C below 2.59 mmol/L [27]. If there is a history of vascular disease it would seem reasonable to be more aggressive and aim to maintain LDL-C <2 mmol/L in line with guidelines in the general population [31]. At present there are no reliable data on whether intervening on other aspects of dyslipidaemia (e.g. triglycerides, HDL-C or Lp(a)) are beneficial in the general population, let alone the transplant population.

Glycaemic control

Many transplant recipients have diabetes mellitus before transplantation and, as stated above, NODAT is a common occurrence post-transplantation, which is associated with a significantly increased risk of cardiovascular disease. There are no trials of glycaemic control in the transplant population with clinical end points. In the general population, the aggregate data from trials of more versus less intensive glycaemic control favours more intensive therapy [32]. Intensive control (which reduced haemoglobin A1c by 0.9%) resulted in a 17% reduction in events of non-fatal myocardial infarction (OR 0.83; 95% CI 0.75–0.93), and a 15% reduction in events of coronary heart disease (OR 0.85; 0.77–0.93). No hypoglycaemic agents are contraindicated by transplantation, and the focus of therapy should be tight glycaemic control rather than on specific agents. Most nephrologists would be comfortable using metformin until estimated GFR (eGFR) <30 mL/min/1.73 m^2, after which caution should be taken.

Antiplatelet therapy

Antiplatelet therapy (chiefly aspirin) is well proven to reduce the risk of cardiovascular events in high-risk patient groups, such as those with symptomatic occlusive arterial disease (e.g. prior myocardial infarction, stroke or transient ishaemic attack). However, its use in the primary prevention of cardiovascular disease is more controversial. In the healthy general population, antiplatelet therapy does modestly reduce the risk of myocardial infarction, but it also increases the risk of intra- and extra-cranial bleeding significantly. In the context of proven safe and effective preventive treatments (e.g. blood pressure and LDL-C-lowering treatments), the absolute benefits of aspirin are likely to be outweighed by the bleeding hazards in low-risk (i.e. cardiovascular risk) patient populations. There is, however, substantial uncertainty in patient groups at moderate risk of cardiovascular disease, which includes patients with diabetes or CKD (including transplant recipients). Most cardiovascular risk factors also increase the risk of bleeding so cannot be used to identify which patients will benefit from aspirin. Direct randomised evidence is therefore required, but at present widespread use of aspirin for primary cardiovascular prophylaxis cannot be justified. However, aspirin is likely to be as effective in secondary prevention in kidney transplant recipients as the general population so should be used in those patients with a history of occlusive arterial disease.

Homocysteine reduction

As stated above, homocysteine appears to be an independent risk factor for cardiovascular disease, with some genetic studies suggesting a causal relationship. However, in the general population, reducing homocysteine has not been shown to reduce the risk of cardiovascular disease. In one large study in a post-myocardial infarction population, reducing homocysteine by 3.8 μmol/L had no impact on the rate of cardiovascular events in almost 7 years of follow-up. The Folic Acid for Vascular Outcome Reduction in Transplantation (FAVORIT) study reported provisional results in 2009 that confirmed that lowering homocysteine in transplant recipients had no impact on cardiovascular disease [33].

Mineral bone disorder

Post-transplant bone disease is discussed in more detail below. It is increasingly recognised that the mineral bone abnormalities observed in CKD are associated with adverse cardiovascular outcomes in addition to fractures and bone disease [34]. Vascular calcification is associated with both serum phosphate and calcium-containing phosphate binder use. There are no specific data in transplant recipients, and in the CKD population it is unclear whether sparing calcium-containing phosphate binders by using sevelamer or other non-calcium containing phosphate binders can prevent the progression of vascular calcification [35]. Current guidelines suggest maintaining serum phosphate in the normal range [36]. The choice of phosphate binder should be guided by the presence of other components of mineral bone disorder, concomitant therapies and side-effect profile.

Summary

Cardiovascular disease is a significant problem for transplant recipients. One year after surgery, death (most likely cardiovascular) with a functioning graft is more likely than graft loss, but it remains an understudied condition. Transplant recipients accrue significant cardiovascular structural damage during the progression of CKD to ESRF, and transplantation does not – at least rapidly – reverse many of these changes and the risks they engender. In addition, immunosuppression has undesirable effects on many cardiovascular risk factors.

With the notable exception of the ALERT study there are no reliable randomised data to guide the treatment and prevention of cardiovascular disease and therefore those caring for these patients must rely on extrapolations from the general population. These would support aggressive control of blood pressure, LDL cholesterol and glucose. If effects observed in the general population could be applied to the transplant population it should be possible to more than halve the risk of cardiovascular disease with careful attention to these risk factors. Transplant clinicians must consider cardiovascular risk carefully from work-up for transplantation through to the long-term follow-up of such patients.

Part 2: Malignancy

The frequency of malignancy is increased in all populations of transplant recipients, with a greater incidence over the general population of approximately 2.7 (SIR). However, the risk varies according to tumour type, from similar incidence rates to those for breast cancer, to rates greater than 15 times for hypernephroma, and over 200 times for squamous cell carcinoma of the skin [37]. At 10 years post-transplantation 10% of the recipients will have developed at least one solid organ tumour, accounting for at least 15% of deaths in UK recipients [38].

Mechanisms leading to neoplasia in transplant recipients

Transplant recipients are exposed to the same genetic and environmental risk factors for the development of malignancy as the general population. However, the presence of the transplanted organ leads to the requirement for long-term immunosuppression to maintain transplant function, which confers an increased risk of opportunistic infection and malignancy. Immunosuppression for other systemic medical disorders such as rheumatoid arthritis has also been shown to lead to an increased incidence of cancer, supporting the hypothesis that immunosuppression is tumourigenic.

Role of immunosuppression

The main objective of immunosuppression is to suppress T-cell-mediated immunity to minimise the immune and inflammatory reaction against the transplanted organ. Unfortunately, many of the commonly used immunosuppressive drugs are non-specific and attenuate a range of cell functions in many cell types. The CNI ciclosporin causes upregulation of transforming growth factor beta (TGF-β) and vascular endothelial growth factor (VEGF), which leads to tumour metastases and angiogenesis in animal models [39]. Azathioprine has been shown to impair repair of ultraviolet-light-induced DNA damage in the skin and CNIs cause a dose-dependent reduction in DNA repair. Many immunosuppressant drugs impair the cell cycle and cell growth in multiple cell types, potentially predisposing to abnormal cell growth. Induction therapy with antithymocyte globulin (ATG) or OKT3 is associated with a significant increased risk of developing post-transplant lymphoproliferative disease (PTLD). Registry and published series of azathioprine and/or CNI-based immunosuppression have only shown an association between duration of immunosuppression risk and malignancy risk and not a relationship with specific immunosuppressive agents [40]. The role of immunosuppression has recently evolved with emerging data on the mammalian target of rapamycin (mTOR) inhibitor sirolimus, which may lead to a reduction in the incidence of cancer. mTOR inhibitors inhibit the growth cycle but importantly also inhibit angiogenesis and may therefore inhibit tumour cell growth and metastasis through upregulation of E-cadherin, which improves cell-to-cell adhesion [39]. In clinical practice mTOR-inhibitors have proven beneficial in the treatment of Kaposi's sarcoma post-transplant. This rare cutaneous tumour's growth is driven by VEGF and the lesion will often regress with conversion of immunosuppression to an mTOR-inhibitor-based regimen [41]. Further evidence comes from a small randomised trial of switching maintenance immunosuppression from a CNI-based regimen to an mTOR-inhibitor regimen in patients with non-melanoma skin cancer (NMSC). There was a small but significant reduction in the incidence of further NMSC in patients switched to the mTOR inhibitor sirolimus compared with those remaining on a CNI-based regimen [42]. It is clear that malignancy is increased post-transplantation, but the causative role of immunosuppression has become more complex with the introduction of mTOR-inhibitors. It is often very difficult to tease out the exact contribution of a given immunosuppressant drug in clinical practice, as the recipient is frequently taking a mixture of two or three immunosuppressive drugs, which may include a drug known to promote malignancy such as ciclosporin and a drug known to reduce malignancy risk such as sirolimus. The variable risk of different cancers post-transplantation suggests that immunosuppression alone cannot explain the increased incidence of tumour development, and additional factors must play a role.

Role of viral infection

Opportunistic viral infections are common in the first year post-transplantation and are frequently the result of reactivation of latent virus in the recipient or new infection from the transplanted organ. Several viral infections are associated with the development of malignancy in individuals receiving maintenance immunosuppressive medication. The most serious example is Epstein–Barr virus (EBV) and its association with PTLD. Human herpes virus 8 (HHV-8) is associated with Kaposi's sarcoma, and polyomavirus infection may be associated with uro-epithelial tumours. There is a clear association between human papilloma virus (HPV) and cervical cancer, but the role of HPV in NMSC is less clear. There are multiple serotypes of HPV and the virus is identified in over 60% of NMSC. However, there is a more definite relationship between actinic keratoses on the skin than warts and subsequent NMSC. The oncogenic virus produces uncontrolled cell division by breaking down the control mechanisms of cell division and preventing the cell from entering apoptosis by encoding FADD 1 like interleukinIB, converting enzyme-like protease inhibited proteins (FLIPs). The resulting transformed cells bearing cell surface viral antigens escape recognition by the recipients suppressed immune surveillance system and can lead to tumourigenesis [43]. A second important mechanism of potential viral-induced cancer is inhibition of the p53 tumour suppressor gene. Normally p53 leads to apoptosis in response to the generation of DNA damage and destruction of potential tumour cells. Ultraviolet-light-mediated DNA damage in the skin may be impeded by direct viral binding to p53 and resultant inhibition allowing the generation of dysplastic cells.

Conventional risk factors

Tobacco smoking is a major risk factor for cancer in the general population. Several studies have confirmed that smoking tobacco also increases risk of cancer in transplant recipients [44]. Genetic factors are also important, and it is common for some recipients to develop more than one type of cancer post-transplantation.

Donor-derived malignancy

Although living and deceased kidney donors are carefully screened for history or signs of malignancy before transplantation proceeds, on very rare occasions a malignancy is transmitted to the recipient at the time of transplantation. In data from the Transplant Tumor Registry in the United States of America, 21 donor-related malignancies were reported in 108,062 transplant recipients [45]. In this circumstance the recipient is often considered for transplant nephrectomy and/or chemotherapy, depending upon the tumour histology.

Key malignancies post-transplantation: presentation and management

The risk of developing many solid organ tumours is only slightly increased over the frequency in the general population. However, it is important to recognise that PTLD, NMSC and hypernephroma (renal cell carcinoma) are all greatly increased in frequency and cause a significant increase in morbidity and mortality in transplant recipients.

Post-transplant lymphoproliferative disorder

EBV is a lymphotropic DNA herpes virus that infects and transforms B-lymphocytes and is attenuated by T-cell-mediated inhibition of viral expansion in immunocompetent individuals. Most adults will have sustained a primary infection and will have latent EBV virus DNA expressed as an episome. T-cell immune surveillance is inhibited by lymphocyte-depleting antibodies (ATG; OKT3) and attenuated by CNIs, which may lead to clonal expansion of EBV-infected B-lymphocytes. A further cytotoxic event can lead to malignant transformation into monoclonal or polyclonal polymorphic B cell lymphoma. PTLD is rare and presents in approximately 2% of kidney transplant recipients, although the risk is greater in those who are EBV naïve at transplantation (×24 RR) and those treated with T-lymphocyte-depleting antibodies (×6 RR). The risk is related to immunosuppressive load, and consequently PTLD rates are much higher in other forms of organ transplantation requiring increased immunosuppression (up to 10% heart–lung transplant recipients are affected). There are two peak periods of incidence with an initial peak within the first 12 months post-transplantation. The second peak occurs more than 10 years post-transplantation, and it is important to maintain a high index of suspicion and low threshold for appropriate investigation to minimise mortality. The clinical presentation can be very varied and frequently does not involve palpable lymphadenopathy. Common presentations include gastrointestinal symptoms frequently with atypical abdominal pain and occasionally obstruction; central nervous system involvement is common and can manifest in a variety of ways ranging from focal neurological symptoms and signs to occult changes in mental state. Any persistent unexplained lymphadenopathy or atypical cutaneous nodule should be biopsied to exclude the diagnosis. It is essential to obtain tissue to confirm the diagnosis, categorise the type of PTLD and determine if the tumour is linked to EBV by staining for viral material by immunohistochemistry with the EBER stain. Labelling for CD20 is useful in predicting response to rituximab. Once confirmed it is important to assess the extent of the disease preferably by a positron emission tomography–computerised tomography (PET-CT) scan at the time of diagnosis, as PTLD is often multi-focal and may involve the transplanted kidney in 20% of cases. In addition, a bone marrow biopsy should be performed to assess extent of systemic involvement and define appropriate management. EBV-positive PTLD is likely to regress with sequential gradual reduction of immunosuppression, whereas EBV-negative and monoclonal forms are much less likely to respond and may require chemotherapy with regimens including anti-B-cell antibodies. Central nervous system localised disease has a much poorer prognosis and may require a combination of surgical debulking and chemotherapy.

In patients responding to gradual reduction of immunosuppression, complete remission can be obtained in 90% with a less than 10% risk of acute rejection. At diagnosis of PTLD it would be appropriate to withdraw completely either azathioprine or mycophenolate mofetil from dual or triple immunosuppressive regimens combined with a CNI while verification of EBV status of the tumour is confirmed. The CNI can subsequently be sequentially reduced over a 6-week period by 10–15% per week in confirmed cases until there is evidence of regression of the PTLD clinically or an adequate antiviral response on T-cell phenotyping.

Non-melanoma skin cancer

NMSC has a cumulative incidence in the UK of 16% with a median time to development of the first tumour of 9 years post-transplantation. The tumours are predominantly squamous cell carcinomas (SCCs) and are often multiple, occur at an earlier age, grow more quickly and metastasise more readily than in the general population. There is a high risk of developing recurrent tumours, with a median time from developing the first tumour to presentation with a second SCC of 11 months [46]. An important risk factor for developing NMSC is exposure to ultraviolet light, and in particular childhood sunburn; other factors include male sex, smoking, age at transplantation and presence of actinic keratoses [46]. In contrast to the general population, post-transplantation cutaneous SCC will metastasise and lead to death in 2% of patients. It is important to remove any unexplained new suspicious skin lesion for histological diagnosis, as many NMSCs have atypical macroscopic appearances in the immunosuppressed. Early lesions may be treated with topical 5-fluorouracil or imiquimod, but larger or progressive lesions will require wide excision and may need adjuvunct radiotherapy. Retinoids can be useful in reducing the frequency of new lesions, but on cessation there is usually a rebound crop of new lesions, so these have limited clinical use. In a randomised controlled trial, reduced ciclosporin exposure resulted in a significant reduction in the rate of NMSC in kidney transplant recipients [47]. More recently, a small randomised trial has shown a significant reduction in the rate of NMSC development in recipients switched from a CNI-based immunosuppression regimen to sirolimus [42]. This observation has recently been confirmed in a large multicentre trial and is a useful approach in individuals who are developing frequent NMSC. Careful consideration to the overall immunosuppression load should be undertaken in any individual with multiple NMSC with a view to cautious immunosuppression reduction and/or substitution with an mTOR-inhibitor. There may be value in combining a switch to an mTOR inhibitor in combination with retinoid therapy, which is to be addressed by a future clinical trial. The high prevalence of NMSC post-transplantation justifies dermatological surveillance of recipients at highest risk, which will vary according to geographical location and skin type. In Northern Europe an annual dermatological skin examination should be undertaken in all those transplanted for more than 10 years or those of Fitzpatrick skin type 1 or 2 (very pale skin that burns easily and tans poorly), recipients aged over 60 or those in an outdoor occupation. More frequent dermatological review should be considered in those with a second kidney transplant if the first transplant lasted for more than 10 years, those with previous cutaneous SCC or any recipient who had frequent childhood sunburn in a tropical climate.

Renal cell carcinoma

Hypernephroma has an increased incidence in ESRF and post-transplantation in the USA has a fifteen-fold increased risk over the general population [37]. The aetiology of hypernephroma is unknown although polyomavirus infection is associated with uro-epithelial neoplasia.

Surveillance for malignancy post-transplantation

The marked increased incidence of particular types of malignancy post-transplantation raises the question as to the potential benefit of prophylactic clinical surveillance strategies to aim to detect early

Table 23.2 Recommendations for surveillance for cancer post-transplantation.

Site (method)	USA	Europe	UK
Skin	Annual screen (all)	Self-awareness	Annual screen (some)
Cervical (smear)	Annual	Annual	3 yearly
Prostate (PSA)	Annual (age >45)	Annual (age >50)	None
Colon (FOB)	Annual	As per general population	3 yearly (age 60–69)
Breast (mammogram)	Annual (age >50)	As per general population	3 yearly (age 50–70)
Ano-genital (clinical exam)	Annual	None	None
Renal (ultrasound)	Annual	None	If indicated

FOB, faecal occult blood; PSA, prostate specific antigen; U/S, ultrasound of native kidneys.

treatable disease. There is already substantial international guidance on cancer screening in the general population and both European and American advice for transplant recipients [27]. In general, standard national guidelines for the general population should apply – for example, regular cervical screening and faecal occult blood testing in the age >60 for the early detection of colon cancer. In addition the physician should maintain a high index of suspicion for PTLD and low index for investigation. Unfortunately, due to the wide variety of potential presentations, it is difficult to screen specifically. By contrast, due to the frequency and often atypical presentations, White patients with skin types 1 and 2 should have annual dermatological surveillance. A full list of current surveillance strategies is shown in Table 23.2. It is important to interpret guidance in the context in the variance of cancer prevalence in different national populations.

Part 3: Bone disease after kidney transplantation

CKD-mineral bone disorder (MBD) encompasses a range of specific bone pathologies (adynamic bone disease, osteomalacia, osteitis fibrosa, osteoporosis), biochemical derangements (abnormal serum phosphate, calcium and parathyroid hormone) and associated complications (e.g. vascular calcification) [34]. CKD-MBD develops almost universally during the progression of CKD, so nearly all patients receiving a kidney transplant will have accrued damage to their bones in one form or another. The effect of transplantation on CKD-MBD is heterogeneous, and there is a lack of good-quality trial data to guide therapy [48]. However, as the number of patients with functioning transplants increases, bone disease after kidney transplantation becomes an increasingly important problem.

Fracture risk and bone mineral density after transplantation

A number of studies have shown that transplant recipients are at increased risk of fracture. An American study showed the risk of being hospitalised for a fracture in the first 3 year post-transplant was more than four times higher compared with the general population [49]. Transplant recipients are also at higher risk than their peers on dialysis: one study of over 100,000 patients placed on the transplant waiting list over a 10-year period found that the adjusted relative risk of hip fracture was 1.34 (95% CI 1.12–1.61) for transplant recipients compared with remaining on dialysis [50].

Fracture rates are highest soon after transplantation, but the risk appears to reduce with time. In the study of hip fracture the excess risk attenuated by about 1% per month so that the risks became approximately equal about 2 years after transplantation [50]. The prevalence of previous fracture has been reported to be as high as 44% in long-term transplant recipient [51]. Fracture rates appear to be higher at all sites; one study found that foot fractures were the most common after solid organ transplantation [52].

Contributory factors for fracture can be subdivided into pre-transplant CKD-MBD, post-transplant and patient-specific (see Table 23.3). One notable omission from this list is BMD. BMD declines rapidly in the first 6–12 months after transplantation [53–55]. After this one study has shown that the rate declines to one similar to the general population [56], whereas other studies have suggested that BMD actually increases [57,58]. However, there is only one study that found that low BMD was predictive of future fracture risk in kidney transplant recipients [59]. Other studies have shown no useful correlation between BMD and fracture risk [51,60], so current international guidelines only recommend measuring BMD in high-risk patients (i.e. those who have received large doses of corticosteroids or with risk factors for osteoporosis who have a

Table 23.3 Contributory factors to post-transplantation bone disease and fractures.

Pre-transplant CKD-MBD	Post-transplant	Patient-specific
Adynamic bone disease	Corticosteroids	Age
Osteomalacia	Hyperparathyroidism	Diabetes mellitus
Osteoporosis	Hypophosphataemia	Smoking
Osteitis fibrosa	Impaired renal function	Physical activity
Mixed bone disease		Duration of RRT career
		Menopausal status

well-functioning graft) [61]. The discordance between BMD and fracture risk is perhaps explained by the complex multifaceted disturbances of bone metabolism that occur after transplantation, compared with the general population in which osteoporosis is the overwhelming pathology.

Pathogenesis of post-transplant bone disease

As shown in Table 23.1 there are numerous contributory factors to post-transplant bone disease. Pre-transplant CKD-MBD will not be discussed here but is clearly significant. The epidemiology of CKD-MBD is changing and low bone turnover – particularly adynamic bone disease – is becoming the predominant form seen in many centres.

Hyperparathyroidism is important both before and after transplantation. Up to 50% of transplant recipients have hyperparathyroidism, and it may take many years for moderate hyperparathyroidism to resolve after transplantation [62,63]. In addition, patients may develop secondary hyperparathyroidism *de novo* after transplantation as graft function declines. Hyperparathyroidism may be detrimental directly, but it also contributes to hypophosphataemia in the early transplant period when the high concentrations of parathyroid hormone meet a functional renal tubule. Hypophosphataemia has been associated with reduced osteoblast activity after transplantation and may therefore contribute to the observed bone disease [64].

Corticosteroids are a major cause of bone disease after transplantation. One study found no association between biochemical or hormonal measures and bone volume and turnover, but did find a negative association between cumulative prednisolone dose and bone volume and turnover [65]. Corticosteroids both stimulate osteoclast activity and inhibit osteoblast activity (directly and via preventing osteoblastogenesis and increasing osteoblastic apoptosis) [66]. Corticosteroids also cause avascular necrosis, which is the most debilitating post-transplant bone complication. It has become less common since CNIs have reduced the cumulative corticosteroid dose used [67]), but one study still suggested it occurs in 4% of transplant recipients by 6 months when examined by magnetic resonance imaging [68]. The data on other immunosuppressants including CNIs, mTOR inhibitors and mycophenolate are inconclusive.

Treatment of bone disease after transplantation

There are three phases of management for post-transplantation bone disease: optimisation of pre-transplant CKD-MBD, preventing early bone loss after transplantation, and long-term preventative therapies. Optimisation of pre-transplant CKD-MBD has been reviewed extensively and is not discussed here further [61]. There are no reliable randomised data on therapies used in CKD-MBD with patient-level outcomes such as fractures and hospitalisations as outcomes, and post-transplant bone disease is no exception.

Preventing early bone loss

Vitamin D-based treatments (native or active vitamin D) have been shown to improve BMD in patients treated with corticosteroids [69]. The trials included in this meta-analysis were not conducted in renal transplant recipients but in patients receiving corticosteroids for a variety of indications. Importantly there is no evidence of an adverse effect of vitamin D treatments on bone. Overall, vitamin D treatment (with or without calcium, compared to placebo or calcium alone) improved BMD by 0.60 (95% CI 0.34–0.85; p < 0.0001). They are therefore recommended in renal transplant recipients for the first 12 months who have an eGFR >30 mL/min/1.73 m^2 and low BMD [61].

Bisphosphonates are more effective than vitamin D at preventing loss of BMD [69]. However, their use is also associated with an increased risk of adynamic bone disease. For example, in a study of intermittent intravenous pamidronate, 50% of participants had reduced bone turnover at baseline, but this was universal in those allocated to receive pamidronate after 6 months [70]. This finding – in combination with the lack of correlation between BMD and clinical events – means that bisphosphonates are not recommended during the first year after transplantation.

Long-term treatment

There is only one study of treating long-term (i.e. >1 year post-transplant) recipients with vitamin D that met the inclusion criteria of international guidelines. This study compared calcitriol (i.e. fully activated 1,25 dihydroxy vitamin D) plus calcium carbonate with no treatment in 45 patients (of whom only 30 completed the trial) [71]. They found no differences between the two groups in histomorphometric analyses, although parathyroid hormone was more suppressed in the active arm.

The data on bisphosphonates are similarly sparse. The largest study compared alendronate with calcitriol (all participants received oral calcium) in 117 patients. BMD improved in both groups by a similar amount [72]. There are no placebo-controlled data to support the use of bisphosphonates in the long-term setting.

General control of CKD-MBD is likely to be more important in the long term, and in the absence of specific evidence it is recommended that the standard guidelines for patients with native kidney function are followed according to the stage of post-transplant CKD. This will include controlling hyperparathyroidism with vitamin D, calcimimetics or surgery and maintaining serum phosphate within the recommended range with dietary restriction and oral phosphate binders.

Summary

Bone disease – manifested as fractures – is common after kidney transplantation, with the highest risk occurring in the first year. During this time there is a substantial loss of BMD, but the pathogenesis of post-transplant CKD-MBD is multifactorial and complex. There are no reliable data to guide therapeutic decisions, so recommendations are based on patients with kidney disease who have not had a transplant or other patients receiving similar therapies.

Part 4: Long-term management and the failing renal transplant

Introduction

Long-term management is essentially the care of a patient with progressive CKD with superimposed risks of immunosuppression. Early transplant loss is now rare, with more than 90% of deceased donor and over 95% of live donor transplants surviving for at least 1 year. Approximately 50% of transplant recipients die with a functioning transplant [73]. This can be regarded as success unless the death is premature, which it often is. In reality all transplants are gradually failing but at different rates. Transplant half-life, the time taken for 50% of patients to lose transplant function, is the quantity usually used to describe long-term outcomes for cohorts of transplant recipients. Current half-life estimates for deceased donor transplants in Europe are 15 years and 20–35 years for live donor transplants (www.ctstransplant.org).

Causes of transplant dysfunction

An elegant review of the pathophysiology of transplant failure is provided in reference [73]. Data from serial protocol biopsies indicate that initial damage affects the tubulointerstitial compartment with progressive fibrosis and loss of tubules, a process that is now labelled as interstitial fibrosis with tubular atrophy [74,75]. This tubulointerstitial damage is multifactorial, with donor factors determining risk as well as post-transplant events. Increasing donor age, pre-existing vasculopathy due to hypertension and ischaemia reperfusion injury due to prolonged cold ischaemia times all result in renal damage. Severe or recurrent acute rejection in the early post-transplant period predisposes to chronic damage. However, mild episodes of early acute rejection where the serum creatinine returns to pre-rejection values appear to have little impact. A major current controversy is the relative importance of CNI nephrotoxicity versus poorly controlled chronic rejection due to insufficient CNI exposure. Data from recipients of non-renal transplants, where 10–20% of CNI treated patients develop severe renal failure within 10 years of transplantation, are supportive of a key role for CNI toxicity [76]. A counterargument to this view is that a lot of these patients have renal disease due to other aetiologies, although confident exclusion of CNI nephrotoxicity in a chronically damaged kidney is an inexact science. There are several reports indicating that the presence of HLA antibody predicts a poor outcome, in particular the presence of donor-specific antibody [77]. Recurrent primary renal disease, hypertension and chronic viral infection are other possible contributors. A fall in GFR is a relatively late event [73], and it is probable that interventions to preserve graft function implemented after the GFR has started to fall are too late to alter the natural history of the progressive chronic renal failure, unless there is clear evidence of an active immunological process that can be modulated.

Screening investigations

Glomerular filtration rate

Precise measurement of GFR requires the use of tracer methods such as iohexol, iothalamate or ^{51}Cr-EDTA. This level of precision is rarely required in routine clinical practice, with the exception of living donor assessment, but has a key role in research studies using renal function as an end point. Serum creatinine is the best established biomarker for estimating GFR in renal transplant recipients. Cystatin C has been used as an alternative in non-transplant populations, but there are insufficient data to recommend routine use in transplant recipients. Measurement of creatinine clearance based on timed urine collections has largely fallen from practice owing to a tendency for inaccuracy in timing of the urine collections leading to inaccurate estimates of GFR. A number of equations have been derived to estimate GFR based on serum creatinine concentration and demographics [78–81]. The estimates apply to a body surface area of $1.73\,\mathrm{m}^2$. The standard MDRD GFR equations should not be used above 60 mL/min, a range that will apply to many well-functioning live donor transplants. However, this range is appropriate for the progressively failing transplant. The MDRD GFR value should be multiplied by 1.21 for individuals who are genetically sub-Saharan African (Black). For descriptive research or audit work including all transplants, use of equations with more consistent performance across the GFR range such as CKD-EPI is probably more appropriate. Current cohorts of transplant patients lose GFR at between 1.5 and 2.0 mL/min per year on average.

Proteinuria

Proteinuria is a screening test for glomerular disease. Although failure of renal tubules to catabolise protein can result in tubular proteinuria, this is uncommon in transplant recipients. A variety of approaches are available to quantify proteinuria. Stick testing measures albumin so does not detect immunoglobulin light chains (Bence-Jones protein) or other globular proteins such as myoglobin. The stick tests are semi-quantitative and make no allowance for urine concentration or dilution that varies with water intake. In general test strips are calibrated as follows but vary from manufacturer to manufacturer and the scale should be checked.
Negative
Trace 150–300 mg/L
+ 300–1000 mg/L
++ 1000–3000 mg/L
+++ 3000–10,000 mg/L
++++ >10,000 mg/L

Normal 24 hour urinary protein excretion is <150 mg/day. However, 24-hour urinary protein measurement has largely been superseded by measurements performed on 'spot' urine samples collected at clinic visits owing to convenience and unreliability of timing of the collections. The protein concentration is expressed as a ratio to the urinary creatinine concentration to correct for dilution or concentration of urine. Albumin/creatinine ratio of 30 mg/mmol equates to a protein/creatinine ratio of 50 mg/mmol or 24 hour protein excretion of 0.5 g. If urinary creatinine is measured in mg/dL, the correction factor is to multiply by 0.088. Albumin/creatinine ratio is more sensitive for detecting low-levels of proteinuria and either test can be used to monitor progression or response to treatment.

In patients with proteinuric primary renal disease, a pre-transplant measurement of proteinuria is invaluable in assessing subsequent changes in urinary protein concentration. Patients with primary FSGS should have measurement of proteinuria daily for 1 week, weekly for 4 weeks, every 3 months for the first year and then annually thereafter [82].

Invisible haematuria

Patients with the potential for recurrence of a nephritic primary renal disease, Immunoglobulin A (IgA) nephropathy, mesangiocapillary glomerulonephritis, anti-glomerular basement membrane disease, or small vessel vasculitis, should undergo urine stick testing for blood once in the first month to determine a baseline, every 3 months during the first year and then annually [82]. In the presence of invisible haematuria, urine microscopy is useful to determine the presence of erythrocyte casts and dysmorphic erythrocytes suggestive of glomerular bleeding. Alternative urological diagnoses including stones and urinary tract malignancy should be considered.

Diagnosis and intervention

The diagnostic pathway for late graft dysfunction is similar to that described in Chapter 22 for early graft dysfunction but with a different spectrum of expected diagnoses. Ultrasound scanning will demonstrate hydronephrosis with ureteric obstruction or an increase in peak systolic velocity in the renal transplant artery to >250 cm/s, suggestive of renal artery stenosis. Investigation and management of these problems is discussed in Chapters 19 and 22. In the absence of an anatomical problem, renal biopsy ought to be performed, although the chances of finding a treatable lesion are significantly less than in the early post-transplant period, which should be taken into account when weighing up the risks versus benefits of biopsy. Biopsy is particularly important for making a diagnosis for patients with potentially treatable primary renal disease. Confirmation of recurrent primary disease will also inform decision-making when considering retransplantation. Occasionally a retrospective diagnosis of primary renal disease is made (e.g. recurrent IgA nephropathy in the transplant when there was no biopsy of the native kidneys). Long-standing transplants are often somewhat resistant to penetration by the biopsy needle and care must be taken that the biopsy needle has actually penetrated the renal capsule before 'firing' the device to avoid a non-diagnostic biopsy. If there is a possibility of recurrent primary disease, the biopsy should be processed for electron microscopy and immunofluorescence/immunohistochemistry as well as conventional light microscopy.

Interstitial fibrosis with tubular atrophy

These are, in effect, the histological changes of an irreversibly damaged kidney that will progress towards failure with multifactorial aetiology. There are no convincing data to indicate that change in immunosuppressive therapy is of benefit after the development of interstitial fibrosis with tubular atrophy (IFTA). The standard measures used in slowing the progression of chronic renal failure should be employed (see below).

Chronic antibody-mediated rejection

A diagnosis of chronic antibody-mediated rejection is based on the typical histological features of: arterial intimal fibrosis without elastosis, duplication of the glomerular basement membrane (transplant glomerulopathy), multilaminated peritubular capillary basement membrane, and interstitial fibrosis) in the presence of donor-specific antibody and C4d labelling of the peritubular capillaries (see Chapter 20). Optimising immunosuppression with tacrolimus, mycophenolate and steroids may result in stabilisation of renal function. Current research efforts are aimed at testing the effectiveness of B-lymphocyte-targeted therapies, including rituximab, intravenous immunoglobulin and plasma exchange [83].

Calcineurin inhibitor nephrotoxicity

The classical features of chronic CNI toxicity are arteriolar hyalinosis with so called 'stripe-fibrosis' of the tubulointerstitial compartment associated with tubular atrophy. The available clinical trial data suggest that while GFR may improve following CNI withdrawal (probably owing to loss of the vasospastic effect), graft survival does not improve, and there may be an inevitable outcome of progressive chronic renal failure when histological changes are established. Withdrawal of the CNI before histological changes develop or in response to an early protocol biopsy showing CNI toxicity is likely to be a more effective strategy [84].

Recurrent glomerular disease

Two of the most common recurrent diseases, focal and segmental glomerulosclerosis (FSGS) and haemolytic uraemic syndrome generally recur during the first month after transplantation and are covered in Chapter 22. The data supporting interventions for late recurrent FSGS including plasma exchange are largely based on early recurrence [85], and optimal management of late recurrence is even less certain. Recent reviews of recurrent disease are provided in references [86,87].

The recurrence rate of IgA nephropathy depends on how it is diagnosed, with a much greater rate of histological recurrence than the rate of graft loss due to IgA nephropathy. Recurrence is more common in younger patients and in those where there was rapid progression of the primary disease. There are no specific therapeutic interventions for IgA nephropathy. There are equivocal data on the use of fish oil in primary IgA nephropathy. This is a potential therapeutic option for transplant recurrence which, while it may not be effective, is at least safe.

Henoch–Schönlein nephritis is a similar disease to IgA nephropathy, with recurrent glomerular IgA deposits in the majority of patients but clinical recurrence in around 22%, leading to graft loss in around 10%. Recurrence is more common in children but carries a poorer prognosis in adults. There is no established effective treatment. The incidence of recurrence of mesangiocapillary glomerulonephritis (MCGN), known as mesangioproliferative glomerulonephritis (MPGN) in the USA, depends on the initial type of disease. Recurrence rate is 20–30% for idiopathic type-I disease and at least 80% for type-II, often leading to graft loss. Optimal management of recurrence is uncertain. The recurrence rate of idiopathic membranous nephropathy has been reported in between 30 and 40% of cases, although primary membranous nephropathy in the transplant is probably more common. There is no established treatment for membranous nephropathy in transplants, but some limited data suggest that rituximab may be effective. Recurrence of lupus nephritis is rare, with the exception of patients with lupus due to deficiency of one of the early components of the classical complement pathway, C2 or C4. Recurrence of antineutrophil cytoplasmic antibody (ANCA)-associated small vessel vasculitis and anti-glomerular basement membrane disease is rare and should be treated in the same way as the primary disease is managed with evidence for high-dose intravenous steroid, cyclophosphamide, plasmapheresis, intravenous immunoglobulin and rituximab.

Primary hyperoxaluria
Primary hyperoxaluria is due to failure of hepatic synthesis of alanine glyoxylate aminotransferase that results in formation of calcium oxalate renal stones and nephrocalcinosis. Simultaneous liver transplantation is curative. In the case of kidney transplantation alone, recurrence is universal. High fluid intake to generate dilute urine reduces stone formation and may prolong transplant survival. Patients with the Gly170Arg mutation respond to treatment with high-dose pyridoxine [88].

Viral nephropathy
Biopsy may show viral inclusion bodies due to BK polyomavirus or cytomegalovirus, which sometimes responds to treatment as outlined in Chapter 14.

General strategies to slow decline in renal function
Although data specifically on the failing transplant are sparse, it is reasonable to apply the principles used in slowing the rate of progression

of CKD in native kidneys. Good control of hypertension is the main intervention with proven benefit. Target blood pressure should be <130/80 mmHg in general with possible benefit from a lower target, e.g. 120/75 mmHg, in patients with significant proteinuria ($\geq$1 g/24 hours). ACE inhibitors and ARBs are probably more effective than drugs from other classes. This will come at the expense of a fall in GFR, which can be difficult to explain to the patient, but there is an expectation of reduction in the gradient of the GFR slope. There is often a temptation to withdraw the ACE inhibitor/ARB as the creatinine starts to rise, which is probably the wrong course of action. If a patient's GFR deterioration is continuing on their previous trajectory, treatment should be continued. As renal function becomes progressively worse with associated acidaemia, hyperkalaemia may become a problem. A low-potassium diet should be implemented initially with drug withdrawal if this is unsuccessful. Introduction of ACE inhibitor/ARB can cause a precipitous fall in GFR in patients with transplant renal artery stenosis. Doppler ultrasound scanning before introduction can often detect this, although the true false negative rate is unknown. Serum creatinine and potassium should be checked 7–14 days after ACE-inhibitor/ARB introduction with drug withdrawal and further investigation in the event of a rise in serum creatinine exceeding 20%. Proteinuria is toxic to renal tubules and reduction may help slow transplant deterioration. ACE-inhibitors/ARBs are more effective than other antihypertensive agents in reducing proteinuria and dual blockade with ACE inhibitor and ARB is superior to either agent alone. Statins may also help to reduce proteinuria.

Compliance/adherence with imunosuppressive therapy

Complete compliance with immunosuppressive therapy is a major challenge even for the best-organised patients, and poor compliance becomes more common with time after transplantation. Polypharmacy is an inevitable problem for transplant recipients, and care should be taken to avoid non-essential medication. Reduced dosing frequency may assist in compliance, but there are no direct supporting data in renal transplant recipients. Poor compliance has been reported to be a major factor in late graft loss due to chronic rejection. Patients need to be reminded that if they stop taking their immunosuppression they will lose their transplant organ. The small number of tolerant patients who have not lost their grafts does not justify equivocation on this. A number of approaches have been tried to assist patients. Education on the reason for taking drugs and possible side effects, with a check that the patient knows which drugs they are taking and the doses, should be part of routine clinic visits. Written medication cards and dosette boxes can be helpful. In the era in which most patients have mobile phones, a daily alarm set for times when medication is due can help ensure adherence to the dosing regimen.

Anaemia

Standard anaemia management guidelines for patients with CKD can be applied to renal transplant recipients. The optimal haemoglobin concentration is 10.5–12.5 g/dL. Erythropoietin deficiency is a diagnosis of exclusion for patients with normochromic normocytic anaemia. Anaemia may be a consequence of treatment with antiproliferative immunosuppressive drugs, including azathioprine, mycophenolate or sirolimus particularly if used in combination. Patients treated with azathioprine are usually macrocytic. Key causes of anaemia that need to be considered are bleeding, in particular into the gastrointestinal tract, which may be occult. Deficiency in iron, vitamin B_{12} or folate should be treated. Haemolysis is an uncommon problem that may be drug-induced. Chronic inflammation, hyperparathyroidism or ACE-inhibitor treatment may be contributory factors.

Gout

The majority (80%) of renal transplant recipients are hyperuricaemic due to a combination of renal impairment and reduced uric acid elimination as a result of CNI treatment. Avoidance of foods high in purines, including meat, fish and beer, can be helpful (www.ukgoutsociety.org/docs/2009FinalDietsheet.pdf). Allopurinol with appropriate limitations on dose, typically 100 mg daily, can be used safely, with the exception of patients on treatment with azathioprine. Allopurinol inhibits the metabolism of azathioprine, leading to accumulation, with the potential for severe haematological toxicity. Although use of low-dose azathioprine with allopurinol has been advocated, it is safest to avoid the combination and switch to an alternative antiproliferative agent such as mycophenolate. Treatment with allopurinol should not be commenced during an acute episode of gout. Uricosuric drugs including sulfinpyrazone can be used to reduce serum uric acid concentrations, and if the patient requires antihypertensive treatment, losartan does have some uricosuric effect. In treating acute episodes of gout non-steroidal anti-inflammatory drugs should be avoided. Low-dose colchicine (0.5 mg three times daily) is usually effective, given until either the pain resolves or the patient develops diarrhoea. If colchicine is either ineffective or not tolerated, a short course of prednisolone is an alternative.

Pregnancy

Ability to achieve successful pregnancy is one of the key aims of renal transplantation in young women. The complication rate for pregnancy in women with well-functioning transplants is remarkably low. A recent meta-analysis found the overall live birth rate in renal transplant recipients and the miscarriage rate of 14% to be similar to that of the general population. Pre-eclampsia (27%), gestational diabetes (8%) and pre-term delivery (46%) were more common than in the general US population. Many transplant pregnancies are small for dates. Both pregnancy and transplant outcomes are better for mothers with serum creatinine <133 µmol/L and 24-hour urinary protein <300 mg at the time of conception. Patients with a well-functioning kidney go through the same physiological changes as those seen in normal pregnancy, with a rise in GFR early on, which falls back to pre-pregnancy levels during the third

trimester. Urinary tract infections are common, affecting t̲
pregnant transplant recipients [89,90]. Occasionally in very la
pregnancy, with descent of the fetus, obstruction can develop with
hydronephrosis and a rise in serum creatinine concentration.

Although none of the immunosuppressive drugs are considered to be
'safe' in pregnancy, there has been no reported increased incidence of
fetal malformations or teratogenicity with azathioprine, corticosteroids,
ciclosporin or tacrolimus and regimens based on these drugs would
generally be regarded as acceptable. They are present in breast milk and
breastfeeding is best avoided. Although blood concentrations in the baby
are low, there is a theoretical risk of drug accumulation due to the
immature cytochrome P450 system. Mycophenolate and sirolimus are
teratogenic and should be avoided.

Ideally, conception should be delayed until 1 year after transplantation
and a non-teratogenic drug regimen, including antihypertensive agents
established prior to conception. Transplantation does not contraindicate
normal vaginal delivery. If a Caesarian section is to be performed, ideally,
a transplant surgeon should be present and consideration given to a
vertical rather than horizontal incision to minimise the potential for
damage of the transplant. Steroid doses should be increased peripartum
to cover the stress of the process. Acute rejection during pregnancy and
post-partum has been reported but is rare. A matched case–control study
from the UK Transplant Pregnancy Registry found no evidence for an
increased rate of renal allograft loss after pregnancy. A univariate analysis
of transplant-related factors found that 2-year renal survival after
pregnancy was significantly lower at 87% in mothers who had drug-
treated hypertension during pregnancy than in those who did not with
100% 2-year graft survival. A trend towards increased serum creatinine
post-pregnancy was identified in mothers with serum creatinine
concentration >150 μmol/L pre-pregnancy [91].

Tapering of immunosuppression

When a transplant has failed with return to dialysis, the risk–benefit ratio
of immunosuppressive therapy changes. However, there is an argument
for continuing some immunosuppression to preserve residual renal
function that can contribute to dialysis adequacy, in particular for
patients on peritoneal dialysis. If a live kidney donor is available with the
prospect for early or even pre-emptive retransplantation,
immunosuppressive therapy should be continued to avoid immunological
sensitisation. A staged approach to immunosuppressive withdrawal is
probably safest. Antiproliferative agents (azathioprine, mycophenolate)
can be stopped immediately, followed by gradual taper of the CNI or
mTOR inhibitor. There are no published data on the optimum rate of
taper, but in our centre we reduce the dose by 25% per week until
withdrawn. Steroids should be the last component to go. In order to
avoid problems due to hypoadrenalism, prednisolone should not be
withdrawn faster than 1 mg per month. In the event of clinical
manifestations of adrenal insufficiency including hypotension or

emia the steroid should be reinstated with attempt at a slower

nsplant nephrectomy

ne decision on whether a failed transplant should be removed is a difficult one, with no consensus as to the best approach, balancing potential mortality and morbidity of graft nephrectomy with risks related to leaving the graft *in situ*. In favour of nephrectomy is removal of a potent immunological stimulus that might result in the generation of HLA antibodies on tapering and withdrawal of immunosuppression. However, all nephrectomy techniques leave some donor vasculature behind, providing an ongoing immunological stimulus. This may have a negative impact on outcomes following retransplantation [92], but this is controversial [93].

The remaining transplant may also serve as a chronic inflammatory stimulus, increasing risk of cardiovascular complications, or may be chronically infected. Patients with a failed graft are more likely to have hypoalbuminaemia, anaemia and raised C-reactive protein [94]. The argument against routine nephrectomy is that it is a major operative procedure in a uraemic patient that carries some risk, with mortality rates of 0–39% in the published literature [95,96]. Failed transplant kidneys often cause no problems on withdrawal of immunosuppressive therapy.

We would recommend the following pragmatic approach. In patients less than one year after transplantation where the patient is likely to be re-transplanted, we would recommend transplant nephrectomy even when graft is asymptomatic. In all other patients, an expectant approach can be adopted with immunosuppressive withdrawal and nephrectomy only in the event of acute graft rejection. This is usually manifest by a painful tender graft with a fall in platelet count and sometimes visible haematuria. The patient may feel systemically unwell with fever. The graft appears oedematous and swollen on ultrasound scanning. In this instance steroid therapy should be reinstituted and plans made for a reasonably urgent nephrectomy, although this does not generally need to be done as an emergency procedure. Other indications for nephrectomy include persistent haematuria, severe hypertension or suspicion of malignancy in the transplant.

Surgical technique for transplant nephrectomy

Reopen the original transplant incision, cutting all the layers until you reach the kidney convexity; cut longitudinally on the convexity, using diathermy. Dissect the upper pole followed by the lateral and medial aspect of the graft, lower pole and the hilum last. Try to keep the capsule on the graft; in some badly scarred cases it might be impossible. Always try to remove all the tissue, leaving the minimum necessary renal vascular tissue on the iliac vessels. Tie off the ureter on the bladder/native ureter surface and cut. Clamp the iliac vessels and cut the graft vessels as short as possible. Having removed the graft, the graft/iliac vessels can be closed using continuous non-absorbable sutures, ideally artery and vein of separately. Careful haemostasis is important; some patients may develop haematoma in the kidney bed. Drainage is recommended. In infected cases, lavage using diluted antiseptic can be used.

Wound closure is important and might be difficult because of scarring. Closing the scarred tissue is more likely to cause a hernia. Even if all the layers cannot be identified, try to close in two layers.

Other late surgical complications

Incisional hernia after kidney transplantation is more likely to happen in patients who are obese, female and aged greater than 50 years. As for any other herniae, this should be surgically treated sooner rather than later as the size of the hernia may increase with time. Although attempts at primary suture are often made, most cases will end up as a hernia mesh repair. Some immunosuppression, in particular the mTOR inhibitors, may affect healing and consideration should be given to conversion to an alternative agent 2 weeks before planned surgery. Cut through the transplant scar; do not try to reach the kidney surface, as you may damage the graft. Dissect the whole hernia ostium. Once having enough 'healthy' fascia all around the hernia gate, measure and place the mesh. The mesh should be sutured as non-tension all around the fascia defect with either continuous or interrupted stitches. Drainage is recommended to prevent seroma with possible infection [97].

References

1. Meier-Kriesche HU, Schold JD, Kaplan B. (2004) Long-term renal allograft survival: Have we made significant progress or is it time to rethink our analytic and therapeutic strategies? *Am J Transplant* **4**, 1289–1295.
2. West M, Sutherland DER, Matas AJ. (1996) Kidney transplant recipients who die with functioning grafts – Serum creatinine level and cause of death. *Transplantation* **62**, 1029–1030.
3. Foley RN, Parfrey PS, Sarnak MJ. (1998) Clinical epidemiology of cardiovascular disease in chronic renal disease. *Am J Kidney Dis* **32** (Suppl 3), S112–119.
4. US Renal Data System. USRDS 2009 Annual Data Report: Atlas of Chronic Kidney Disease and End-Stage Renal Disease in the United States. Bethesda: National Institutes of Health, National Institute of Diabetes and Digestive and Kidney Diseases; 2009.
5. London GM. (2003) Cardiovascular calcifications in uremic patients: clinical impact on cardiovascular function. *J Am Soc Nephrol* **9** (Suppl 4), S305–S309.
6. Kasiske BL, Chakkera HA, Roel J. (2000) Explained and unexplained ischemic heart disease risk after renal transplantation. *J Am Soc Nephrol* **11**, 1735–1743.
7. Wolfe RA, Ashby VB, Milford EL, *et al.* (1999) Comparison of mortality in all patients on dialysis, patients on dialysis awaiting transplantation, and recipients of a first cadaveric transplant. *N Engl J Med* **341**, 1725–1730.
8. Kasiske BL, Anjum S, Shah R, *et al.* (2004) Hypertension after kidney transplantation. *Am J Kidney Dis* **43**, 1071–1081.

9. Montanaro D, Gropuzzo M, Tulissi P, *et al.* (2005) Effects of successful renal transplantation on left ventricular mass. *Transplant Proc* **37**, 2485–2487.
10. Perico N, Ruggenenti P, Gaspari F, *et al.* (1992) Daily renal hypoperfusion induced by cyclosporine in patients with renal transplantation. *Transplantation* **54**, 56–60.
11. Yavuz A, Tuncer M, Gurkan A, *et al.* (2004) Cigarette smoking in renal transplant recipients. *Transplant Proc* **36**, 108–110.
12. Patel RK, Mark PB, Johnston N, *et al.* (2008) Renal transplantation is not associated with regression of left ventricular hypertrophy: A magnetic resonance study. *Clin J Am Soc Nephrol* **3**, 1807–1811.
13. Brown JH, Murphy BG, Douglas AF, *et al.* (1997) Influence of immunosuppressive therapy on lipoprotein(a) and other lipoproteins following renal transplantation. *Nephron* **75**, 277–282.
14. Hricik DE, Bartucci MR, Mayes JT, *et al.* (1992) The effects of steroid withdrawal on the lipoprotein profiles of cyclosporine-treated kidney and kidney-pancreas transplant recipients. *Transplantation* **54**, 868–871.
15. Kuster GM, Drexel H, Bleisch JA, *et al.* (1994) Relation of cyclosporine blood levels to adverse effects on lipoproteins. *Transplantation* **57**, 1479–1483.
16. Artz MA, Boots JM, Ligtenberg G, *et al.* (2003) Improved cardiovascular risk profile and renal function in renal transplant patients after randomized conversion from cyclosporine to tacrolimus. *J Am Soc Nephrol* **14**, 1880–188.
17. Lentine KL, Rocca-Rey LA, Bacchi G, *et al.* (2008) Obesity and cardiac risk after kidney transplantation: experience at one center and comprehensive literature review. *Transplantation* **86**, 303–312.
18. Arnadottir M, Hultberg B, Wahlberg J, *et al.* (1998) Serum total homocysteine concentration before and after renal transplantation. *Kidney Int* **54**, 1380–134.
19. Montori VM, Basu A, Erwin PJ, *et al.* (2002) Posttransplantation diabetes: A systematic review of the literature. *Diabetes Care* **25**, 583–592.
20. Webster AC, Woodroffe RC, Taylor RS, *et al.* (2005) Tacrolimus versus ciclosporin as primary immunosuppression for kidney transplant recipients: Meta-analysis and meta-regression of randomised trial data. *BMJ* **331**, 810–820.
21. Kasiske BL, Klinger D. (2000) Cigarette smoking in renal transplant recipients. *J Am Soc Nephrol* **11**, 753–759.
22. Aalten J, Christiaans MH, de Fijter H, *et al.* (2006) The influence of obesity on short- and long-term graft and patient survival after renal transplantation. *Transpl Int* **19**, 901–907.
23. Turnbull F. (2003) Effects of different blood-pressure-lowering regimens on major cardiovascular events: Results of prospectively-designed overviews of randomised trials. *Lancet* **362**, 1527–1535.
24. Turnbull F, Neal B, Pfeffer M, *et al.* (2007) Blood pressure-dependent and independent effects of agents that inhibit the renin-angiotensin system. *J Hypertens* **25**, 951–958.
25. Ninomiya T, Perkovic V, Gallagher M, *et al.* (2008) Lower blood pressure and risk of recurrent stroke in patients with chronic kidney disease: PROGRESS trial. *Kidney Int* **73**, 963–970.
26. Cross NB, Webster AC, Masson P, *et al.* (2009) Antihypertensives for kidney transplant recipients: Systematic review and meta-analysis of randomized controlled trials. *Transplantation* **88**, 7–18.

27. Kidney Disease: Improving Global Outcomes (KDIGO) Transplant Work Group. (2009) KDIGO clinical practice guideline for the care of kidney transplant recipients. *Am J Transplant* **9** (Suppl 3), S1–155.
28. Holdaas H, Fellstrom B, Jardine AG, *et al.* (2003) Effect of fluvastatin on cardiac outcomes in renal transplant recipients: A multicentre, randomised, placebo-controlled trial. *Lancet* **361**, 2024–2031.
29. Baigent C, Landray MJ, Reith C, *et al.* (2011) The effects of lowering LDL cholesterol with simvastatin plus ezetimibe in patients with chronic kidney disease (Study of Heart and Renal Protection): A randomised placebo-controlled trial. *Lancet* **377**, 2181–2192.
30. Baigent C, Keech A, Kearney PM, *et al.* (2005) Efficacy and safety of cholesterol-lowering treatment: Prospective meta-analysis of data from 90,056 participants in 14 randomised trials of statins. *Lancet* **366**, 1267–1278.
31. JBS 2: Joint British Societies' guidelines on prevention of cardiovascular disease in clinical practice. (2005) *Heart* **91** (Suppl 5), 1–52.
32. Ray KK, Seshasai SR, Wijesuriya S, *et al.* (2009) Effect of intensive control of glucose on cardiovascular outcomes and death in patients with diabetes mellitus: A meta-analysis of randomised controlled trials. *Lancet* **373**, 1765–1772.
33. Bostom AG, Carpenter MA, Kusek JW, *et al.* (2011) Homocysteine-lowering and cardiovascular disease outcomes in kidney transplant recipients: Primary results from the folic Acid for vascular outcome reduction in transplantation trial. *Circulation* **123**, 1763–1770.
34. Moe SM, Drueke T, Lameire N, *et al.* (2007) Chronic kidney disease-mineral-bone disorder: A new paradigm. *Adv Chronic Kidney Dis* **14**, 3–12.
35. Navaneethan SD, Palmer SC, Craig JC, *et al.* (2009) Benefits and harms of phosphate binders in CKD: A systematic review of randomized controlled trials. *Am J Kidney Dis* **54**, 619–637.
36. Kidney Disease: Improving Global Outcomes (KDIGO) CKD-MBD Work Group. (2009) KDIGO clinical practice guideline for the diagnosis, evaluation, prevention, and treatment of Chronic Kidney Disease-Mineral and Bone Disorder (CKD-MBD). *Kidney Int* **113**, S1–130.
37. Kasiske BL, Snyder JJ, Gilbertson DT, *et al.* (2004) Cancer after kidney transplantation in the United States. *Am J Transplant* **4**, 905–913.
38. Briggs JD. (2001) Causes of death after renal transplantation. *Nephrol Dial Transplant* **16**, 1545–1549.
39. Guba M, von Breitenbuch P, Steinbauer M, *et al.* (2002) Rapamycin inhibits primary and metastatic tumor growth by antiangiogenesis: Involvement of vascular endothelial growth factor. *Nat Med* **8**, 128–135.
40. Opelz G, Dohler B. (2004) Lymphomas after solid organ transplantation: A collaborative transplant study report. *Am J Transplant* **4**, 222–230.
41. Stallone G, Schena A, Infante B, *et al.* (2005) Sirolimus for Kaposi's sarcoma in renal-transplant recipients. *N Engl J Med* **352**, 1317–1323.
42. Salgo R, Gossmann J, Schofer H, *et al.* (2010) Switch to a sirolimus-based immunosuppression in long-term renal transplant recipients: reduced rate of (pre-)malignancies and nonmelanoma skin cancer in a prospective, randomized, assessor-blinded, controlled clinical trial. *Am J Transplant* **10**, 1385–1393.
43. Hanahan D, Weinberg RA. (2000) The hallmarks of cancer. *Cell* **100**, 57–70.
44. Danpanich E, Kasiske BL. (1999) Risk factors for cancer in renal transplant recipients. *Transplantation* **68**, 1859–1864.

45. Kauffman HM, McBride MA, Cherikh WS, *et al.* (2002) Transplant tumor registry: Donors with central nervous system tumors1. *Transplantation* **73**, 579–582.

46. Ramsay HM, Fryer AA, Reece S, *et al.* (2000) Clinical risk factors associated with nonmelanoma skin cancer in renal transplant recipients. *Am J Kidney Dis* **36**, 167–176.

47. Dantal J, Soulillou JP. (2005) Immunosuppressive drugs and the risk of cancer after organ transplantation. *N Engl J Med* **352**, 1371–1373.

48. Weisinger JR, Carlini RG, Rojas E, *et al.* (2006) Bone disease after renal transplantation. *Clin J Am Soc Nephrol* **1**, 1300–1313.

49. Abbott KC, Oglesby RJ, Hypolite IO, *et al.* (2001) Hospitalizations for fractures after renal transplantation in the United States. *Ann Epidemiol* **11**, 450–457.

50. Ball AM, Gillen DL, Sherrard D, *et al.* (2002) Risk of hip fracture among dialysis and renal transplant recipients. *JAMA* **288**, 3014–3018.

51. Durieux S, Mercadal L, Orcel P, *et al.* (2002) Bone mineral density and fracture prevalence in long-term kidney graft recipients. *Transplantation* **74**, 496–500.

52. Ramsey-Goldman R, Dunn JE, Dunlop DD, *et al.* (1999) Increased risk of fracture in patients receiving solid organ transplants. *J Bone Miner Res* **14**, 456–463.

53. Julian BA, Laskow DA, Dubovsky J, *et al.* (1991) Rapid loss of vertebral mineral density after renal transplantation. *N Engl J Med* **325**, 544–550.

54. Almond MK, Kwan JT, Evans K, *et al.* (1994) Loss of regional bone mineral density in the first 12 months following renal transplantation. *Nephron* **66**, 52–57.

55. Mikuls TR, Julian BA, Bartolucci A, *et al.* (2003) Bone mineral density changes within six months of renal transplantation. *Transplantation* **75**, 49–54.

56. Brandenburg VM, Ketteler M, Heussen N, *et al.* (2005) Lumbar bone mineral density in very long-term renal transplant recipients: Impact of circulating sex hormones. *Osteoporos Int* **16**, 1611–1620.

57. Carlini RG, Rojas E, Weisinger JR, *et al.* (2000) Bone disease in patients with long-term renal transplantation and normal renal function. *Am J Kidney Dis* **36**, 160–166.

58. Grotz WH, Mundinger FA, Gugel B, *et al.* (1995) Bone mineral density after kidney transplantation. A cross-sectional study in 190 graft recipients up to 20 years after transplantation. *Transplantation* **59**, 982–986.

59. Akaberi S, Simonsen O, Lindergard B, *et al.* (2008) Can DXA predict fractures in renal transplant patients? *Am J Transplant* **8**, 2647–2651.

60. Grotz WH, Mundinger FA, Gugel B, *et al.* (1994) Bone fracture and osteodensitometry with dual energy X-ray absorptiometry in kidney transplant recipients. *Transplantation* **58**, 912–915.

61. KDIGO. Chapter 5: Evaluation and treatment of kidney transplant bone disease. (2009) *Kidney Int* **76** (S113), S100–S110.

62. Torres A, Rodriguez AP, Concepcion MT, *et al.* (1998) Parathyroid function in long-term renal transplant patients: Importance of pre-transplant PTH concentrations. *Nephrol Dial Transplant* **13** (Suppl 3), 94–97.

63. Heaf J, Tvedegaard E, Kanstrup IL, *et al.* (2003) Hyperparathyroidism and long-term bone loss after renal transplantation. *Clin Transplant* **17**, 268–274.

64. Moorhead JF, Wills MR, Ahmed KY, *et al.* (1974) Hypophosphataemic osteomalacia after cadaveric renal transplantation. *Lancet* **1**, 694–697.

65. Monier-Faugere MC, Mawad H, Qi Q, *et al.* (2000) High prevalence of low bone turnover and occurrence of osteomalacia after kidney transplantation. *J Am Soc Nephrol* **11**, 1093–1099.

66. Weinstein RS, Jilka RL, Parfitt AM, *et al.* (1998) Inhibition of osteoblastogenesis and promotion of apoptosis of osteoblasts and osteocytes by glucocorticoids. Potential mechanisms of their deleterious effects on bone. *J Clin Invest* **102**, 274–282.

67. Metselaar HJ, van Steenberge EJ, Bijnen AB, *et al.* (1985) Incidence of osteonecrosis after renal transplantation. *Acta Orthop Scand* **56**, 413–415.

68. Lopez-Ben R, Mikuls TR, Moore DS, *et al.* (2004) Incidence of hip osteonecrosis among renal transplantation recipients: A prospective study. *Clin Radiol* **59**, 431–438.

69. Amin S, LaValley MP, Simms RW, *et al.* (1999) The role of vitamin D in corticosteroid-induced osteoporosis: A meta-analytic approach. *Arthritis and rheumatism* **42**, 1740–1751.

70. Coco M, Glicklich D, Faugere MC, *et al.* (2003) Prevention of bone loss in renal transplant recipients: A prospective, randomized trial of intravenous pamidronate. *J Am Soc Nephrol* **14**, 2669–2676.

71. Cueto-Manzano AM, Konel S, Freemont AJ, *et al.* (2000) Effect of 1,25-dihydroxyvitamin D3 and calcium carbonate on bone loss associated with long-term renal transplantation. *Am J Kidney Dis* **35**, 227–236.

72. Jeffery JR, Leslie WD, Karpinski ME, *et al.* (2003) Prevalence and treatment of decreased bone density in renal transplant recipients: A randomized prospective trial of calcitriol versus alendronate. *Transplantation* **76**, 1498–1502.

73. Chapman JR, O'Connell PJ, Nankivell BJ. (2005) Chronic renal allograft dysfunction. *J Am Soc Nephrol* **16**, 3015–3026.

74. Nankivell BJ, Borrows RJ, Fung CL, *et al.* (2003) The natural history of chronic allograft nephropathy. *N Engl J Med* **349**, 2326–2333.

75. Sis B, Mengel M, Haas M, *et al.* (2010) Banff '09 meeting report: Antibody mediated graft deterioration and implementation of Banff working groups. *Am J Transplant* **10**, 464–471.

76. Ojo AO, Held PJ, Port FK, *et al.* (2003) Chronic renal failure after transplantation of a nonrenal organ. *N Engl J Med* **349**, 931–940.

77. Lachmann N, Terasaki PI, Budde K, *et al.* (2009) Anti-human leukocyte antigen and donor-specific antibodies detected by luminex posttransplant serve as biomarkers for chronic rejection of renal allografts. *Transplantation* **87**, 1505–1513.

78. Cockcroft DW, Gault MH. (1976) Prediction of creatinine clearance from serum creatinine. *Nephron* **16**, 31–41.

79. Nankivell BJ, Gruenewald SM, Allen RD, *et al.* (1995) Predicting glomerular filtration rate after kidney transplantation. *Transplantation* **59**, 1683–1689.

80. Levey AS, Bosch JP, Lewis JB, *et al.* (1999) A more accurate method to estimate glomerular filtration rate from serum creatinine: A new prediction equation. Modification of Diet in Renal Disease Study Group. *Ann Intern Med* **130**, 461–470.

81. Levey AS, Stevens LA, Schmid CH, *et al.* (2009) A new equation to estimate glomerular filtration rate. *Ann Intern Med* **150**, 604–612.

82. KDIGO Clinical Practice Guideline for the Care of Kidney Transplant Recipients. (2009) *Am J Transplant* **9** (Suppl 3), S1–S155.

83. Archdeacon P, Chan M, Neuland C, *et al.* (2011) Summary of FDA antibody-mediated rejection workshop. *Am J Transplant* **11**, 896–906.

84. Diekmann F, Campistol JM. (2006) Conversion from calcineurin inhibitors to sirolimus in chronic allograft nephropathy: Benefits and risks. *Nephrol Dial Transplant* **21**, 562–568.
85. Hickson LJ, Gera M, Amer H, *et al.* (2009) Kidney transplantation for primary focal segmental glomerulosclerosis: Outcomes and response to therapy for recurrence. *Transplantation* **87**, 1232–1239.
86. Ponticelli C, Glassock RJ. (2010) Posttransplant recurrence of primary glomerulonephritis. *Clin J Am Soc Nephrol* **5**, 2363–2372.
87. Ponticelli C, Moroni G, Glassock RJ. (2011) Recurrence of secondary glomerular disease after renal transplantation. *Clin J Am Soc Nephrol* **6**, 1214–1221.
88. Cochat P, Liutkus A, Fargue S, *et al.* (2006) Primary hyperoxaluria type 1: Still challenging! *Pediatr Nephrol* **21**, 1075–1081.
89. Deshpande NA, James NT, Kucirka LM, *et al.* (2011) Pregnancy outcomes in kidney transplant recipients: A systematic review and meta-analysis. *Am J Transplant* **11**, 2388–2404.
90. Armenti VT, Constantinescu S, Moritz MJ, *et al.* (2008) Pregnancy after transplantation. *Transplant Rev* **22**, 223–240.
91. Sibanda N, Briggs JD, Davison JM, *et al.* (2007) Pregnancy after organ transplantation: A report from the UK Transplant pregnancy registry. *Transplantation* **83**, 1301–1307.
92. Khakhar AK, Shahinian VB, House AA, *et al.* (2003) The impact of allograft nephrectomy on percent panel reactive antibody and clinical outcome. *Transplant Proc* **35**, 862–863.
93. Messa P, Ponticelli C, Berardinelli L. (2008) Coming back to dialysis after kidney transplant silure. *Nephrol Dial Transplant* **23**, 2738–2742.
94. Ayus JC, Achinger SG, Lee S, *et al.* (2010) Transplant nephrectomy associates with improved survival in patients with failed renal allograft. *JASN* **21**, 374–380.
95. Ayus JC, Achinger SG. (2005) At the peril of dialysis patients: ignoring the failed transplant. *Semin Dial* **18**, 180–184.
96. Lair D, Coupel S, Giral M, *et al.* (2005) The effect of a first kidney transplant on a subsequent transplant outcome: An experimental and clinical study. *Kidney Int* **67**, 2368–2375.
97. Mahdavi R, Mehrabi M. (2004) Incisional hernia after renal transplantation and its repair with propylene mesh. *Urol J* **1**, 259–262.

24 Living donor follow-up

Robert Elias and Jiří Froněk

Living donor follow-up

The postoperative follow-up of living donors fulfils two main roles. The first and obvious role is to ensure the well-being of the donor. The second role is to provide a clear understanding of the consequences of donor nephrectomy. Although this second role does not benefit the individual being monitored directly, it is crucial for the well-being of living donor transplant programmes as a whole and for individuals who may consider donation in the future.

Typical follow-up

Typical follow-up includes:
- peri-operative inpatient management
- post-surgery outpatient review at 2 weeks
- review at 1 year post-surgery
- invitation to attend transplant unit for annual check-up
- request for health and renal data at least every 5 years.

Donor well-being: the long-term consequences of kidney donation

Living kidney donors allow physical harm to be done to themselves in order to benefit another person. The predictable 'harm' of a nephrectomy – namely the trauma of surgery, surgical wounds and loss of a kidney – is accompanied by other risks. These risks can be categorised into:
- peri-operative and early complications of nephrectomy
- long-term consequences of unilateral nephrectomy.

Peri-operative and early complications of donor nephrectomy are summarised in Chapter 7. Here we consider the long-term consequences of kidney donation.

Handbook of Renal and Pancreatic Transplantation, First Edition. Edited by Iain A. M. MacPhee and Jiří Froněk.
© 2012 John Wiley & Sons, Ltd. Published 2012 by John Wiley & Sons, Ltd.

Data limitations

A persistent concern with data about long-term outcomes after donation is that there is no suitable comparison group. Survival after donation is comparable to that of matched controls from the general population, and the risk of developing end-stage renal failure after donation is less than for someone in the general population. Potential donors will be reassured by this information. But favourable comparison with the general population is not the same as saying that donation will not affect their own survival or increase their own risk of end-stage renal failure. An ideal comparison group for donors would be a group of people who pass (or would pass) screening tests for kidney donation but then do not go on to donate. Potential donors who are not used for donation for reasons other than being declined on medical grounds could form such a group. The absence of data for such a comparison limits our understanding of how, precisely, the risk of end-stage renal failure (and indeed any other outcome) is modified by kidney donation. Studies of donor outcomes are also often limited by a lack of data. Despite repeated calls for the formation of registries, long-term follow-up of donors remains patchy. Some problems associated with long-term data collection are discussed below.

Outcomes

Survival

Surgical mortality from living kidney donation is approximately 3 per 10,000 donors [1]. Long-term mortality after kidney donation is similar to that of matched controls in the general population [2]. It has been claimed that kidney donors live longer, on average, than members of the general population [3]. This would be consistent with the fact that they are usually carefully screened in order to donate and so form a highly selected subset of the healthy population. Recent larger studies, however, have not confirmed a survival advantage or disadvantage.

Risk of end-stage renal failure

A study of 3698 kidney donors who donated kidneys in the United States between 1963 and 2007 found that 11 donors had developed end-stage renal failure, on average 22.5 years after donation [2]. This gave an estimated incidence of end-stage renal failure in donors as 180 per million people per year, compared with an overall adjusted incidence rate of 268 per million people per year in the White population of the United States.

A study of 1112 donors who underwent nephrectomy in Sweden between 1965 and 2005 found that at least six had developed end-stage renal failure at a median of 20 years after donation [4]. Based on a population incidence of end-stage renal failure of 125 per million people per year, the authors estimated that the incidence of end-stage renal failure in donors was just under three times higher than might be expected in an equivalent population. The population incidence quoted is, however, half of that in the American study.

A meta-analysis [5] has suggested a prevalence of end-stage renal failure among donors of less than 0.2%, which is lower than the two studies quoted above.

Careful selection from a healthy population means that one would expect lower rates of end-stage renal failure among donors when compared to the general population. This is tempered, however, by the possibility that:

- even with careful screening, relatives of people with end-stage renal failure as a result of certain diseases may be at higher risk of developing kidney failure
- nephrectomy does indeed increase the risk of end-stage renal failure.

Changes in glomerular filtration rate and urinary protein excretion

Removal of one kidney typically results in compensatory functional hypertrophy in the remaining kidney. Glomerular filtration rate (GFR) will, of course, drop immediately after nephrectomy but will then improve, usually within weeks, as the compensation takes effect.

There has been ongoing debate as to whether the compensatory hypertrophy of reduced renal mass results in progressive deterioration of renal function as a result of hyperfiltration. This deterioration would be manifested by increasing proteinuria and decreasing GFR. Provisos about the poor availability of prospective data for long-term follow-up of donors hold here, as for all measures.

In a systematic review and meta-analysis, Garg *et al.* [5] examined 48 studies from 27 countries, which followed a total of 5048 donors for an average of 7 years. They found:

- an average of 7 years after donation, the average GFR was 86 mL/min and the average 24-hour urine protein was 154 mg/day
- 12% of donors developed a GFR between 30 and 59 mL/min
- 0.2% of donors developed a GFR less than 30 mL/min
- urinary protein excretion was higher in donors than in controls and became more pronounced with time
- the average difference in GFR between donors and controls was 10 mL/min.
- initial decrease in GFR was not accompanied by accelerated losses over that anticipated with normal ageing.

A more recent study of 255 donors and matched controls found that GFR in donors was, on average, 63.7 mL/min compared with 81.6 mL/min in controls [2]. However, the urinary albumin to creatinine ratio was lower in donors than in controls.

The possibility that there might be increased rates of proteinuria observed after donation warrant further investigation, given the known association of proteinuria with worse renal and cardiovascular outcomes. Nonetheless, it appears that those outcomes are no worse, and perhaps even better, for donors than for the general population.

Estimated GFR and chronic kidney disease classifications

Given the inevitable reduction of GFR as a result of nephrectomy, a variable proportion of donors will have a measured or estimated GFR of less than 60 mL/min. This means that they will be labelled as having chronic kidney disease (CKD). Depending on definition and time of measurement, this label has been applied to between 6 and 90% of donors [6]. The measurement of estimated GFR (eGFR) and the use of the 'chronic kidney disease' label for anyone with significant proteinuria or an eGFR of less than 60 mL/min is now ubiquitous in the United Kingdom. There has been a great deal of controversy about the potential for over-medicalisation in this system. There is an important, and as yet unanswered question, as to the extent to which the reduction of eGFR that results from a nephrectomy in an otherwise healthy person should prompt the same concerns as a similar reduction in someone with a pathological cause of decline in renal function. In other words, should donors who have an eGFR of less than 60 mL/min after their nephrectomy be labelled as having CKD? Classifying them as such raises the same questions as are rehearsed below about placing an expectation on donors about follow-up. The label of CKD transforms a donor from their previously fit status to someone who has a 'disease'. This may have diverse consequences, ranging from impacting on anxiety levels, being called for regular reviews in primary care, and affecting insurance premiums.

The absence of underlying disease obviously distinguishes donors from others with CKD. But there is no clear evidence yet as to whether the cardiovascular risks associated with CKD are relevant to donors with reduced eGFR.

Hypertension

Long-term data on donors' blood pressure after donation is limited. A meta-analysis in 2006 of 48 studies from 28 countries, which followed a total of 5145 donors, suggested that here may be a 5 mmHg increase in blood pressure within 5–10 years of donation over that anticipated with normal ageing [7]. Of 3698 donors at the University of Minnesota between 1963 and 2007, 255 agreed to measurement of their GFR. And among that group of 255, the prevalence of hypertension was 32% (24.7% were receiving antihypertensive medication and 7.5% were newly diagnosed). The mean systolic and diastolic blood pressures were 122 and 73 mmHg, respectively. Independent risk factors for hypertension were age and higher body mass index (BMI). These were also risk factors for a GFR of less than 60 mL/min [2]. The increasing rates of living donor transplantation and willingness to consider donors with hypertension and high BMIs suggest an imperative to continue to collect data on blood pressure after donation. This may be especially true in those countries where the incidence of obesity and diabetes are also rapidly increasing.

Outcomes for marginal donors

Short-term data suggest that donation is safe for donors who have easily controlled hypertension (using one or two agents) and who otherwise complete standard work-up for donation. A study of 24 White donors with hypertension controlled by angiotensin receptor blocker with or without a diuretic showed no adverse effects compared with other donors up to 1 year after donation. So far, there is very little long-term data on outcomes for donors who are hypertensive at the time of donation or who have a high BMI. Risks must be carefully discussed with all potential donors. It is equally important to discuss the uncertainties and lack of data about outcomes for donors who might be considered 'marginal'. The extent to which a potential donor should be allowed to take risks raises interesting questions about clinical and patient autonomy (see Chapter 25 on the ethics of transplantation).

Quality of life and overall health status

Just as psychological assessment forms a key part of pre-donation assessment, it is essential to consider the donor's psychological well-being after donation. Physical and mental health scores after donation are generally reported to be better than in the general population. Donors are expected to have 'a normal life span, a health status that is similar to that of the general population, and an excellent quality of life' [2].

Population data do not provide all the answers in terms of providing care after donation. A small proportion of living kidney transplants will not be successful. The physical outcome – and even the long-term mental outcome – for the donor may be good, but the psychological impact of an unsuccessful transplant should not be underestimated. Here is yet another illustration of the importance of a continuing relationship between the transplant team and the donor. Impersonal requests for follow-up data, for example, risk prompting the donor for information at a time when their recipient is sick or has recently died.

Pregnancy outcomes after donation

Women of childbearing age routinely donate kidneys and in some populations are the largest group of kidney donors. Fetal and maternal outcomes of pregnancy after kidney donation are comparable to those reported in the general population. However, there is evidence to suggest that outcomes for pregnancies after donation are not as good as outcomes for pregnancies before donation. A retrospective study of over 1500 female donors found increased rates of fetal loss, prematurity, gestational diabetes, gestational hypertension, pre-eclampsia and proteinuria in pregnancies after donation compared with pregnancies before donation [8]. Age may play a confounding role, as might ascertainment bias in a closely monitored group, but post-donation reduction in renal function remains a plausible cause of increased risk. Although the risks do not exceed those for the general population, the apparently increased risk in a carefully selected population warrants further investigation. If it were needed, here is another reason to insist on prospective national registries for all kidney donors.

Racial variation

There is some evidence that Black and Hispanic donors may have an increased risk of hypertension, diabetes mellitus and CKD after donation compared with White donors [9]. The extent to which these risks reflect background population risks as opposed to risks associated with nephrectomy is not clear. Again, further prospective data are urgently required to clarify the safety of donation for these groups (and other ethnic groups) whose potential recipients may already have lower levels of transplantation (from both living and deceased donors) than White patients.

Data collection

Registries

There have been and continue to be repeated calls for national and supra-national registries for living donor follow-up [10,11,12]. Good-quality prospective data are the only way of reassuring donors, recipients, clinicians and policy-makers about the safety of living donation – and the only way of providing clear estimates of the risks and likely outcomes for donors. This is particularly important when considering the use of more 'marginal' living donors. For example, some current policies allow people with hypertension controlled with one antihypertensive agent to donate a kidney. Only prospective data collected over years will provide confirmation that this policy is reasonable. The need for registries providing prospective data illustrates the fact that policies regarding donation are not strictly 'evidence-based'. New drug treatments or surgical interventions generally require significant bodies of experimental and randomised controlled trial data before they can be put into routine use. It is simply not possible to collect data of that kind for kidney donation. The UK Transplant Registry established the Living Donor Registry in 2000 (it is now held by NHS Blood and Transplant.) Data are collected on discharge from hospital and at 1, 2, 5 and 10 years, and every 5 years thereafter. The requested dataset includes:

- transfer to another unit or loss to follow-up
- death
- serum creatinine, haemoglobin, GFR (measured or estimated)
- blood pressure
- urine dipstick and quantification of proteinuria
- serious medical condition since last follow-up
- antihypertensive drugs prescribed since last follow-up
- whether the donor has returned to previous levels of activity [13].

   Regular follow-up with collection of this kind of dataset would reassure the transplant team that the donor is being well looked after, as well as providing regular data about outcomes to inform the broader programme. There are, however, important challenges to be met.

Challenges

Burden on the donor

Is it reasonable to place any kind of requirement for follow-up on the donor?

A fit and healthy person who has donated a kidney might, very reasonably, wish to return to their life without experiencing undue concerns about their ongoing health. They will have been offered the most up-to-date information about the likely impact of nephrectomy on their health. They, and the health-care team, would usually proceed with transplantation on the basis that there is only a very small chance of there being a significant long-term impact on their well-being. There is therefore an important question as to how much the mere fact of trying to monitor a donor in the long-term might have a negative impact on them. An annual review of blood pressure, proteinuria and renal function has the potential to cause anxiety as much as reassurance. Although health-care teams no doubt believe that an annual check-up is not particularly onerous (and may indeed be recommended for anyone, not just donors), care should be taken to respect the wishes of the donor. Potential donors should be made aware that routine, regular follow-up is a necessary part of kidney donation. The donor should be informed that their own safety and the safe running of the transplant programme places a requirement on transplant teams to monitor the health of donors after transplantation. But this requires an important disclosure to donors. Transplant teams must explain the limitations in the data about outcomes and the need for ongoing investigation. Of course, it is hoped that ongoing prospective data collection will continue to confirm the safety of living donor nephrectomy. But that in itself would pose a challenge to donor follow-up. The safer the procedure, the less imperative there is for any individual to go along with long-term monitoring, despite the need for transplant teams to constantly audit outcomes.

Organisational and logistical challenges

Even if the donor is willing, systems need to be put in place to share information between renal units, between primary care and renal units, and indeed between facilities in different countries. Many donors now travel from different countries or from distant parts of the same country to donate a kidney. They often have work or family commitments that make returning to the transplant centre difficult, even if the cost and logistics of travelling large distances do not. Clinicians will be all too familiar with the difficulties of coordinating surveillance and management of patients between clinical teams within the same hospital or between neighbouring primary- and secondary-care facilities [14]. The challenges of managing a triangular relationship between transplant team, donor and a health-care team local to the donor should not be underestimated. And it is worth reiterating that the challenge may be exacerbated by the donor being (usually) fit and well and disinclined (or simply having no good reason to remember) to interact with a health-care system. Many transplant teams find that a dedicated clinic for donor follow-up run by a nurse practitioner provides optimal outcomes.

Responsibilities towards all potential donors

Organ donation programmes carry a responsibility towards all patients who are screened for donation, not just those who go on to donate. Thorough screening of potential donors inevitably results in the identification of abnormalities, ranging from the probably insignificant, such as unusual anatomy of the renal vasculature, through to the discovery of malignant tumours. Where necessary, referral to other teams for investigation and treatment should be prompt. The transplant team must be satisfied that abnormalities discovered during work-up for donation are appropriately followed up. This might be difficult if, for example, a renal cell carcinoma is discovered in a donor who has travelled from overseas on a short visa. The transplant team also has a responsibility to ensure that incidental findings of no or of limited clinical significance are discussed with the potential donor. A key issue that remains to be resolved internationally is financial provision for lifelong health care for donors from states without socialised medicine or with limited provision. If a kidney donor from a country with no dialysis provision were to develop end-stage renal failure, would the transplanting centre have a responsibility to provide dialysis?

There may also be a significant psychological impact on a potential donor who is not permitted to donate, for whatever reason. A parent, for example, might be devastated not to be able to help their child by donation.

Conclusion

Living kidney donation is considered safe for individuals who have been appropriately screened, although it is not without risks.

Long-term regular follow-up of donors is:
- preferable for monitoring and intervention (if necessary) to secure the donor's well-being
- imperative to audit the safety of living donation, especially where more marginal donors are being considered.

Long-term follow-up of donors requires:
- early involvement of the potential donor to design and agree a follow-up programme
- coordination between transplant centre and donor's preferred place of care
- care to attend to psychological as well as physical health
- awareness of the impositions (financial, practical and emotional) of follow-up on the donor
- systematic data collection of an agreed dataset
- national and/or supra-national registries.

References

1. Segev DL, Muzaale AD, Caffo BS, *et al.* (2010) Perioperative mortality and long-term survival following live kidney donation. *JAMA* **303**, 959–966.
2. Ibrahim HN, Foley R, Tan L, *et al.* (2009) Long-term consequences of kidney donation. *N Eng J Med* **360**, 459–469.
3. Fehrman-Ekholm I, Elinder CG, Stenbeck M, *et al.* (1997) Kidney donors live longer. *Transplantation* **64**, 976–978.
4. Fehrman-Ekholm I, Norden G, Lennerling A, *et al.* (2006) Living kidney donors developing end-stage renal disease. *Transplant Proc* **38**, 2642–2643.
5. Garg AX, Muirhead N, Knoll G, *et al.* (2006) Proteinuria and reduced kidney function in living kidney donors: A systematic review, meta-analysis, and meta-regression. *Kidney Int* **70**, 1801–1810.
6. Barri Y, Parker T III, Kaplan B, *et al.* (2009) Primum non nocere: Is chronic kidney disease staging appropriate in living kidney transplant donors? *Am J Transplant* **9**, 657–660.
7. Boudville N, Prasad GV, Knoll G, *et al.* (2006) Meta-analysis: Risk for hypertension in living kidney donors. *Ann Intern Med* **145**, 185–196.
8. Ibrahim HN, Akkina SK, Leister E, *et al.* (2009) Pregnancy outcomes after kidney donation. *Am J Transplant* **9**, 825–834.
9. Lentine KL, Schnitzler MA, Xiao H, *et al.* (2010) Racial variation in medical outcomes among living kidney donors. *N Eng J Med* **363**, 724–732.
10. Manyalich M, Ricart A, Martinez I, *et al.* (2009) EULID Project: European living donation and public health. *Transplant Proc* **41**, 2021–2024.
11. Mjøen G, Øyen O, Holdaas H, *et al.* (2009) Morbidity and mortality in 1022 consecutive living donor nephrectomies: Benefits of a living donor registry. *Transplantation* **88**, 1273–1279.
12. Emara M, Raqheb A, Hassan A, *et al.* (2008) Evidence of a need to mandate kidney transplant living donor registries. *Clin Transplant* **22**, 525–531.
13. NHS Blood and Transplant Kidney Living Donor Assessment Follow-Up Form K-LIV-F12 (Version 20/08/08)
14. Mandelbrot DA, Pavlakis M, Karp SJ, *et al.* (2009) Practices and barriers in long-term living kidney follow-up: a survey of U.S. transplant centres. *Transplantation* **88**, 855–860.

25 Ethics of transplantation

Robert Elias and Rehana Iqbal

Introduction

The first ethical challenge to clinicians involved in transplantation is to appreciate that 'ethics' permeates every aspect of their practice. Every interaction with a potential donor or recipient, every clinical decision, every reading of a randomised controlled trial is shaped by values. The information and attitudes that we communicate to our patients reflects a complex combination of societal attitudes towards death and dying, personal experience of clinical practice and interpretation of available evidence.

Consent, confidentiality and shared decision-making are key concepts that the General Medical Council use to describe vital components of good clinical practice. In this chapter we first briefly describe those concepts and highlight some of the difficulties involved in employing them in complicated real-life decisions about transplantation.

We then identify crucial areas of contention that arise in deceased donor and living donor transplantation. Our emphasis is unashamedly on issues that arise in the day-to-day work of clinicians; hence the weight given to questions of consent and confidentiality.

Key concepts

Consent

We have rightly come a long way from the days when a signature on a consent form was thought to constitute consent to a procedure. There are many reasons why it is important to understand the difference between the formal processes that have been put in place to encourage clinicians to seek consent and actually achieving 'informed consent'.

When providing a blood sample, a patient can consent implicitly, perhaps by proffering an arm. But that consent does not necessarily extend to the tests that might be done on the blood sample. Nor does it extend to consent to disclosure of the information found during those tests. The many tests that accompany work-up of both recipients and

Handbook of Renal and Pancreatic Transplantation, First Edition. Edited by Iain A. M. MacPhee and Jiří Froněk.
© 2012 John Wiley & Sons, Ltd. Published 2012 by John Wiley & Sons, Ltd.

donors for transplantation – HIV tests, HLA crossmatching that might question paternity, complex scans that might uncover hidden anatomical abnormalities of uncertain prognostic significance – have the potential to ask searching questions of the clinical team and their patients about how to deal with uncertainty, where to draw the boundaries of risk, and whether, when and how to disclose information.

The following statements are accompanied by a brief discussion that alludes to the complexity that underlies even apparently straightforward statements about consent.

A patient can change their mind

No decision is entirely binding until a course of action has been followed. The vast machinery of people, resources and technology that go towards providing a transplant service can be outweighed by a change of mind in a patient, even as they are being wheeled into theatre.

Clinical teams should (and do) take precautions to ensure that those involved in transplantation have ample opportunity to change their minds. But decisions to proceed to transplant are not always black and white, and are not usually exclusively in the hands of the recipient and donor. The constraints of working with a scarce resource (deceased donor kidneys) can limit the information given to patients.

Decisions should be made free from coercion

The momentum of a vast medical system can raise expectations and provide an environment in which it could be difficult to express a change of heart. There is another interesting question as to what constitutes coercion within a family or among friends. At what point does the weight of expectation within a family become coercion for a sibling who, it is assumed, will be happy to donate a kidney?

Consent for a major, life-changing operation is not something that is obtained at a single time, in a single setting

Consent is a process, not an event. Ultimately, in order for a transplant to take place, there must be a point at which the recipient and donor give their agreement to the procedure taking place. But arriving at that point involves a long process of coming to understand what is involved, what the alternatives are, and what impact the decision will have on their lives.

There is no such thing as 'fully informed consent'

No consent can be 'fully' informed, in the sense of being exhaustively informed. There is too much information about outcomes, about what it will be like to experience one mode of treatment or another, for anyone to be exhaustively informed. The concept of 'fully informed consent' is problematic, and now obsolete. Consent should be 'adequately' informed. This, of course, acknowledges the significant grey areas that abound in determining what is and what is not adequate. And the growing movement in favour of patient-centred medicine stresses the need for patient involvement in determining what constitutes adequate consent for them. In other words, the clinician should seek to establish what constitutes adequate information and involvement for each patient, realising that decision-making varies from one patient to another. One person may want to know a huge amount of intricate detail; another may ask the clinical team to make decisions on their behalf, and ask for only broad details.

Confidentiality

Confidentiality plays a fundamental role in the creation of a trusting relationship between clinicians and patients. The UK General Medical Council guidance on confidentiality does, however, emphasise that: 'appropriate information sharing is essential to the efficient provision of safe, effective care, both for the individual patient and for the wider community of patients'.

And: 'Confidentiality is an important duty, but it is not absolute. You can disclose personal information if:
- it is required by law
- the patient consents – either implicitly for the sake of their own care or expressly for other purposes
- it is justified in the public interest' [1].

Shared decision-making

Shared decision-making describes the process whereby the clinical expertise of health-care providers is combined with the personal 'expertise' of the patient. Clinicians are experts in the investigation and management of disease. Patients are experts in the experience of illness and their own preferences. Patient expertise has traditionally been neglected in favour of a paternalistic approach. Although the aim of shared decision-making seeks to redress the balance, it remains unclear how it can best be achieved in many clinical situations.

'Whatever the context in which medical decisions are made, you must work in partnership with your patients to ensure good care. In so doing, you must:
- listen to patients and respect their views about their health
- discuss with patients what their diagnosis, prognosis, treatment and care involve
- share with patients the information they want or need in order to make decisions
- maximise patients' opportunities, and their ability, to make decisions for themselves
- respect patients' decisions' [2].

Deceased donor transplantation

Scarcity and resource allocation

Deceased donor organ allocation forms a particularly visible form of rationing because of the severe shortage of donor organs and the obvious needs of people who can be clearly identified because they are on a waiting list. An Organ Donation Taskforce undertook a comprehensive review of organ donation in the UK in 2008 and is readily accessible online [3].

The way in which deceased donor organs are allocated has been described in Chapter 8. We will not embark on a detailed discussion of the ethics surrounding organ allocation here, which warrants a book of its own. We will instead briefly comment on two ethical issues that gain prominence because of the shortage and consequent rationing of organs.

Marginal donors

The chronic shortage of donor organs has meant that higher-risk donors and 'marginal' deceased donor organs are being considered for transplantation. Guidelines suggest that it is acceptable for someone with hypertension controlled with one agent to donate a kidney. But there is inevitable pressure to allow potential donors to take greater risks for loved ones who perhaps stand little chance of receiving a deceased donor organ. The boundaries between what is acceptable in clinical practice and what is expected of donors are shifting and interconnected. The emotional bond that motivates people to donate can also be a coercive force on them. The ability and willingness to consider higher-risk procedures can only make it more difficult to disentangle the two.

More marginal deceased donor organs include those from non-heartbeating donors (donation after circulatory death) and those from diabetic donors or with impaired renal function at the time of death. It is vital that the desire to provide more organs for more people does not prevent an honest appraisal of whether it is in this recipient's best interests to receive this organ. And as knowledge of outcomes becomes more complex and the variety of available organs becomes greater, so the ways in which patients are involved in decisions about transplantation must diversify.

Patient obligations

Scarcity of organs makes it all the more dispiriting when a patient loses a kidney because they have not been taking their medication, have not been attending follow-up or have been somehow harming themselves.

There is a need for careful psychological evaluation of potential recipients. But there is no magic formula that will predict whether someone will not meet the demands of post-transplant medication and follow-up. A previously poor attender might value their transplanted kidney all the more precisely because haemodialysis was intolerable for them.

The scarcity of donor organs places a great deal of pressure on clinicians and patients to ensure that they are used as well as possible. Does that mean, however, that those people with 'cleaner' lifestyles, or with the lowest rates of 'did not attend' clinic appointments, should score more points on the waiting list?

Definition of death

It seems unnecessary, on the face of it, to stress that death is the point at which a patient can become a deceased organ donor. But the transition from patient to donor can pose awkward ethical questions for families and clinicians.

- The majority of donors die in highly medicalised settings, such as intensive-care units, where the point at which death occurs may not be obvious. For donors after circulatory death, a diagnosis of death after cardio-respiratory arrest is similarly essential. It is vital that clinicians and families have confidence in a clear code of practice so that there can be no doubt about the diagnosis of death. There are clear guidelines from the Academy of Medical Royal Colleges [4] on the diagnosis and confirmation of death.
- Once a decision has been made to withdraw treatment, or death is seen as inevitable, the question arises as to whether it is acceptable to manage the process of treatment withdrawal and death in order to ensure the best possible outcome for planned organ retrieval. There may also be investigations that would be helpful for organ donation which would not otherwise be done. Treating the patient differently for organ donation sits uncomfortably for some clinicians. If there is clear consent from the patient for organ donation, then preparation for donation may well be in their best interests. But consent for donation is not always clearly expressed. Indeed, some would argue that being on the organ donor register – perhaps having registered many years before – falls short of what would usually be considered consent.

Patient information and consent

Deceased donor transplantation generates particular challenges for ensuring that patients are adequately informed and given the opportunity to consent to their treatment.

A delay of months or years from activation on the transplant waiting list to transplantation is usual. The process of working up for transplantation, discussing the pros and cons, and being deemed fit for transplantation can therefore be significantly removed from the transplant operation itself. This poses significant logistical problems for transplant teams, often spread over large geographical areas, to ensure that everyone on the waiting list is fit to be transplanted. It is crucial that anyone called into hospital for a transplant should be fit to receive it. If a potential recipient is found to be unfit at that stage, transplantation of a precious organ might be delayed (with consequent reduced chance of success) or even prevented altogether.

Just as it is vital to ensure that the waiting list is kept up to date in terms of clinical information, so it is vital that the consent and information needs of potential recipients are continuously met. This challenge is perhaps less noticed than the purely clinical one. It is common for patients to be called into hospital for a transplant and not remember any specific discussion about the process of transplantation or the risk–benefit balance of transplantation against other options.

The need to reappraise the risks and benefits of transplantation will vary from person to person on the waiting list. A young person's attitude to transplantation may vary little over a number of years. But an older man with co-morbidities may find that he has adjusted to life on dialysis since joining the waiting list. The benefits of transplantation may become less obvious to him over time.

Individual needs and population needs

Separation of what is 'clinical' and 'non-clinical' when it comes to weighing up risks and benefits is not possible. Evidence of the likely outcomes of interventions needs to mesh with people's experiences of their lives to provide a decision about what to do. But deceased donor transplantation provides an outright challenge to patient autonomy when it comes to deciding about individual kidneys.

In the UK, a national matching system allocates donor kidneys based on an algorithm that gives weight to how long potential recipients have been waiting for a transplant, how well they match the kidney and how well matched they are to the donor's age, among other factors (see Chapter 8). Once the kidney is allocated and the potential recipient is called into hospital to receive the kidney, the focus is on checking that the potential recipient is fit to go ahead with the procedure and informing them (again) what is involved. It is not usual practice to discuss with the potential recipient specific details about the donor and the nature of the donor kidney.

Information about the donor kidney could potentially be highly relevant to a patient's decision as to whether to proceed with transplantation. Whereas someone who is highly sensitised might not stand a good chance of getting another opportunity for a transplant, a young person who is not sensitised might want to gamble in favour of a better kidney next time, should they be offered a 'marginal' organ on this occasion.

At present, these deliberations do not typically involve the potential recipient. The need to use a limited resource efficiently means that decisions about allocation are taken centrally, or by local clinicians, but the patient is not involved. The process of taking individual patients through a detailed breakdown of risks and benefits associated with receiving the particular organ that is available at that moment would be too time- and resource-intensive to allow for optimal use of organs. As with a patient who is found not to be fit for transplantation, a patient who decides not to receive an organ potentially jeopardises the use of that organ for others.

There is a challenge here to involve the patient as much as possible, without threatening the welfare of all those on the transplant waiting list. And there is a question as to how the use of more marginal donor organs does and should affect the information given to patients [5].

Living donor transplantation

In living donor kidney transplantation, the process of transplantation is planned. There is therefore usually more certainty about what is going to happen and when it will happen. The likely events, outcomes and risks can more easily be communicated in a planned and timely way. But living kidney donation gives rise to its own distinct ethical challenges.

Confidentiality, consent and trust

The relationships of people who donate kidneys to the health-care system and to their recipients are complex. Organ donors are unusual in subjecting themselves to risk of mortality and morbidity from a previously healthy state. They voluntarily become patients. In the case of kidney donors, they are often cared for around the time of the operation and afterwards by the same team who care for their recipient.

In the process of being assessed and prepared for possible kidney donation, potential donors are counselled by a clinician who has no direct responsibility for the care of the potential recipient. This separation of responsibility serves three main purposes.

- To prevent concerns about the well-being of the person with end-stage renal failure from interfering with an assessment of the donor's psychological and physical fitness to donate.
- To protect the process of informed consent. The doctor with responsibility for the donor can focus on ensuring that the donor is adequately informed and consents to the procedure without coercion. Since the Human Tissue Act came into effect in the UK in 2006, an independent assessor must interview any proposed donor and their recipient separately and prepare a report to assist the Human Tissue Authority in deciding whether to approve the transplantation.
- To protect the confidentiality of both donor and recipient. Despite this, there is usually some sharing of information. The donor is counselled about the likelihood of success of the procedure and possible complications. Outcomes of the procedure will, in part, depend on characteristics of the recipient. For example, co-morbidities other than kidney failure may increase the risk of peri-operative death. And the disease causing kidney failure can sometimes recur in the transplanted kidney.

The sharing of information between donor and recipient is not usually controversial: patients with diabetes, for example, do not typically object to the diagnosis of diabetes being shared with their potential donor. That sharing of information assists communication with the potential donor about the risks and benefits of transplantation because a detailed, contextualised picture can be built up for them. But not all potential recipients are happy to disclose their medical details. It is common for people with HIV disease, for example, not to disclose their diagnosis, even to close family and friends. Would it then be reasonable to ask someone to donate a kidney without them knowing their recipient's diagnosis of HIV?

There is a tension between confidentiality and consent. It is preferable for a recipient to allow disclosure of confidential medical information so that a potential donor can be adequately informed. But it is not always necessary for a potential donor to know clinical information that the recipient would rather keep confidential. HIV forms an interesting test case because renal transplantation in HIV disease is relatively new. Although short-term outcomes are good, the longer-term outcomes are unknown. It is certainly challenging to describe the potential outcomes of transplantation in the context of HIV disease without referring to HIV. But for a donor who has been told and accepts that the clinical information they will be given about their recipient will necessarily be incomplete, it should be possible.

Teams who undertake transplants for people with HIV disease do often insist on disclosure of the diagnosis between donor and recipient if the transplant is to go ahead. There are two main reasons for this.

The first is the belief that consent cannot be informed consent if information that would change the donor's decision is withheld from them. This is straightforwardly true for information about outcomes, such as the risk of recurrence of primary disease in the transplant. This is less obvious for information that is not overtly 'clinical'. It is not the role of the clinical team to disclose details that they might know about an extra-marital affair, even if that information would change the mind of the potential donor about donating. It would certainly be impossible to proceed if the potential donor had stated that they would not dream of donating an organ to someone with HIV. But what of the mother who says that she would like to donate to her daughter regardless? Should we still insist on disclosure of the diagnosis, despite the daughter's desire not to?

The important ethical realisation at this point is that 'informed consent' is a blunt tool. It can take you so far, but no further. The question that the team must ask of themselves about, for example, a wife who is going to donate without knowing about her husband's affair, or the mother who will give to her daughter without knowing about her HIV, is whether it is the right thing to do. And deciding whether it is the right thing to do hinges on far more than whether 'informed consent' can be achieved.

The second reason revolves around the importance of trust. Trust forms a vital part of the work of transplant teams. Donors and recipients must trust the team to take good care of them. The team looks for evidence of a trusting relationship between donor and recipient. Failure to disclose information about a diagnosis such as HIV may not always preclude the possibility of informed consent, but it almost certainly leads the team to question the nature of the relationship between donor and recipient. This is of particular concern where, as in living kidney donation, the recipient stands to gain so much and the donor is putting him/herself at risk.

In an evermore legalistic world, trust is a difficult concept to pin down. And clinicians must be very careful to disentangle genuine concerns about the relationship between recipient and donor from personal or cultural views that do not match those of the pair.

Incidental findings

We have already commented on the fact that potential kidney donors are unusual in exposing themselves to morbidity and mortality (albeit at very low risk) from a healthy state. In addition to the morbidity and mortality associated with the procedure itself, the investigations involved in being 'worked up' to donate a kidney might engender anxiety without significant benefit for the donor. The discovery of a small renal stone or an adrenal adenoma in the donor might be important for the transplant team to know, for example, but induce only anxiety in the donor.

There is also the potential to make findings with potentially huge consequences for the donor and recipient but without direct relevance to the technical process of transplantation. For example, HLA tissue typing sometimes reveals that a father and child are not genetically related. What then? Is it for the transplant team to disclose that information, or can they allow the transplant to go ahead without saying anything?

There is a wide variety of opinion on this matter, both anecdotally and in the literature. Commentators agree that it is a genuine ethical dilemma. On the one hand it might be argued that donor and recipient cannot be adequately informed about the procedure if the information about paternity is not disclosed. On the other hand, the information can be seen as incidental to the procedure and the potential to cause harm by disclosure is huge.

Again, the issue of trust is crucial here. There is scope for a long debate about informed consent in this case and for weighing up the potential risks and benefits of disclosure. But it is difficult to see how any definite rule can be set. Knowledge of the people involved, the microscopic detail of the clinical situation, the family and relationships is surely vital in assessing what is the right thing to do. In some ways, the easy option would be to stipulate that there can be no valid consent without disclosure of information about misattributed paternity, or to sidestep the issue altogether by finding a spurious reason why the transplant cannot go ahead. But this may not be the right thing to do for the donor and recipient.

There is not space here to rehearse detailed arguments about misattributed paternity. However, the very real problem that it increasingly poses (it is estimated to occur in up to 0.5% of all living kidney transplants [6]) suggests three recommendations.

- Do not undertake tests unless they will affect clinical management.
- Give patients adequate information prior to any tests about what will be tested and what information will be disclosed. Explaining to donor and recipient that you may discover information about their genetic relationship may provoke anxiety but will help you understand what information they would like to receive after the test.

• Know in advance how your team will deal with difficult ethical scenarios such as this: who will decide what to do and how.

Risk, autonomy and coercion

There has been a vigorous swing in Western medicine over recent decades from medical paternalism to 'patient-centred' medicine. Advanced care planning and advanced refusals of treatment have taken centre stage in much media coverage of medicine. In the UK, however, it remains a fundamental principle that patients cannot insist on receiving a certain treatment. A competent person can refuse any treatment, and can provide instructions for what they would want should they become incompetent. Since the Mental Capacity Act, a competent person can, for the first time in the UK, appoint someone else to consent on their behalf should they become incompetent. But none of this amounts to the ability to demand treatment. That remains at the clinical team's discretion.

Case study

Mr S is a 65-year-old man with diabetes and ischaemic heart disease. He wants a transplant. He is currently receiving haemodialysis, having failed peritoneal dialysis after 5 years, and having had a previous deceased donor renal transplant that lasted for 10 years. He has good vascular access through an arterio-venous fistula. But he hates haemodialysis. He finds that he is exhausted after every session. He is desperate to travel and visit his family overseas. His 37-year-old son is willing to donate a kidney. He is fit and well. There is no reason to think that he would not be able to donate a kidney.

Mr S unfortunately has significant ischaemic heart disease. The cardiology team, in conjunction with the renal transplant team, have estimated that his peri-operative mortality risk is approximately 50%. Mr S and his son are aware of this. They both remain extremely keen to proceed with transplantation. Mr S says that a life on dialysis is no life at all and that the 50% risk is worth taking. His son accepts that risk as well. For him, the possibility of a year or two's better quality of life for his father makes it worth taking the risk of losing not only his kidney but also his father.

This case raises a number of interesting questions.

Clinical autonomy and patient autonomy

One of the main reasons why the clinical team might not agree to transplantation in this case is because it represents a wasteful, or at least sub-optimal use of resources. If the patient were requesting a deceased donor kidney, there would be a clear argument that the organ could be better used elsewhere. This, however, is a directed living donation. The organ is not available for anyone else. And if we imagine for a moment that resources are unlimited, should the clinical team agree to go ahead?

The clinical team may still decline to do the transplant, even if resources are unlimited. The clinical decision that it is not right to do the transplant outweighs the potential recipient and donor pair's wishes. There might be a number of reasons for this.

* Despite his opinion, the team feel that it is not in the best interests of the potential recipient to go ahead.

This position throws up the interesting question of whether the team can know what is in someone's best interests better than the individual patient. On the one hand, the patient, after all, is the expert in their own experience of life. They know what they are living through. If they are competent to make decisions having understood all the information that the team wish to share with them then they, surely, have priority over the team in deciding what is in their best interests. And if that is the case, there cannot be a best interests argument for denying them a risky transplant. (It is important here to remember that the competence of someone to make a decision is not in any way contingent on them making what someone else would consider a wise or sensible decision. Put another way: a decision that is foolish or with which the clinical team disagree is not a reason to question someone's competence to make that decision.)

On the other hand, although the patient is the expert in their experience of their illness and of their life, the clinical team holds a great deal of expertise in the management of renal failure and transplantation. The ambition of 'shared decision-making' is to bring together the differing expertises of patient and clinicians to come to a decision. The idea of shared decision-making acknowledges that neither patient nor clinical team has absolute priority in making decisions, partly because the complete sharing of expertise is not possible. Inhabiting the life of a patient is not possible, no matter how empathic the clinician. And clinicians know that patients struggle to come to terms with the realities of illness, often changing their attitudes to death and disability along the way.

* The team feels that the risks to the potential donor cannot be justified despite his stated wishes.

The clinical team sits in a very unusual relationship with the donor. They will cause him harm for the benefit of someone else. Even where there is also clear benefit to the donor in giving a kidney, this relationship sits far outside the usual territory of medicine. Although the risks of donating a kidney are small, they are significant. So care is taken to ensure that the overall benefit of donation massively outweighs the risk. One reason to decline to transplant in this case is that the risk to the donor (although the same as in any transplant) is high when compared to the potential benefits.

Of course, the same question about competence and autonomy arises. If the donor is competent and well informed by the team and would still like to go ahead, why should the clinical team prevent him from doing so? Reasons for refusing to go ahead in this case – other than the question of resource allocation – are not transparent. The case becomes even more difficult if the estimated risks of surgery are reduced for the father. At what estimated rate of cardiac risk for the father does the team, reluctantly perhaps, agree to go ahead?

• Undertaking risky procedures can jeopardise the transplant programme as a whole.

Appropriate use of resources is not the only way in which the decision-making about individual cases is affected by wider concerns. Public trust in transplantation is nurtured by the success of the transplant programme. Furthermore, potential living donors (directed or altruistic) and the families of deceased donors want to see the safe and responsible use of organs.

The morale of the clinical team is also an important consideration. Discussion of ethics infrequently touches upon the emotional life of clinicians when perhaps it should. The work undertaken by transplant teams is technically, intellectually and emotionally challenging. On the one hand, it is not unreasonable that clinicians should seek out environments in which they believe that their work is important and valuable. On the other hand, those labels 'important' and 'valuable' must surely be defined primarily by reference to the experiences of patients.

The multidisciplinary team

We have been talking about 'the clinical team' but that team is made up of a large number of people from different disciplines and professions. The functional and efficient running of that team is fundamental to good quality, ethical decision-making. Keeping details about patients on the waiting list up to date and keeping those patients adequately informed requires clear communication, often from multiple centres of patient care to and from the transplanting centre.

The separation of responsibility for donor and recipient in living donation presents challenges. Confidentiality is crucial and medical details should not be disclosed. However, unnecessary tests for the donor can be avoided if the recipient is not fit for transplant, and the recipient similarly needs to know if a transplant is not possible from a particular donor.

It is usually the same surgical team who looks after the donor and recipient. Often, the only difference in terms of 'separation of care' is that the physician looking after the donor is not the same as the physician looking after the recipient. This raises the question of who, exactly, makes decisions about whether to proceed to transplantation. It is the surgeon and the anaesthetist in theatre who take responsibility for the procedure itself. But it is the broader transplant team who give the go ahead for transplantation. Any member of the team must feel able to voice concerns. The process of confirming that transplantation is a reasonable course of action and that both donor and recipient have been informed and have consented without coercion must be robust.

Just as there can be differences of opinion within clinical teams, there can also be differences between transplant teams. One centre might be prepared to offer a transplant to someone who another centre considers too high a risk. Again, robust procedures are needed to ensure that every potential donor and recipient are treated fairly and transparently, no matter where they live.

Conclusion

We have mentioned only a few of the very many important and fascinating ethical issues that arise in transplantation. There are many more to explore, including questions that arise from paired, pooled, domino and altruistic donation (briefly described in Chapters 10 and 17) and from culturally diverse attitudes to organ donation. We have also put aside the vast issues around money, including arguments about donor compensation, the creation of a market for organs, and health tourism.

New ethical issues will continue to arise in transplantation faster than they can be described. The more 'normal' paired or ABO incompatible or marginal donors become in clinical practice, for example, the more complex and vexing the ethical issues are likely to be. No two clinical situations are identical and doing what is right requires careful attention to the detail as much as to overriding principles.

We have highlighted some of the controversies that abound in the hope that structured thinking about these problems will facilitate robust and transparent ethical decision-making in the future.

Key references

1. General Medical Council. (2009) *Confidentiality*. Available online from: www.gmc-uk.org/guidance/ethical_guidance/confidentiality.asp.
2. General Medical Council. (2008) *Consent: Patients and Doctors Making Decisions Together*. Available online from: www.gmc-uk.org/guidance/ethical_guidance/consent_guidance_index.asp.
3. Department of Health. (2008) *Organs for Transplants: A report from the Organ Donation Taskforce*. Available online from: http://www.dh.gov.uk/en/Publicationsandstatistics/Publications/PublicationsPolicyAndGuidance/DH_082122.
4. Academy of Medical Royal Colleges. (2008) *A Code of Practice for the Diagnosis and Confirmation of Death*. Available online from: http://www.aomrc.org.uk/publications/reports-guidance.html.
5. Replies to Halpern SD, *et al.* (2008) Informing candidates for transplantation about donor risk factors. *N Engl J Med* **359**, 1182–1183.
6. Young A, Kim SH, Gibney EM, *et al.* (2009) Discovering Misattributed paternity in living kidney donation: Prevalence, preference and practice. *Transplantation* **87**, 1429–1435.

Index

Notes: Pages numbers in *italics* refer to Figures; those in **bold** to Tables

ABO blood groups, 273
ABO-incompatible kidney
    transplantation, 271–9
  blood transfusion following, 278–9
  immunosuppression, 272
  postoperative titre monitoring,
    274–5, 277
  results, 271–3, **279**
  splenectomy, 271
Acceptable Mismatch (AM)
    programme, 155
accessory artery anastomosis, 298
ACE inhibitors *see* angiotensin-
    converting enzyme (ACE)
    inhibitors
acute antibody-mediated rejection
    (acute AMR), 321–3
acute cellular rejection *see* acute T-cell-
    mediated rejection (aTCMR)
acute cellular (T-lymphocyte-
    mediated) rejection, 265, 324–6
acute cystitis, 343
acute pyelonephritis, 343
acute rejection, 388, 422
    treatment, 265–6
    ultrasound, 300
    grading, 325
    acute tubular necrosis (ATN), 300–1,
        307, 388
    adefovir, 368
adenovirus infection, 373–5
    adult polycystic kidney disease, 26
adynamic bone disease, 421
albumin/creatinine ratio, 424
albumin spot-analysis, potential live
    kidney donors, 43
alemtuzumab, 247–8, 263, 280
alendronate, 421
alfacalcidol, 395

allopurinol
    azathioprine and, 255
    gout, 396, 428
    interactions, **250**
Alport syndrome, 26–7
amantadine, 374
amphotericin-B
    aspergillosis, 349, 350
    candidiasis, 349
    cryptococcosis, 351
amyloidosis, 27
anaemia, 427–8, 395
analgesia, early post-transplant period,
    394
angiotensin-converting enzyme (ACE)
    inhibitors
    ABO-incompatible kidney
        transplantation, 275
    left ventricular systolic dysfunction,
        14
    post-transplant hypertension,
        397–8, 427
angiotensin II receptor blockers
    (ARBs), 14, 397–8, 427
ano-genital cancer, **418**
anterior subcostal extraperitoneal live
    donor nephrectomy, 117, 136–7
anthracycline-based chemotherapy,
    362–3
antibiotics
    deceased donor kidney
        transplantation, 160
    interactions, **250**
    live donor nephrectomy, 238
    pancreas transplantation
        prophylaxis, 198
    urinary tract infection, 343
    see also individual drugs
antibodies, therapeutic, **246**

Handbook of Renal and Pancreatic Transplantation, First Edition. Edited by
Iain A. M. MacPhee and Jiří Froněk.
© 2012 John Wiley & Sons, Ltd. Published 2012 by John Wiley & Sons, Ltd.

antibody-incompatible kidney
    transplantation, 271–85
antibody-mediated rejection (AMR),
    265, 321–323, 333
anticoagulation, pancreas
    transplantation, 198–9
antidiuretic hormone (ADH)
    brainstem-dead donors, 83, 87–8
antifungals, **250**
antiglomerular basement membrane
    disease, 25, 426
antihypertensive drugs, 219, 409
anti-lymphocyte globulin (ALG),
    246–7
antimalarial agents, 376
antineutrophil cytoplasmic antibody
    (ANCA)-associated vasculitis, **22,**
    25, 426
antiphospholipid antibodies, 25
antiplatelet therapy
    cardiovascular risk reduction, 15,
        411–12
antiproliferative agents, 255–9
antireflux ureterocystoneostomy, 290
antiretrovirals, immunosuppression
    and, 266, 372
antithymocyte globulin (ATG), 245,
    246–7, 372, 413
    acute cellular (T-lymphocyte-
        mediated) rejection, 265
    antibody-mediated rejection, 265
Anxiety, 17, 443
aorto-iliac disease, 17
appendix removal, 290
area under the concentration-time
    curve (AUC),
    immunosuppression, 243–4
arrhythmias, 404
arterial pressure measurement
    deceased donor kidney
        transplantation, 161
    pancreatic transplantation
        anaesthesia, 229–30
arterial stiffness, transplant recipients,
    404
arteriovenous fistula (AVF)
    kidney transplant patients, 220
    pancreatic transplantation, 229
    post-transplant management, 400
    ultrasound, 306
aspergillosis, 345, 349–50
aspiration risk, 220
aspirin
    cardiovascular risk reduction,
        411–12
    coronary revascularisation, 15
    deceased donor kidney
        transplantation, 160

renal transplant biopsy, 390–1
    thromboprophylaxis, 394
asymptomatic bacteriuria, 343
asymptomatic candiduria, 343
ATG see antithymocyte globulin (ATG)
Atherosclerosis, 166–7, 192, 403–4
atherosclerotic reno-vascular disease,
    donors, 42
atracurium, 221, **222**
atrial filbrillation, chronic, 16
autonomic storm, 81
autonomy, 237, 456–7
avascular necrosis, 420
azathioprine, **249, 250,** 255–6, 413

bacterial infections, 342–8
    see also individual infections
bacteriuria
    asymptomatic, 343
    potential live kidney donors, 43–4
balloon dilation, ureteric obstruction,
    387
Banff classification scheme, 317, **318,**
    319–31
Banff pancreas classification scheme,
    331–3
bariatric surgery, 19
barotrauma, 239
basal cell carcinoma, **29**
basiliximab, 246, 275
belatacept, 261–263
beta-blockers, 14, 160, 398
beta cells, 203
bile duct, multiorgan heartbeating
    donation, 94
bipolar disorder, 17
bisphosphonates, 421
BK polyoma virus, 304, 366–7
bladder
    drainage, pancreas transplantation,
        194
    paediatric renal transplantation, 288
bladder augmentation, 169–70
bladder cancer, **29**
blood clots, ureteral obstruction, 304
blood pressure, 220, 408–9, 427
blood transfusion
    post-ABO-incompatible kidney
        transplantation, 278–9
    post-transplant, 395
Boari flap, 387
body mass index (BMI)
    National Pancreas Allocation
        Scheme, 151
    pancreatic donors, 208
    potential live kidney donors, 35
    potential transplant recipient, 18–19
    transplant contraindication, 19

bone disease, post-transplantation *see* post-transplant bone disease
bone marrow biopsy, 416
bone mineral density, post-transplantation, 419–20
bortezomib, 265
brachiocephalic arteriovenous fistulae, 400
bradycardia, laparoscopic live donor nephrectomy, 239
brain death, 80–84
brain-directed therapies, 79–80
breast cancer
    post-transplantation surveillance, **418**
    recurrence-free waiting time, **28**
breastfeeding, 266
British Transplantation Society live donor selection guidelines, 235
bupivacaine, **222**, 223

caesarian section, 429
calcineurin inhibitors (CNIs), 248–55
    antiretroviral interactions, 373
    bioavailability, 251
    blood concentration measurement, 244
    children, 291
    generic preparations, 264
    interactions, **250**, 251, 264, 373
    light microscopic toxic findings, 327–8
    minimisation, 263–5, 292
    nephrotoxicity, 251, 390, 396, 422, 425
    new-onset diabetes after transplantation, 251, 407
    post-transplant dyslipidaemia, 406
    post-transplant hypertension, 405
    side effects, **254**
    toxicity, 251, 327–8, 388
    vasospasm induction, 388
    see also individual drugs
calcineurin inhibitors (CNIs)-free regimens, 263
calcitriol, 421
calcium, serum
    ABO-incompatible kidney transplantation, 275
    immediate postoperative period, 382
calcium carbonate, 421
calcium channel blockers, 16, **250**, 398
calcium-phosphate product, 395–6
Campath-1H *see* alemtuzumab
Candida albicans, 348
candidiasis, 348–9
candiduria, asymptomatic, 343
capacity, 17

carbamazepine, **250**
carbapenem, 343
carbothorax, 240
cardiac output measurement, 230
cardiovascular assessment, potential recipients, 12–17, 30
cardiovascular disease, 49, 403–36
caspofungin, 349, 350
Castleman's disease, 365
catheter angiography, 310–313
    antegrade pyelography, 312–13
    antegrade ureteric stenting, 312–13, *313*
    contrast media nephrotoxicity, 311
    nephrostomy, 312–13
    post-biopsy haemorrhage, 311–12
    renal transplant artery stenosis, 312
    vascular thrombosis, 311
Cattell-Braasch manoeuvre, 92–3, 104
CD25 antibody, 246
cell-saver, 395
central venous catheter, 160, 399
central venous pressure (CVP)
    deceased donor kidney transplantation, 160–161
    pancreatic transplantation anaesthesia, 229, 230
    renal transplantation anaesthesia, 221, 222
cephalosporin, 343
cerebrovascular disease, post-transplant, 16
cervical cancer
    post-transplantation surveillance, **418**
    recurrence-free waiting time, **29**
chickenpox *see* varicella
children
    steroids, 291
    organ allocation, 149, 150, 154–5
    post-transplant lymphoproliferative disorder, 293
    renal transplantation *see* paediatric renal transplantation
chimerism, 5
cholecystectomy, 94
chronic active antibody-mediated rejection, 323–4
chronic active T-cell-mediated rejection, 326–7, 333
chronic antibody-mediated rejection, 425
chronic kidney disease-mineral bone disease (CKD-MBD), 418
chronic rejection, 305

ciclosporin, 251–2
  blood concentration measurement, 252
  cosmetic impact, 252
  HIV, 372
  interactions, **250**
  pancreas transplantation, 197–8
  pharmacokinetic properties, **249**
  post-transplant dyslipidaemia, 406
  side effects, **254**
  therapeutic range, 252
  toxicities, 252
cidofovir, 356, 364–5, 374
cigarette smoking *see* smoking
cinacalcet, 395–6
ciprofloxacin, 376
cirrhosis, 20, 371
cisatracurium
  pancreatic transplantation anaesthesia, 229
  renal transplantation anaesthesia, 221, **222**
clarithromycin, **250**
clopidogrel
  deceased donor kidney transplantation, 160
  percutaneous coronary intervention, 15–16
  renal transplant biopsy, 391
Clostridium difficile infection, 339–41, 346
CO_2 insufflation, 239
coagulopathy dissemination, 83–4
cocciodiomycosis, 353
Cockcroft–Gault formula, 39
cognitive impairment, potential renal transplant recipient, 17
colchicine, 396, 428
Collaborative Islet Transplant Registry (CITR), 206, 214
collagenase, islet isolation, 209, *210*
colloids, 222, 230
colorectal cancer, **28**
colour Doppler ultrasound (CDU), 299
combined epidural–general anaesthesia, 228–229
combined laparoscopic/open live donor nephrectomy techniques, 126
combined liver and bone marrow transplant, first, 5
combined spinal–epidural anaesthesia (CSE), 228.
common bile duct, 97
common iliac artery, 165
community-acquired infections, 336

complement-dependent cytotoxicity (CDC), 60, 280
  HLA allosensitisation detection, 63–4
  HLA-I transplantation, 281
complement-dependent lymphocytotoxic crossmatch (CC-XM) assays, 67–8
  Amos wash technique, 67–8
  positive pretransplant donor, 71
computerised tomography (CT)
  abscess formation, 309
  nephrolithiasis, potential live kidney donors, 45
  pancreatic islet transplantation, 213
  Pneumocystis pneumonia, 351, *352*
  pneumonia, 344–5
  post-renal transplantation imaging, 307–9
  post-transplant lymphoproliferative disorder, 361
computerised tomography angiography (CTA), 309
  potential live kidney donors, 41, *42*
  renal graft torsion, 309
  renal vein thrombosis, 309
conception, 429
confidentiality, 449, 453–5
consent, 447–9, 451–5
constipation, post-transplant, 383–4
contraception, 399
coronary angiography, 14, 192
coronary artery disease (CAD)
  management algorithm, *15*
  pancreas transplantation, 192
coronary revascularisation, 14
corticosteroids, 261
  avascular necrosis, 420
  lipid metabolism effects, 406
  new-onset diabetes after transplantation (NODAT), 407
  paediatric kidney transplantation, 292
  polyomavirus-associated nephropathy, 367
  post-transplant bone disease, 420
  toxicity, 261
  see also individual drugs
co-trimoxazole
  infection prophylaxis, 335–6
  listeriosis prophylaxis, 345
  nocardiosis, 345, 346
  Pneumocystis pneumonia, 352–3, 373
  side effects, 353
  urinary tract infection prophylaxis, 344
CP-690,550 (Tasocitinib), 262
creatinine, 382, 423

critical care, 80
crossmatching, 220
   HLA-I transplantation, 280
   pancreas transplantation, 196
cryptococcal antigen, 351
cryptococcomas, 351
cryptococcosis, 350–351
crystalloids, 230
CT see computerised tomography (CT)
cutaneous cryptococcosis, 350
cutaneous ureterostomy, 170
CYP3A5*1 allele, 254
cystatin C, 423
cystitis
   acute, 343
   haemorrhagic, 201
cystogram, 233
cytokine-release syndrome, 246, 247
cytomegalovirus hyperimmunoglobulin
   (CMVIg), 273
cytomegalovirus (CMV) infection,
   353–6
   children, 293
   donor screening, **338**
   histopathology, 329
   pancreas transplantation, 198
   pre-emptive therapy, 354–5
   prevention, 354–5
   treatment, 355–6
cytotoxic crossmatch, 3

daclizumab, 246
dapsone, 353
deceased donor (DD)
   classification, 159
   infection screening, 337
deceased donor after brain death
   (DBD), 146–50
deceased donor kidney transplantation,
   159–72
   abnormal urinary tract continuity,
    169–70
   bench reconstruction, 162
   bladder augmentation, 169–70
   consent, 451–2
   definition of death, 451
   diseased artery anastomosis, 166–7
   dual kidney transplantation,
    170–171
   ethics, 449–52
   extravesical uretero-cystoneostomy,
    165, 168
   graft preparation, 161–3
   hockey-stick approach, 163
   hospital admission assessment, 160
   ileal conduit, 170
   incisions, 163
   inferior epigastric vessels, 164

   intravesical ureteroneocystostomy,
    168
   kidney graft reperfusion,
    167–8
   lower urinary tract dysfunctions, 169
   lower urinary tract reconstruction,
    168–70
   multiple artery anastomoses, 166–7
   nephrectomy and, 163–4
   neurogenic bladder, 169
   patient information, 451–2
   recipient preparation, 159–61
   renal artery anastomosis, 162, 162–3,
    165, 166
   renal vein–iliac vein anastomosis,
    164–5, 165
   right renal vein elongation,
    161–2, 162
   second warm ischaemia period, 162
   ureter-ureter anastomoses, 168–9
   vascular anastomoses, 164–7
   venous anastomoses, 164–6
   venous hypertension, 166
deceased donor retrieval, 91–107
declined kidney scheme, UK, 150
decoy cell shedding, 366
delayed graft function, 319
dense deposit disease (type II
   mesangioproliferative
   glomerulonephritis), **22**, 24
depression, 17
desflurane, 229
desmopressin acetate (1-deamino-8-$_D$-
   arginine vasopressin DDAVP), 83,
   391
diabetic autonomic neuropathy, 228
diabetes insipidus, 83
diabetes mellitus
   complications, 204
   diagnosis, 19
   islet beta cell failure, 203
   potential live kidney donors, 47–8
   type 1 see type 1 diabetes mellitus
   type 2 see type 2 diabetes mellitus
   WHO diagnostic criteria, **48**
diabetic peripheral neuropathy
   kidney–pancreas transplant benefits,
    231
   pain, 230–231
diagnostic imaging, post-transplant see
   post-transplant diagnostic
   imaging
diaphragm
   laparoscopic live donor
    nephrectomy, 239
   multiorgan heartbeating donation,
    92
dietary advice, 399, 408

digital subtraction angiography (DSA), 41

diltiazem, 398, **250**

dipstick test, 43–4, 423

dithiothreitol (DTT), 68

diuretics, 222

diverticulitis, post-transplant, 20

DNA-based HLA typing, 60–1

dobutamine stress echocardiography, 13

donor(s)
  crossmatching *see* pre-transplant donor crossmatch
  hepatitis B-positive, 369–70
  infections, 50
  malignancy, 50
  optimisation *see* donor optimisation
  pre-transplant infection screening, 337, **338**
  see also living donor kidney transplantation

donor after brainstem death (DBD), 159

donor after circulatory death (DCD), 102–5
  classification, **102**, 102–3
  controlled donors, 102, **102**, 103–5
  death diagnosis, 102, 451
  definition, 159
  Eurotransplant Kidney Allocation System, 157
  graft vascular injury, 104, *105*
  kidney allocation UK, 150
  no-touch period, 103
  organ preservation, 103–5, *105*
  organ procurement, 103–5, *105*
  pancreas procurement, 209
  uncontrolled donors, **102**, 103

donor-derived malignancy, 415

donor optimisation, 84, **86–8**, 89

donor organs
  histopathology, 319

donor-specific antibodies (DSA), 279–83
  HLA-I transplantation, 280, *283*, 388
  hyperacute rejection, 321

dopamine, 160

Doppler ultrasound
  post-transplant, 381
  pre-renal transplant dysfunction, 385

double-balloon triple-lumen (DBTL) catheter, 103

double filtration plasma exchange (DFPE)
  ABO-incompatible kidney transplantation, 275–6
  HLA-I transplantation, 281

double ureter, 169

doxycycline, 376

dried blood spots, immunosuppression, 245

drug eluting stents (DESs), 15

drug-induced allergic interstitial nephritis, 325

drug-induced toxic changes, 305, 327–8

dual kidney transplantation, 170–1

dual perfusion, 104

duodenoduodenostomy, 194–5

dysautonomia, 231

dyslipidaemia, 405–6

echinocandins, 349

echocardiography, 13

eculizumab
  antibody-mediated rejection, 265
  haemolytic uraemic syndrome, 389

Edmonton protocol, 5, 206

efavirenz, 373

elderly donors, 156

electrolytes, immediate postoperative period, 382

electron microscopy (EM), 319

en-bloc transplantation
  children, *289*, 290–291
  organ recovery, 290
  thrombi formation, 290–291

endarterectomy, 167

endoscopic live donor nephrectomy techniques, 111, 119
  intraperitoneal *vs.* extraperitoneal, 137
  open techniques *vs.*, 115–17, 136–7
  pure *vs.* hand-assisted, 129
  see also individual approaches/ techniques

endotracheal tube (ET), 237

end-stage renal disease (ESRD)
  children, 287
  elderly, 18
  malignancy development risk factors, 27–8
  pancreas transplantation, 207
  psychological aspects, 17

end-to-end vascular anastomosis, 1

entecavir, 369

enzyme-linked immunosorbent assay (ELISA)
  Clostridium difficile infection, 346
  HLA allosensitisation detection, 64

epidural anaesthesia, 228.

Epstein–Barr nuclear antigen (EBNA), 360–1

Epstein–Barr virus (EBV), 359–63
  donor screening, **338**
  post-transplant lymphoproliferative disorder, 330, 415

Epstein–Barr virus (EBV)-specific CTL clones, 363
equity, organ allocation, 146
erythrocytosis, post-transplant, 395
erythromycin
    interactions, **250**
    Legionella species infection, 347
erythropoiesis-stimulating agents, 394–5
erythropoietin deficiency, 428
Escherichia coli, 342
Escherichia coli 0157 toxin, 389
ethambutol, 347
ethics, 447–59
    appropriate use of resources, 458
    deceased donor transplantation, 449–52
    marginal deceased donors, 450
Eurotransplant countries, 141–5
Eurotransplant Kidney Allocation System (ETKAS), *153*, 152–7
    Acceptable Mismatch programme, 155
    blood group rules, 156, **156**
    donation after circulatory death, 156
    highly urgent patients, 154
Eurotransplant pancreas allocation system, 157–8
    blood group rules, 158
    highly immunised patients, combined kidney pancreas transplant, 157
    special urgency for vascularised pancreas transplantation, 157
Eurotransplant Senior Program (ESP), 156
Everolimus, 259–261
    interactions, **250**
    pharmacokinetic properties, **249**
    see also sirolimus
exercise ECG, 13
expanded criteria donors (ECDs), 159
explicit consent (opting-in system), 145
extended Kocher manoeuvre, 92
external iliac artery
    living donor kidney transplantation, 176, *176, 177*
    radiological anatomy, 298
external iliac vein
    deceased donor kidney transplantation, 164
    living donor kidney transplantation, 178, *178, 179*
extracorporeal membrane oxygenation (ECMO), 103
extracorporeal membrane oxygenation (ECMO)-assisted NHBD technique, 103

extravesical uretero-cystoneostomy, *165*, 168
ex-vivo organ perfusion systems, 78

femoral pulses, 12
fentanyl
    early post-transplant period, 394
    pancreatic transplantation, 229
    patient-controlled analgesia, 223
    renal transplantation, 221, **222**
fibrinogen, 276
finger-assisted (mini-open) approach live donor nephrectomy, 118
fingerprick sampling, immunosuppression monitoring, 245
flank incision live donor nephrectomy *see* lumbotomy approach live donor nephrectomy
flow cytometry, antibody screening, 64–5
flow cytometry crossmatch (FC-XM), 67, 71, 280
fluconazole, 343, 349
flucytosine, 351
fluids, postoperative, 190, 382, 383
fluoroquinolones, 347–8
5-fluorouracil, 417
focal and segmental glomerulosclerosis (FSGS), 23
    recurrence, **22**, 23–4, 388–9, 425
Foscarnet, 356, 364–5
fractionator, 276
fracture risk, post-transplantation, 419–20, **419**
fresh frozen plasma, 276
functional residual capacity, laparoscopic live donor nephrectomy, 239
fungal infections, 348–53
furosemide, 290

gallbladder stones, 20
gamma cells, 203
ganciclovir, 198, 355–6, 363–5, 374
gastric neuropathy, 231
gastroduodenal artery, 97
gastro-oesophageal reflux, 228
gastroparesis, 220, 228, 231
general anaesthesia, 220
geographical equity, organ allocation, 146
glomerular filtration rate (GFR), 39–40
    potential live kidney donors, 39–40
    standard MDRD equations, 423
glomerulonephritis, recurrence, 20–21
glucose, postoperative period, 382
glucose tolerance, 406–7

GlycoSorb ABO columns, 271–2, *272*
golden triangle, 161
gout, 396, 428
graft pancreatitis, 199–200
graft torsion, 309
grapefruit juice, **250,** 251
greater omentum, multiorgan
    heartbeating donation, 94
grey-scale ultrasound, 299
gum hypertrophy, ciclosporin-induced,
    252

haemoglobin, 160, 220, 230, 382
haematological cancers, **29**
haematological disorders, brainstem-
    dead donors, 83–4
haematoma, 304, 309
haematopoietic stem cell
    transplantation, 62
haematuria, 44
haemodynamic instability, brainstem
    death, 80
haemolytic uraemic syndrome (HUS)
    atypical, **22,** 25–6
    de novo (post-transplant
        microangiopathy), 389
    genetic mutations, 25–6
    recurrence, **22,** 25–6, 389, 425
haemorrhage
    computerised tomography, 309
    post-biopsy, 311–12
    ultrasound, 306
haemorrhagic cystitis, 201
hand-assisted laparoscopic
        extraperitoneal live donor
        nephrectomy, *111–4,* 122–6, 139
hand-assisted laparoscopic live donor
        nephrectomy, 121–2
hand-assisted laparoscopic
        retroperitoneoscopic live donor
        nephrectomy *see* hand-assisted
        laparoscopic extraperitoneal live
        donor nephrectomy
heartbeating brain-dead multiorgan
        donor, 77–90, **85–8**
    multiorgan *see* heartbeating
        multiorgan donation
heartbeating multiorgan donation,
        92–102
heart failure, 404
Henoch-Schönlein nephritis, 23, 426
heparin
    ABO-incompatible kidney
        transplantation, 275
    deceased donor kidney
        transplantation, 160
    multiorgan heartbeating donation,
        95

pancreatic transplantation, 232
    thromboprophylaxis, 394
hepatic portal system, 211
hepatitis B virus , 367–70
hepatitis B vaccine, **340**
    donor screening, **338**
    HIV co-infection, 373
    post-transplant recurrence, 368
    potential renal transplant recipient,
        20
hepatitis C virus (HCV), 370–1
    donor screening, 337, **338**
    HIV co-infection, 373
hepatitis e antigen (HBeAg), 368
hereditary systemic amyloidosis, 27
herpes simplex virus (HSV) infection,
        356–7
herpes zoster (shingles), 357–8
herpes zoster ophthalmicus, 358
high-density lipoprotein cholesterol
        (HDL-C), 406, 408
highly sensitised patients (HSPs), organ
        allocation, 149
highly urgent (HU) patients, 154
hip fractures, 419–20
histidine–tryptophan–ketoglutarate
        (HTK) solution, 209
histocompatibility, 55–75
histopathology *see* transplant
        histopathology
histoplasmosis, 353
HIV, 371–3
    CD4+T-cell count, 372
    donor disclosure, 453–4
    donor screening, 337, **338**
    immunosuppression, 266
    opportunistic infection prophylaxis,
        373
    pancreas transplantation, 193
    recipients, ethical issues, 454
    rejection rates, 372
    vaccination, 373
HIV-associated nephropathy (HIVAN),
        371
HLA alloantigens, sensitisation to, 63
HLA allosensitisation detection, 63–5
    cell-based assays, 63–4
    clinical applications, 65–71
    solid-phase assays, 64–5
HLA-I transplantation, 279–83, **281–2,
        283**
    crossmatching, 280, 281
    donor-specific antibodies, 280, *283,*
        388
    IVIg protocols, 279–80
    pretransplant immunoadsorption
        (protein A), 280
    sensitisation event, 280

HLA matching, 62–3, 147
HLA mismatch, children, 288
HLA polymorphism, 56–60
HLA-specific antibody screening
    post-kidney transplantation, 71–3
    pretransplant, 65–6
    repeat transplant, 66
HLA system, 55–60
    antigenic protein epitopes, 66
    phenotype prevalence, 57, **58–9**
HLA typing
    DNA-based, 60–1
    kidney transplantation, 61–2
    methodology, 60–1
    mismatch grade, 61–2
    pancreas transplantation, 61–2
    paternity findings, ethical issues, 455
    serological, 60
HMG-CoA reductase inhibitors
    (statins), 410
Homocysteine, 406, 412
horseshoe kidney transplantation,
    171–2
human anti-chimeric antibody
    (HACA) response, 246
human herpesvirus 6 (HHV-6)
    infection, 363–4
human herpesvirus 7 (HHV-7)
    infection, 363–4
human herpesvirus 8 (HHV-8)
    infection, 364–5
human immunodeficiency virus (HIV)
    see HIV
human papilloma virus (HPV), **341**,
    414
Human Tissue Act, 453–5
human T-lymphotrophic virus
    (HTLV), **338**
hydronephrosis, 386
hyperacute rejection (HR), 69,
    321, 385
    donor-specific antibodies, 321
    light microscopic findings, 321
hypercoagulability screening, 193
hyperkalaemia, 253, 382
hyperlipidaemia, sirolimus-induced,
    260
hypernatraemia, brainstem-dead
    donors, 85
hypernephroma (renal cell carcinoma),
    417
hyperoxaluria, primary, 426
hyperparathyroidism, 395–6, 420
hypertension
    ciclosporin-induced, 252
    live kidney donation
        contraindication, 46–7
    living donor follow-up, 440

paediatric kidney transplantation,
    294
post-transplant, 397–8, 405
hypogastric artery, 166
hypoglycaemic agents, 397
hypoperfusion, brainstem-dead donors,
    82
hypophosphataemia, 253, 396, 430
hypotension, brainstem-dead donors,
    85
hypothalamic failure, 82–3
hypothalamo-pituitary axis failure, 83
hypothermia, brainstem death, 82–3
hypovolaemia, brainstem-dead donors,
    83, 85

idiopathic membranous nephropathy,
    426
ileal conduit, 170, 186–7
iliac vessel angiogram, 192–3
imidazole antifungals, **250**
imiquimod, 417
ImmuKnow assay, 245
immunisation, transplant recipients,
    339, **340–1**
immunoadsorption (IA), 275, *277*
    ABO-incompatible kidney
        transplantation, 271–2, *272*
    post-transplantation, 277
    rituximab and, 272–3
immunogenetics, 55–75
immunoglobulin A nephropathy
    (IgAN), 21–3, **22**, 426
immunohistochemistry (IH)
    microscopy, 319
immunological risk assessment, 68–71,
    72
immunosuppression, 243–70
    acute rejection treatment, 265–6
    antibody induction, 245–6
    antiretroviral interactions, 266, 372
    breastfeeding, 266
    children, 291–2
    compliance/adherence, 265–6, 427
    complications, 243
    co-stimulatory blockade, 261–2
    drug interactions, **250,** 264
    generic preparations, 264–5
    lytic induction, 246
    monitoring, 243–5
    pancreas transplantation, 197–8, 229
    pancreatic islet transplantation,
        212–14
    pharmacodynamic monitoring, 245
    pregnancy, 266, 429
    small-molecule drugs, 248, **249, 250**
    steroid minimisation, 262
    targets, **244**

immunosuppression (*cont'd*)
   therapeutic drug monitoring, 243–5
   see also individual drugs
impaired fasting glucose (IFG), 47–8,
   48
impaired glucose tolerance (IGT),
   47–8, **48**
implantation biopsy, 319
incisional hernia, 431
infection, 335–79
   diagnosis, 335
   donor screening, 337, **338**
   histopathology, 328–30
   paediatric kidney transplantation,
      293–4
   pre-transplant screening, 337–9
   see also individual infections
infectious mononucleosis, 360
infective endocarditis, 345
inferior epigastric artery, 165, 167,
      175–6
inferior mesenteric artery, heartbeating
      donation, 93
inferior mesenteric vein, organ
      procurement, 96
inferior vena cava
   deceased donor kidney
      transplantation, 165–6
   kidney retrieval en-bloc, 98
   multiorgan heartbeating donation,
      92, 93, 95
   non-heartbeating donation, 102
influenza, 373–5
Influenza vaccine, **340**
informed consent
   high-risk deceased donors, 337
   potential live kidney donors, 34
infrarenal abdominal aorta, 93
inherited kidney disease, 45
instant blood-mediated inflammatory
      reaction (IBMIR), 206
insulin-dependent diabetes mellitus
      (IDDM) *see* type 1 diabetes
      mellitus
insulin replacement, 203
interferon, 20, 371
internal iliac artery
   living donor kidney transplantation,
      179–80
   paediatric renal transplantation, 289
International Pancreas Transplant
      Registry, 191
interstitial fibrosis and tubular atrophy
      (IF/TA), 327, 425
intestinal segments, bladder
      augmentation, 169–70
intra-abdominal infections, 344
   pancreas transplantation, 198

intracranial pressure (ICP), 79–80
intrauterine devices (IUD), 399
intravenous urogram (IVU), 41
intravesical ureteroneocystostomy, 168
inulin clearance, 39
invisible haematuria, 424
ischaemia-reperfusion injury, 319, *320*
ischaemic reperfusion pancreatitis, 200
islet burn-out, 213
islet cell transplant *see* pancreatic islet
      transplantation
islet of Langerhans, 203
   cryopreservation, 211
isoflurane, 221
isoniazid, 347, 348
Israel Penn International Tumour
      Transplant Registry, 28

JC virus, 366–7
JJ ureteric stent, 387

Kaposi's sarcoma (KS), 260, 364–5, 414
kidney
   abnormalities, potential live kidney
      donors, 42–3
kidney allocation *see* organ allocation
kidney-only retrieval, 98–9
   back-table preparation, 99, *100*, *101*
kidney retrieval en-bloc, 98–100
   non-heartbeating donation,
      104–5
kidney stones *see* nephrolithiasis
kidney transplantation *see* renal
      transplantation
kinase inhibitors, 262

Lamivudine, 20, 368–9
laparoscopic live donor nephrectomy,
      239–40
laparoscopic transperitoneal live donor
      nephrectomy, 119–20
laparotomy, heartbeating donation, 92
laudanosine, 221
left ventricular hypertrophy (LVH),
      12–14, 405
left ventricular systolic dysfunction
      (LVSD), 14
Legionella pneumophila infection,
      346–7
lesser omentum, multiorgan
      heartbeating donation, 93
leukaemia, **29**
lidocaine, 392
lifestyle advice, 399, 408
linezolid, 346
liquid chromatography-based assays,
      244
Listeria monocytogenes, 345

lithium, 17
live donor(s), potential
    age, 45–6
    co-morbidity, 45–8
    confidentiality, 34
    diabetes mellitus, 47–8
    family history, 49
    follow-up *see* living donor
        follow-up
    hypertension, 46–7
    infection screening, 50, 51, 337
    information, 34–5
    informed consent, 34
    medical evaluation, 36–53
    obesity, 46
    peri-operative risks assessment,
        48–9
    renal abnormalities, 42–3
    renal anatomy assessment, 37–43,
        235
    renal function assessment, 37–43
    screening investigations, 36, 38
    smoking, 46
    thromboembolic risks, 38, 49
    transmission risk factors, 50
live donor nephrectomy, 109–40
    anaesthesia *see* live donor
        nephrectomy anaesthesia
    approaches, comparison of, 128–39
    complications, 138–9, 237
    consent, 237
    donation contraindications, 236
    donation psychology, 237
    draping, 111, *114*
    early complications, 138
    endoscopic *see* endoscopic live donor
        nephrectomy techniques
    incision, *111, 112*
    kidney graft cold perfusion, 138
    laparoscopic, 236
    morbidity, 138
    mortality, 138
    open techniques *see* open live donor
        nephrectomy techniques
    operative field preparation, 110
    patient information, 110
    patient positioning, 111, *112, 113,*
        114, 238
    pre-operative preparation, 110–111
    renal vessel handling, 137
    renal vessel length, 137
    risks, 138–9
    shaving, 111
    skin markings, 110–111, *112*
    surgical technique, 236
    ureter handling, 137
    urinary catheter, 111
    warming mats, *114*

warm ischaemic time, 138
    see also individual approaches/
        techniques
live donor nephrectomy anaesthesia,
    235–41, **240**
liver, en-bloc procurement, 95–6, *96*
liver biopsy, 370–371
liver-pancreas en-bloc procurement,
    95–6
    back-table division, 97
    non-heartbeating donation,
        104, *105*
liver puncture, 215
living donor follow-up, 437–45
living donor islet transplant, 21
living donor kidney transplantation,
    173–90
    arterial anastomosis, 179–83
    arteriotomy, 180, *180, 181*
    bench-table kidney graft
        preparation, 173, *174*
    biopsy, 189
    blood vessel dissection, 174–7, *176,*
        177
    children, 288
    coercion, 456
    donor counselling, 453–5
    donor-recipient information sharing,
        453–4
    drainage, 189
    ethics, 453–6
    four-corner technique venous
        anastomosis, 178, *179*
    ileal conduit, 186–7
    iliac vessel dissection, 175, *176*
    incidental findings, 455
    incision, 174–7, *176*
    internal iliac artery end-to-end
        anastomosis, 179–80
    kidney graft perfusion, 173, *174*
    lymphatics, 176, *177*
    multiple artery bench
        reconstruction, pros/cons, 181
    multiple artery *in-vivo*
        reconstruction, 181–3, *182, 183*
    postoperative care, 189–90
    recipient infection screening, 51
    renal vessel assessment, 173, *175*
    reperfusion, 183
    revascularisation, 177–83
    spermatic cord, 175
    two-corner technique venous
        anastomosis, 178, *179*
    ureteric anastomosis, 183–8
    ureteric complication prevention,
        188, *188*
    uretero-cysto anastomosis, antireflux
        mucosal tunnel, 184–5

living donor kidney transplantation
    (cont'd)
  uretero-cysto anastomosis, simple,
    one layer, 183–4, *184, 185, 186,
    187, 188*
  uretero-uretero anastomosis, 185–6
  ureter to skin anastomosis, 187–8
  vascular slings, 176, 177, *177, 178*
  venous anastomosis, 177–8, *178, 179,
    180*
  wound closure, 189, *189*
Living Donor Registry, 442
loin incision live donor nephrectomy
    see lumbotomy approach live
    donor nephrectomy
long-term complications management,
    403–36
  screening investigations, 423–4
losartan, 428
low-density lipoprotein cholesterol
    (LDL-C), 406, 409–11
lower urinary tract dysfunction, 169
lower urinary tract obstruction, 387
lumbar arteries, 93
lumbotomy approach live donor
    nephrectomy, 115–17, *133*
Luminex
  HLA allosensitisation detection, 65
  HLA-I transplantation, 280
  median fluorescence intensity, 65
lung cancer, **28**
lupus nephritis recurrence, **22,** 25, 426
lymphocele, 164, 386, 393
  ultrasound, 304–5
lymphocytotoxicity *see* complement-
    dependent cytotoxicity (CDC)
lymphoma, **29**
lytic induction, 246

Maastricht classification, **102**
machine perfusion, 99
magnesium, 382
magnetic resonance angiography
    (MRA)
  post-transplant diagnostic imaging,
    309–10
  potential live kidney donors, 41–2
magnetic resonance imaging (MRI),
    309–10, 351
major histocompatibility complex *see*
    HLA system
malaria, 376
malignancy, transplant recipients,
    413–18, **418**
mammalian target of rapamycin
    (mTOR) inhibitors, 259–61
  blood concentration measurement,
    244

Kaposi's sarcoma, 414
  malignancy incidence reduction, 260
  see also individual drugs
mannitol
  paediatric renal transplantation, 290
  pancreatic transplantation, 230
marginal deceased donors, ethics, 450
marginal living donors, 440–442
Masson's technique, 171
MDRD study formula, 39
melanoma, **29**
membrane co-factor protein (MCP)
    mutations, 389
membranoproliferative
    glomerulonephritis (MPGN),
    recurrent, 24
membranous nephropathy (MN),
    recurrent idiopathic, 24–5
Mental Capacity Act, 456
6-mercaptopurine, 255
mesangiocapillary glomerulonephritis
    (MCGN), **22,** 426
mesangioproliferative
    glomerulonephritis (MPGN), **22,**
    24, 426
metabolic disorders, brainstem-dead
    donors, 83–4
metal stents, 313, *313*
metformin, 397, 411
methylprednisolone
  ABO-incompatible kidney
    transplantation, 275
  acute cellular rejection, 265
  brainstem-dead donors, 88
metronidazole, 346
microalbuminuria, 43
midazolam, 221, **222**
mineral bone disorder, 412
mini-open (finger-assisted) live donor
    nephrectomy, 118
minors, as live kidney donors, 45–6
mismatch probability (MMP), 153
Mitrofanoff procedure with flap-valve
    mechanism, 170
Model for End-stage Liver Disease
    (MELD) score, 155
morphine, 394
mouth ulcers, sirolimus-induced, 260
MRI *see* magnetic resonance imaging
    (MRI)
mTOR inhibitors *see* mammalian
    target of rapamycin (mTOR)
    inhibitors
multidisciplinary team, 458–9
multiple myeloma, 27
muromonab-CD3, 245, 247
mycobacterial infection, 347–8
Mycobacterium tuberculosis, 347

mycophenolate, 197–8, 213, 256–9, 264, 272, 291
  HIV, 372
  interactions, 257
  optimal dose, 257
  pharmacokinetics, **249**, *256*, 256–7
  teratogenicity, 266, 429
mycophenolate mofetil (MMF), see mycophenolate
mycophenolate sodium (MPS), see mycophenolate
mycophenolic acid (MPA), 256, 257
  AUC algorithms, 258
  elimination, 398
  gastrointestinal toxicity, 258–9
  myelosuppression, 258
  therapeutic drug monitoring, 257–8
  toxicities, 258–9

nasogastric tubes, 229
National Kidney Allocation Scheme (NKAS), 146–50
National Organ Retrieval Service, 142, 143
National Pancreas Allocation Scheme, 151–2
natural orifice transluminal endoscopic surgery (NOTES) live donor nephrectomy, 128
necrotic tissues, 344
nephrectomy
  live donor *see* live donor nephrectomy
  post-biopsy bleeding, 393
nephrolithiasis, 44–5
nephrostomy, 312–13
nephrotic syndrome, 388
neuraminidase inhibitors, 374
neurogenic bladder, 169
neurogenic hypotension, brainstem death, *81*, 82
neurogenic pulmonary oedema, brainstem death, 82
new-onset diabetes after transplantation (NODAT), 251, 253, 262, 396–7, 406–7
nifedipine, 398
nocardiosis, 345–6
non-heartbeating donor (NHBD) see donor after circulatory death (DCD) ,
non-melanoma skin cancer (NMSC), 414, 416–17
non-obstructive dilatation, 303–4
non-steroidal anti-inflammatory drugs (NSAIDS), 238, 394
non-tuberculous mycobacterial (NTM) infection, 347

nosocomial colonisation, 339
nuclear medicine (NM), 307, *308*
nucleos(t)ide analogue, 369
nystatin, 198, 349

obesity
  potential live kidney donors, 46
  potential renal transplant recipient, 18–19
  transplant outcomes, 408
oestrogen-only combined oral contraceptives, 399
OKT3 *see* muromonab-CD3
ondansetron, 223
open live donor nephrectomy techniques, 111, 115–18, 236
  see also individual techniques
opiates, 238
opting-in system (explicit consent), 145
opting-out system (presumed consent), 145
oral glucose tolerance test, 48
organ allocation, 141–58
  deceased donor, HLA mismatches, 67
  ethics, 449–50
organ retrieval, 143
organ sharing, 141–58
oseltamivir, 374
outpatient follow-up, 384
oxalosis, primary, **22**, 26
oxaluria, secondary, 26
oxfloxacin, 348

p53 tumour suppressor gene inhibition, 415
paediatric renal transplantation, 287–96
  appendix removal, 290
  arterial anastomosis, 289, *289*
  bladder, 288
  catch-up growth, 292
  contraindications, 287–8
  corticosteroids, 292
  en-bloc transplantation, 171, *289*, 290–1
  end-to-end anastomosis, 289, *289*, 290
  growth and, 288, 292
  growth hormone use, 292–3
  immunosuppressive treatment, 291–2
  incision, 289
  infection, 293–4
  malignancy, 293
  morbidity, 292–4
  patient survival, 287
  pre-emptive transplantation, 288

paediatric renal transplantation
(cont'd)
  pre-transplant bilateral nephrectomy,
    287
  pre-transplant recipient preparation,
    288
  recipient age and, 288
  retroperitoneal approach, 289, *289*
  steroid withdrawal, 291
  surgical technique, 288–91
  temperature control, 288–9
  therapeutic regimen non-
    compliance, 294
  transperitoneal approach, *289,*
    289–90
  transplant survival, 287
  ureter re-implantation, 290
  vaccinations, 288, 294
Page phenomenon, 312
pamidronate, 421
pancreas
  Banff classification *see* Banff
    pancreas classification scheme
  biopsy handling, 331
  en-bloc procurement, 95–6, *96*
  histopathology, 331–3
pancreas after kidney transplantation,
  191
  indications, 193–4
pancreas allocation
  pancreatic islet transplantation,
    208–9
  priority, 208
pancreas graft thrombosis, 200–201
pancreas retrieval, en bloc excision, 209
pancreas transplantation, 191–202
  anaesthesia *see* pancreatic
    transplantation anaesthesia
  anastomotic leakage, 201
  antibiotic prophylaxis, 198
  anticoagulation, 198–9
  arterial anastomosis, 194, 196
  bladder drainage, 194, 201
  bladder-drained graft leaks, 201
  complications, 204
  diagnostics, 191–4
  duodenum shortening, 195–6
  enteric anastomosis, 194
  enteric-drained graft leaks, 201
  exocrine anastomosis, 197
  exocrine drainage, 194
  graft monitoring, 232–3
  graft placement, 194
  graft preparation, 195–6
  graft survival, 191, 197
  HLA typing, 61–2
  immunosuppression, 197–8
  incision, 196

  indications, 191–4
  intra-abdominal infections, 198
  intraoperative medication, 197–9
  islet cells *see* pancreatic islet
    transplantation
  pancreatic islet transplantation *vs.,*
    205
  peri-operative morbidity/mortality,
    227
  portal venous anastomosis, 194
  portal-venous and enteric drainage,
    195
  postoperative complications,
    199–201
  postoperative treatment, 199
  pre-transplant assessment, **192,**
    192–3
  recipient preparation, 196
  reperfusion, 196–7
  surgery therapy, 194–5
  surgical access, 196
  surgical preparation, 195–6
  surgical technique, 196–7
  systemic-venous and bladder
    drainage, 195
  systemic-venous and enteric
    drainage, 194–5
  thrombotic disorder screening, 193
pancreas transplantation after living
  donor kidney transplantation
  (PALK), 191
pancreatic abscess, 199
pancreatic islet transplantation, 203–18
  autotransplantation, 215–16
  central isolation laboratory, 211
  clinical outcomes, 214–15
  complications, 215
  C-peptide production, 214
  cryopreservation, 211
  donors, 208
  early graft loss, 205
  exclusion criteria, 208
  immunological rejection, 205
  immunosuppression, 212–14
  immunosuppression-related
    complications, 215
  indications, 207–8
  insulin independence rate, 214
  islet culture, 210–11
  islet graft imaging, 213
  islet infusion, 211
  islet isolation, 209–10, *210*
  islet mass, 211
  islet quality assessment, 210–211
  mini-laparotomy with infusion
    catheter introduction, 212
  pancreas allocation, 208–9
  pancreas procurement, 208–9

pancreas transplantation *vs.,* **205**
post-transplant islet function
  assessment, 213
post-transplant management,
  212–14
recipient selection, 207–8
rejection diagnosis, 213
repeat, 212
stem cells, 216
transplant procedure, 211–12, *212*
pancreatic pseudocyst, 199
pancreatic transplantation *see* pancreas
  transplantation
pancreatic transplantation anaesthesia,
  227–33
  cardiovascular status assessment, 227
  combined epidural–general
    anaesthesia, 228–9
  difficult intubation, 228
  fluid management, 230
  intensive care management, 232–3
  monitoring, 229–30, 232
  pain management, 230–231
  peri-operative anaesthesia planning,
    228–30
  pre-medication, 227–8
  regional anaesthesia, 228.
  see also individual drugs
pancuronium, 229
paracetamol, 223, 238, 394, 396
parachuting technique, 180
parainfluenza, 373–5
partial occluding clamps, 289
partial portal thrombosis, 215
patient-controlled analgesia (PCA), 223
patient expertise, 449
patient information, live kidney
  donors, 34
patient self-operated parenteral system,
  analgesia, 394
pauci-immune glomerulonephritis, 25
PCR typing using sequence-specific
  oligonucleotide probes (PCR-
  SSOP), 61
PCR typing using sequence-specific
  primers (PCR-SSP), 60–1
PCR with sequence-based typing
  (PCR-SBT), 61
peak systolic velocity (PSV), 299
penicillin, 343
pentamidine, 352
peptic ulceration, 19–20
percutaneous balloon dilatation, 313
percutaneous coronary intervention
  (PCI), 15
percutaneous nephrostomy, 386
perfluorocarbon, 209
perinephric abscess, 304

perinephric collections, 304–5, *305*
peripheral nerve stimulator, 221
peripheral vascular disease, potential
  recipients, 12, 16–17
peritoneal cooling, 103
peritoneal dialysis catheters, 399
peritonitis, 199
phenytoin, **250**
phosphate, 382
phosphate binders, 396, 412
physiotherapy, post-transplant, 384
plasma exchange
  ABO-incompatible kidney
    transplantation, 276–7
  antibody-mediated rejection, 265
  HLA-I transplantation, 281
plasmapheresis
  focal and segmental
    glomerulosclerosis, 24
  haemolytic uraemic syndrome, 389
*Pneumocystis jiroveci (Pneumocystis
  carinii) pneumonia,* 351–3
pneumonia, 344–5
pneumoperitoneum, 239
pneumovax vaccine, **340**
polyclonal immunoglobulin
  preparations, 245
polyomavirus hominis 1 (BK) *see* BK
  virus
polyomavirus hominis 2 (JC) *see* JC
  virus
polyomavirus infection, 366–7
polyomavirus nephropathy (PVN)
  diagnosis, 366–7
  differential diagnosis, 330
  histopathology, 329, *329, 330*
  immunosuppression reduction, 367
  kidney biopsy, 367
  prevention, 366–7
  retransplantation, 367
  risk factors, 366
  treatment, 366–7
polypharmacy, 398, 427
polyuria, 383
portal vein, 196
positron emission tomography–
  computerised tomography
  (PET-CT), PTLD, 213,
  361, 416
post-biopsy haemorrhage, 311–12
post-operative nausea and vomiting
  (PONV), 223
postreperfusion graft pancreatitis, 200
post-transplant bone disease, 418–22
post transplant imaging: transplant
  complications, **298**
  see also individual imaging techniques
post-transplant erythrocytosis, 395

post-transplant lymphoproliferative
disorder (PTLD), 359–63
belatacept, 262
children, 293
diagnosis, 293, 360–1
differential diagnosis, 331
Epstein–Barr virus, 330, 415
histopathology, 330–1, 361, **362**
immunosuppression reduction/
cessation, 361–2, 416
immunotherapy, 363
management, 415–16
peak periods of incidence, 416
pre-emptive strategies, 363
presentation, 359–60, 415–16
prevention, 363
recurrence-free waiting time, **29**
staging, 360–1
surgery, 362
post-transplant management
contraceptive advice, 399
dialysis access, 399–400
dietary advice, 399
early events timeline, **385**
early recurrent disease, 388–93
early surgical complications, 393
first three months, 381–401
immediate postoperative period
monitoring, 381–2, **382**
immediate post-transplant
monitoring algorithm, 382–3
lifestyle advice, 399
outpatient follow-up, 384
prescribing, 398–9
post-transplant microangiopathy (*de
novo* haemolytic uraemic
syndrome), 389
potassium-free solutions, 222
potential renal transplant recipient *see*
renal transplant recipient (RTR),
potential
povidone iodine, 96
pp65 antigenaemia assay, 354
pravastatin, 410
prednisolone, 261
gout, 396
pharmacokinetic properties, **249**
withdrawal, 429
pre-emptive transplantation, children,
288
pregnancy, 428–9
immunosuppression, 266, 429
living donor follow-up, 441
urinary tract infection, 429
prescribing, post-transplant, 398–9
presumed consent (opting-out), 143–5
pre-transplant donor crossmatch,
66–70

pre-transplant plasmapheresis (PP),
271–3
primary effusion lymphoma, 365
primary hyperoxaluria, 426
primary non-function, 319
probiotics, 346
progesterone-only contraceptives, 399
propofol
live donor nephrectomy anaesthesia,
237
pancreatic transplantation
anaesthesia, 229
renal transplantation anaesthesia,
222
prostate cancer, **29, 418**
protease inhibitors, 372–3
proteinuria
assessment techniques, 43
focal and segmental
glomerulosclerosis, 23
glomerular disease screening test,
423–4
living donor follow-up, 439
potential live kidney donors, 43
pre-transplant measurement, 424
reduction, 427
protocol biopsy, 390, 422
pseudoaneurysm (PSA)
catheter angiography, 312
ultrasound, 306
psychological defence mechanisms, 17
psychosis, 17
pulmonary artery, multiorgan
heartbeating donation, 95
pulmonary embolism, 49
purines, 428
pyelography, catheter angiography,
312–13
pyelonephritis, acute, 343
pyelo-pyelo anastomoses, 168–9
pyelo-ureter anastomoses, 168–9
pyrazinamide, 347
pyridoxine therapy
mycobacterial infection, 348
primary oxalosis, 26
pyuria, 43–4, 342

rabbit anti-human thymocyte
immunoglobulin
(Thymoglobuline), 247
radial fistulae, 400
Ramsay Hunt syndrome, 358
rapamycin *see* sirolimus
rapid antigen testing, respiratory
viruses, 374
rapid sequence intubation (RSI)
technique, 220
recurrent glomerular disease, 425–6

renal anatomy assessment
  imaging techniques, 41–2
  potential live kidney donors,
    37–43
renal artery anastomosis
  deceased donor kidney
    transplantation, *165,* 166
  paediatric renal transplantation, 289
  triangulation technique, *165,* 166
renal artery stenosis (RAS)
  catheter angiography, 312
  stenting *vs.* angioplasty, 312
  ultrasound, 301, *302*
renal artery thrombosis
  surgical correction, 311
  ultrasound, 301
renal biopsy *see* renal transplant biopsy
renal cancer, **28,** 417, **418**
renal dilatation, 303
renal disease, post-transplant
  recurrence, 20–7, **22**
renal function
  age-related decline, 40
  decline, strategies to slow, 426–8
  potential live kidney donors,
    37–43
  split function measurement, 40
renal transplantation
  anaesthesia *see* renal transplantation
    anaesthesia
  antibody-incompatible, 271–85
  children *see* paediatric renal
    transplantation
  contraindications, 11
  deceased donor *see* deceased donor
    kidney transplantation
  dialysis prior to, 219
  early complication, **298**
  early graft loss, 9–10
  elderly, 18
  ethics *see* ethics
  HLA typing, 61–2
  late complications, **298**
  late surgical complications, 431
  living donor *see* living donor kidney
    transplantation
  outcomes, HLA matching and,
    62–3
  patient positioning, 220
  postoperative complication
    frequency, **298**
  potential recipients *see* renal
    transplant recipient (RTR),
    potential
  pre-emptive, 10
  psychological aspects, 17
  radiological anatomy, 297–9
  resources rationing, 143–5

renal transplantation anaesthesia,
  219–25
  aspiration risk, 220
  cannulation, 220
  checklist, **223–5**
  drug doses, **222**
  immunosuppresant administration,
    222
  induction, 221
  lines, 220–1
  maintenance, 221–2
  monitoring, 220–1
  normothermia maintenance, 222
  pain treatment, 223
  peri-operative fluid management,
    222
  post-anaesthesia care, 223, **225**
  post-operative fluid therapy, 223
  pre-assessment, 219–20
  pre-operative management, 220
  see also individual drugs
renal transplant biopsy, 390–3
  early graft dysfunction, 424
  handling, 318–19
  post-biopsy bleeding, 393
  potential live kidney donors, 44
  staining, 318–19
renal transplant dysfunction *see*
  transplant dysfunction
renal transplant failure, 422–32
renal transplant recipient (RTR),
  potential
  assessment, 9–31
  cardiovascular assessment *see*
    cardiovascular assessment,
    potential recipients
  co-morbid disease, 9
  infection screening, 337–9
  lifestyle, 18–19
  malignant disease-free waiting
    period, 27–8, **28–9**
  obesity, 18–19
  peri-operative mortality, 9
  pre-operative serological testing,
    339
  previous infections, 11, 338
  previous malignancy, 11,
    27–8
  psychological assessment, 17
  recurrent renal disease,
    20–27
  smoking, 19
  underlying renal disease cause, 11
  viral hepatitis, 20
  waiting list management, 30
renal tumour, incidental, live donors,
  42–3
renal vein, kidney retrieval, 99, *100*

renal vein–iliac vein anastomosis
  deceased donor kidney
    transplantation, 164–5, *165*
  triangulation technique, 164–5
renal vein thrombosis
  CT angiography, 309
  ultrasound, 301
rescue allocation, 156–7
respiratory disease, potential recipients,
    19, 219
respiratory syncytial virus, 373–5
respiratory viruses, 373–5
retinoids, 417
ribavirin, 20, 371, 374
rifampicin, 347–8
rimantadine, 374
Ringer's solution, 222
ritonavir, 266
rituximab, 248
  ABO-incompatible kidney
    transplantation, 271, 272–3
  antibody-mediated rejection, 265
  dosing regimen, 248
  HLA-I transplantation, 279, 280
  immunoadsorption and, 272–3
  post-transplant lymphoproliferative
    disease, 362, 363
  pretransplant plasmapheresis and,
    273
robotic-assisted laparoscopic live donor
    nephrectomy, 135–6
rocuronium, 229
ropivacaine, 228–9, 231

salt intake, 408
Schwann cell abnormalities, 231
secondary amyloidosis, 27
serological HLA typing, 60
seromuscular colocystoplasty, 170
serum sickness, 247
sevoflurane, 221, 229
shared decision-making, 449, 457
shingles (herpes zoster), 357, 358
Simulect *see* basiliximab
simultaneous pancreas-kidney (SPK)
    transplantation, 191–3
  organ allocation, 151
sirolimus, 259
  cancer incidence reduction, 414
  diabetogenicity, 260
  haematological toxicity, 260
  interactions, **250**
  Kaposi's sarcoma, 365
  pancreas transplantation,
    197–8
  pancreatic islet transplantation, 213
  pharmacokinetic properties, **249**
  post-transplant dyslipidaemia, 406

teratogenicity, 266, 429
  therapeutic range, 260–1
sirolimus pneumonitis, 260
skin cancer
  post-transplantation surveillance,
    418
  recurrence-free waiting time, **29**
smoking
  excess graft loss, 19
  malignancy, transplant recipients,
    415
  potential live kidney donors, 46
  potential renal transplant recipient,
    19
smoking cessation, 399, 408
'smudge cells,' 374
Sotrastaurin, 262
specialist nurses in organ donation
    (SN-ODs), 143
spinal anaesthesia, pancreatic
    transplantation, 228.
spleen, 97
splenectomy, 271
spot urine samples, 424
squamous cell carcinoma (SCC), **29,**
    416
Staphylococcus aureus, 345
statins (HMG-CoA reductase
    inhibitors), 410
stem cells, 216
sternotomy, heartbeating donation, 92
steroid minimisation strategies,
    children, 291
steroids
  acute cellular (T-lymphocyte-
    mediated) rejection, 265
  interactions, **250,** 264
  late withdrawal, 262
  minimisation, 262
  new-onset diabetes after
    transplantation (NODAT), 262
  pancreas transplantation, 198
  withdrawal, children, 291
  see also corticosteroids; *individual
    drugs*
stomach, bladder augmentation, 170
stress-induced cardiomyopathy
    (brainstem-dead donors), 81, 87
stress radionuclide myocardial
    perfusion images, 13
stripe-fibrosis, 425
stroke, 409
structural heart disease, 404
subclinical rejection, 390
substance abuse, 17
succinylcholine, 229
sudden cardiac death (SCD), 404
sufentanil, 228–9

sulfamethoxazole (SMX), 198
sufentanil, 231
sulfinpyrazone, 428
superior mesenteric artery-patch, 96, 96
suprarenal abdominal aorta, 93–4
Swan–Ganz catheter, 230
syphilis, **338**
systemic lupus erythematosus, 25
systemic primary amyloidosis, 27

tacrolimus, 252–4
    cosmetic effects, 253
    ethnic differences, 254
    HIV-infected patients, 266
    immunoassay, 254
    interactions, **250**, 264
    neurotoxicity, 253
    new-onset diabetes after
        transplantation (NODAT), 397
    pancreas transplantation, 197–8
    pancreatic islet transplantation, 213
    pharmacokinetic properties, **249**
    side effects, **254**
    steroid withdrawal, 262
    toxicities, 253
takotsubo cardiomyopathy see stress-
    induced cardiomyopathy
Tasocitinib (CP-690,550), 262
99mTc-MAG, 307
telbivudine, 368
temperature probes, 221
tenofovir, 369
testicular cancer, **29**
tetanus, diphtheria, acellular pertussis
    (DTP) vaccine, **340**
6-thioguanine, 255
thiopentone, 221, **222**
thiopurine-S-methyltransferase
    (TPMT), 255
    deficiency, 255–6
thoracic epidural analgesia (TEA), 231
thrombolysis, 311
thromboprophylaxis, 394
    pancreatic transplantation, 232
thrombotic disorders
    brainstem-dead donors, 83
    pancreas transplantation, 193
thrombotic microangiopathy (TMA),
    323
Thymoglobuline (rabbit anti-human
    thymocyte immunoglobulin), 247
thyroid cancer, **29**
time zero biopsy, living donor kidney
    transplantation, 189
T-lymphocyte-mediated (acute
    cellular) rejection, 265
tobacco smoking see smoking

total parental nutrition, 232
toxin-binding resins, 346
toxoplasma, **338**
tramadol, 394
transoesophageal echocardiography
    probe (TOE), 230
transplant arteriopathy (TA), 320
transplantation
    history, 1–6
    kidney see renal transplantation
    organ supply maximisation, 6
    pancreatic see pancreas
        transplantation
transplant coordinators, 89, 91
transplant dysfunction
    causes, 422–3
    diagnosis, 384–5, 386, 424–5
    glomerular filtration rate, 384
    management, 384–5, 424–5
    post-renal, 385
    pre-renal, 385
    renal, 387–8
transplant glomerulopathy, 323
transplant half-life, 422
transplant histopathology, 317–34
    Banff classification see Banff
        classification scheme
    kidney, 317–31
    pancreas, 331–3
    recurrent and de novo disease, 330
transplant nephrectomy, 430–1
transplant pyelonephritis, 343, 389
transplant recipients
    donor kidney, information about,
        452
    fever, 341
    immunisation, 339, **340–1**
    malignancy see malignancy,
        transplant recipients
    potential see renal transplant
        recipient (RTR), potential
transplant services organisation,
    141–58
Transplant Tumor Registry, 415
travellers, advice for, 375–6
travellers' diarrhoea, 376
triazoles, 349, 350
trimethoprim (TMP)
    pancreas transplantation, 198
    Pneumocystis pneumonia
        prophylaxis, 353
triple hormone replacement therapy,
    83
tubulitis, 324, 324
tubulointerstitial damage, 422
24-hour urine collection, proteinuria,
    43, 424
two-layer method, 209

type 1 diabetes mellitus, 191–2, 203
    peri-operative morbidity/mortality,
        227
type 2 diabetes mellitus,191–2, 203

UK General Medical Council
    confidentiality guidance, 449
UK National kidney allocation scheme,
    146–50
UK Transplant Pregnancy Registry, 429
ultrasound
    acute rejection, 300
    acute tubular necrosis, 300–301
    cental vein cannulation, 220
    chronic rejection, 305
    contrast agents, 306–7
    drug toxicity, 305
    early complications evaluation,
        300–307
    early graft dysfunction, 424
    hepatitis C virus, 370
    increased pulsatility index, 300
    increased resistive index, 300
    infections, 305
    late complications, 305–6
    lymphocele, 304–605
    normal appearance, 299
    postoperative living donor kidney
        transplantation, 190
    post-transplant diagnostic imaging,
        299–300
    renal artery stenosis, 301, *302*
    renal artery thrombosis, 301
    renal vein thrombosis, 301
    reversed/reduced diastolic flow, 300
    tumours, 306
    ureteric complications, 301–3
    ureteric obstruction, 306, 386
    urinary obstruction, *303,* 303–4
    urine leak, 304
    urinoma, 304
ultrasound-guided renal biopsy, 306
    post-biopsy complications, 306
United Network for Organ Sharing
    (UNOS) pancreas transplantation,
    191
University of Wisconsin (UW)
    solution, 209
uraemic cardiomyopathy, 405
ureteral anastomosis, radiological
    anatomy, 298
ureteral kinking, 304
ureteral necrosis, 307
ureteral obstruction, 303, 304
ureteral stenosis, 307
ureteral stones, 304
ureteric leaks, 313
ureteric obstruction, 306, 385–7

ureteric stenosis, 304
ureteric stenting, 312–13, *313*
ureterocystoplasty, 170
ureterostoma, 170, 187–8
uretero-uretero anastomosis, 185–6
ureters
    kidney retrieval en-bloc, 99
    procurement, *101*
    re-implantation, children, 290
ureter to skin anastomosis, 187–8
ureter-ureter anastomoses, 168–9
urethral catheter, 161
uricosuric drugs, 428
urinary catheter
    live donor nephrectomy, 111
    pancreatic transplantation, 233
    removal, 384
urinary microscopy, haematuria, 44
urinary obstruction, ultrasound, *303,*
    303–4
urinary protein excretion, 43
urinary tract infection (UTI), 342–4
    pancreas transplantation, 198, 201
    potential live kidney donors, 43–4
    pregnancy, 429
    prevention, 344
urine leaks, 304, 387
urine output, postoperative, 190, 383
urinoma, 304
urogenital cancer, **28**

vaccination
    contraindications, 375
    history, transplant recipients, 339
    HIV patients, 373
    paediatric renal transplantation, 288,
        294
    pre-travel, 375–6
    recommended/contraindicated,
        340–1
valaciclovir, 355, 357, 358
valganciclovir, 198, 355
valganciclovir, children, 293
valvular calcification, 16
valvular heart disease, 16
vancomycin, 346
vancomycin-resistant *Enterococcus
    faecium* (VRE) infections, 339
varicella zoster, 293, 357–9
varicella zoster vaccine, **340**
varicella zoster immune globulin
    (VZIG), 294, 359
vascular acute rejection (grade III acute
    T-cell-mediated rejection), 325
vascular calcification, 412
vasoparalysis, 81, 82
vasopressin *see* antidiuretic hormone
    (ADH)

vasopressors
  renal transplantation, 222
  severe brain injury, 79–80
  subendocardial ischaemia, 79–80
vasospasm, calcineurin inhibitor-
    induced, 388
venous anastomosis, radiological
    anatomy, 298
venous gas embolism, 239
venous iliacal bifurcation, 98
venous thrombosis
  catheter angiography, 311
  pancreatic graft failure, 193
verapamil
  interactions, **250**
  post-transplant hypertension, 398
vesico-ureteric reflux, 342
viral capsid antigen (VCA), 360
viral hepatitis, potential recipients, 20
viral infection, 336, 353–75
  chronic, 336
  post-transplant malignancy, 414–15
  see also individual infections
viral nephropathy, 426
vitamin B₆ *see* pyridoxine therapy
vitamin D-based treatment, 421

volatile anaesthesia, 221
voriconazole, 349, 350

waiting lists, patient risk/benefits
    reappraisal, 451–2
warfarin
  end-stage renal disease, 16
  renal transplant biopsy, 391
warm ischaemic time (WIT), 119, 138
weight gain, 399, 408
Wilm's tumour, **29**
World Health Organization
    Nomenclature Committee for
    'Factors of the HLA System,' 57
wound complications, 393
wound dehiscence, 393
wound drain removal, 384
wound infections, 344, 393
wound site, postoperative management,
    383

xenotransplantation, 6
  pancreatic islets, 216
X-map see Luminex

zanamivir, 374